The Royal Marsden CANCER COOKBOOK

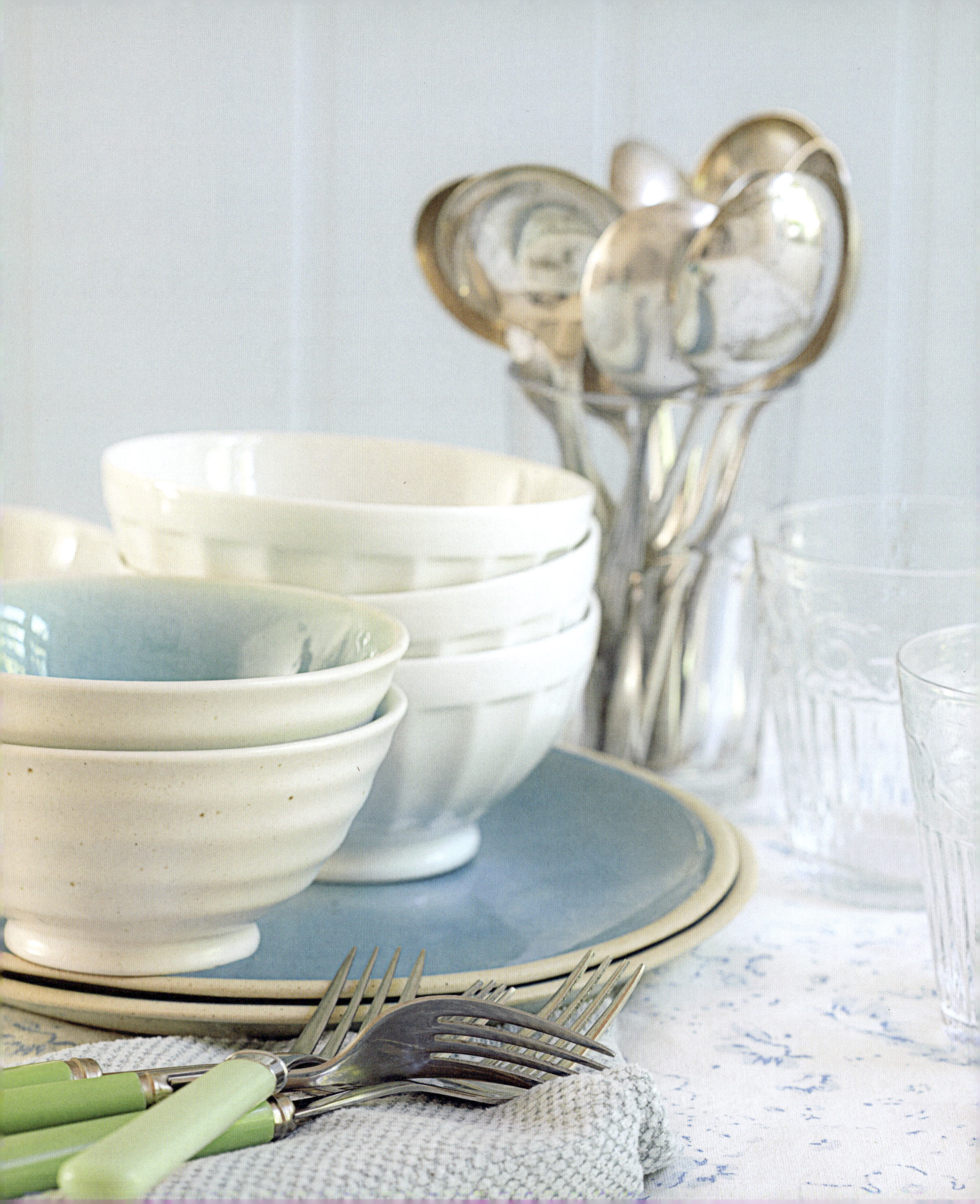

The Royal Marsden CANCER COOKBOOK

Nutritious recipes during and after cancer treatment, to share with friends and family

Catherine Phipps

Introduction and edited by Dr Clare Shaw PhD RD
Consultant Dietitian at The Royal Marsden NHS Foundation Trust

Photography by Georgia Glynn Smith

Cover photograph by Cara Cormack

Kyle Books

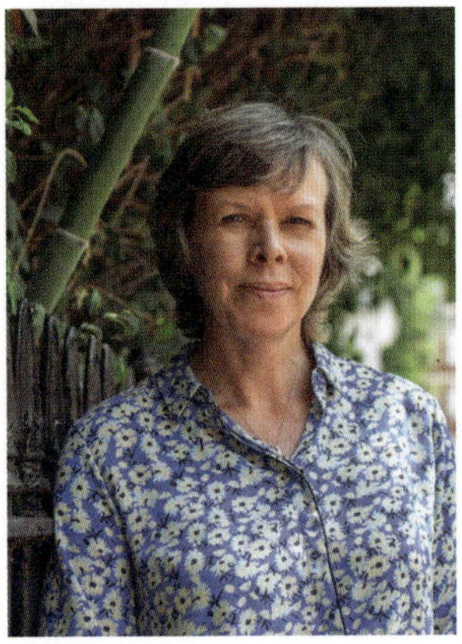

Acknowledgements

I would like to thank the patients at The Royal Marsden NHS Foundation Trust for their excellent ideas over the years, many of which are included in this book.

In addition I would like to thank Lucy Eldridge for reading the manuscript, Kate Jones for her expertise on activity and exercise, Justine Hofland for her excellent questions and Joanne Adcock for her analysis of the recipes. Catherine Phipps and others have translated the nutritional principles into delicious recipes, which have been beautifully photographed by Georgia Glynn Smith. Kyle Books have been a pleasure to work with during the production of this book. Last, but not least, thank you to my husband Robert whose support is unwavering.

Dr Clare Shaw PhD RD

50% of the royalties from this book will be donated to The Royal Marsden Cancer Charity.

Imagine a future beyond cancer. At The Royal Marsden we're dedicated to making this happen.

We're a world-leading cancer centre who pioneer new treatments that save lives, using our research every day to provide the very best in diagnosis, treatment and care for our patients.

The revolutionary way we treat people in our hospitals has far-reaching impact, nationally and internationally.

By supporting The Royal Marsden you are investing in a future beyond cancer for you and for everyone you know.

The Royal Marsden Cancer Charity
For a future beyond cancer

www.royalmarsden.org
Registered Charity No. 1095197
A charitable company limited by guarantee
Registered in England No. 4615761

INTRODUCTION

By Dr Clare Shaw PhD RD

Eating well when you have cancer

One in two people in the UK born after 1960 will be given a diagnosis of cancer during their lifetime. Such news is life-changing and brings many physical, psychological and emotional challenges for people living with the disease and facing cancer treatment. It will also have a profound effect on the family, friends and carers of the person with cancer. It may raise many questions about what has caused the cancer and whether lifestyle or, indeed, diet has contributed to its development. There is a wealth of research about diet and the causes of cancer, which is gradually forming a general picture of how what we eat affects our health, particularly during growth, development and into our adult lives.

This book is not about diet and the causes of cancer. Its aim is to help people who are being treated for the disease and who are experiencing changes in body weight, appetite, ability to taste and swallow, the way their digestive system works or how full or nauseous they feel. These unpleasant effects are all common before or during treatment and can make eating more difficult. It can be hard to know what to eat or how to continue with a good, healthy diet and at the end of treatment people may have lost or gained weight and need to rethink their eating patterns.

For many people, a diagnosis of cancer leads them to reconsider their diet and how it can be improved, or they may want to ensure they can continue to eat the right balance of foods. It is very important to get support from the team of doctors, nurses and other health care professionals looking after you, including dietitians and physiotherapists. There may be times during or after treatment when people are required to follow a special diet. A registered dietitian will be able to provide expert advice on why a special diet is needed, how to follow it and ways to ensure it contains all the vital nutrients to aid recovery.

This book aims to help you navigate through the facts and myths about what you should eat when you are being treated for cancer. It contains the information you need about the foods that are right for you and will inspire you to eat delicious healthy food that will support and nourish you. These recipes are for you and all your family and friends to enjoy sharing.

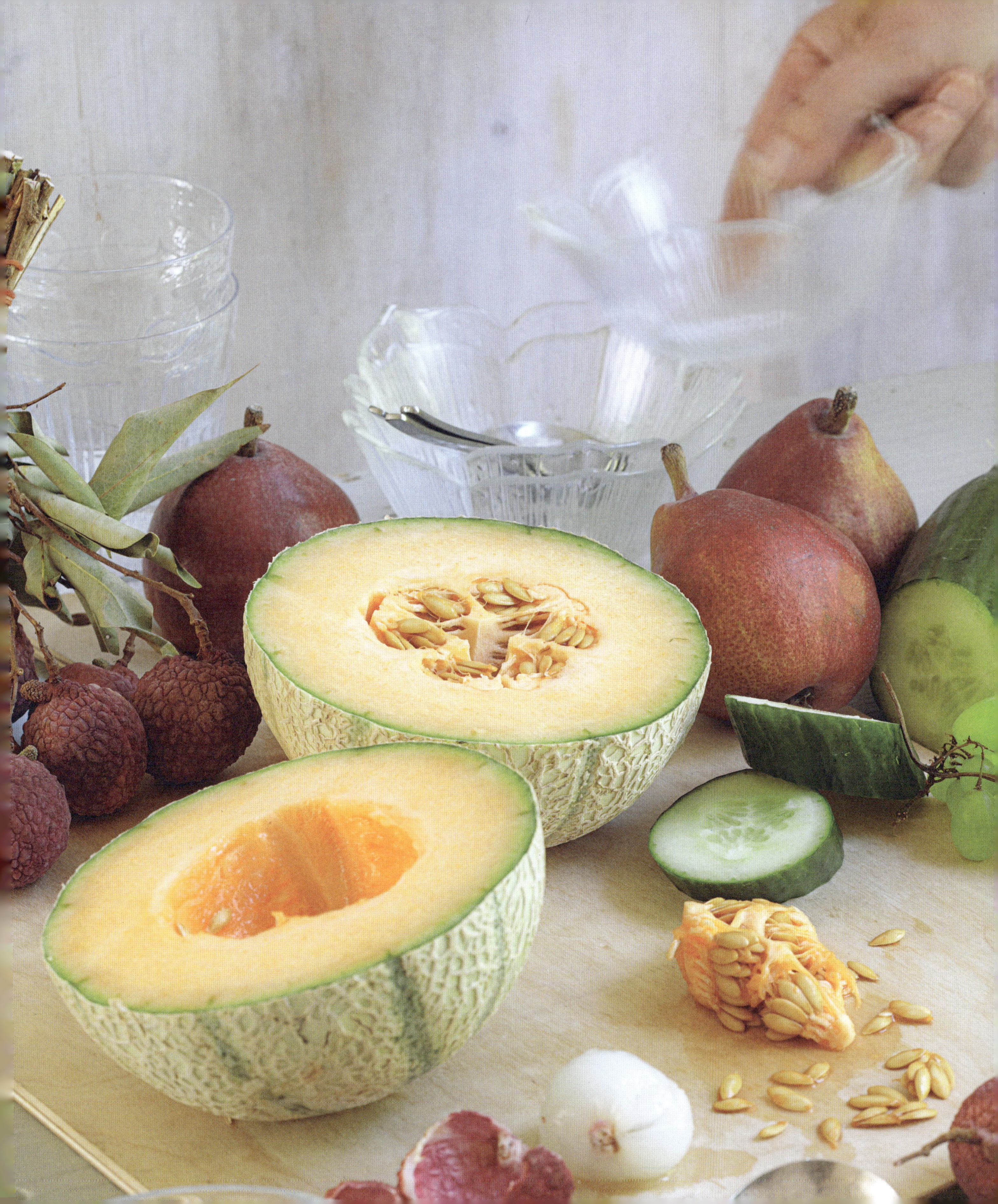

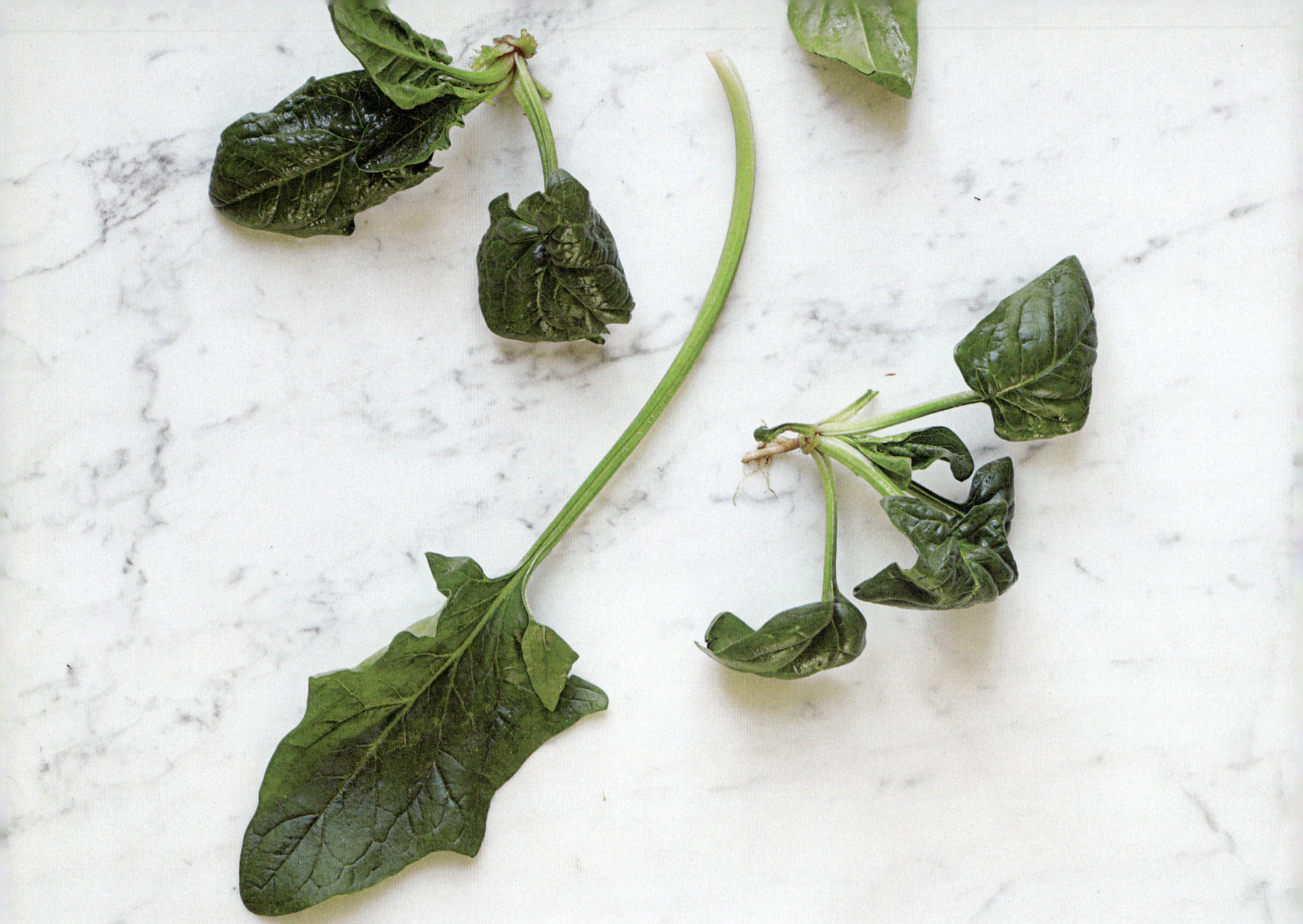

Cancer and cancer treatments

Cancer occurs when the usual process of cell growth and cell death goes out of control. All the cells of the body have a lifecycle where they grow, develop and eventually die. When this cycle is disrupted, abnormal cells can grow, forming a tumour. Cancer can develop in any organ of the body and there are over 200 types of cancer affecting certain parts of the body – the lung, bowel, stomach, breast (predominantly in women), prostate (in men), brain or skin. Cancer may occur in circulatory systems, such as the blood, or lymphatic systems. And, unless checked, cancer can spread from the initial site (the primary tumour) to other areas (secondary tumours or metasteses) of the body. Cancer treatments are used to remove or contain and destroy the cancer; often a combination of the different treatments may be used.

How do cancer treatments affect diet?

All cancer treatments affect normal cells, tissues and organs in the body and, depending on the type of treatment, may cause specific symptoms such as nausea, sickness, diarrhoea, sore mouth and taste changes. Some treatments may affect the way you feel by causing tiredness, hair loss, fatigue, loss of appetite or may actually make it difficult for you to eat, particularly if the treatment is targeting your mouth, stomach or digestive tract. Surgery is a traumatic and stressful event for the body and may change the need for certain nutrients after an operation. Any cancer treatment can also make eating more difficult due to loss of appetite or other side effects. For many people, the normally pleasurable experience of eating diminishes and so eating a healthy diet becomes more difficult.

Surgery

Surgery may be used at various times following diagnosis of cancer. People may require invasive surgery to remove the cancer itself or to alleviate symptoms, for example, to help the digestive system work. The time leading up to surgery may be very stressful, as you are worried about the operation itself and how you will recover. The stress or the surgery may affect the way that you eat for a number of reasons. Eating well is a vital part of the recovery process to help tissues heal and help you to regain strength. Surgery may cause:

- Periods when you are unable to eat
- Reduced appetite and fatigue
- Taste changes
- Periods when the digestive system does not work as well as usual
- Particular difficulties with eating following treatment to the mouth, stomach or bowel

Radiotherapy

This is usually given as a course of treatment over a number of weeks, or may be used in shorter doses to help with symptoms. Radiotherapy uses high-energy rays to destroy cancerous cells. It may be given on its own or in combination with drugs (chemotherapy). The radiotherapy is non-specific: it will affect both the cancer cells and the normal tissues around the site of the treatment. It may cause:

- Inflammation around the site of the treatment, for example, if applied to the mouth, gullet (oesophagus), stomach or bowel, and may make swallowing or digestion difficult
- Reduced appetite
- Fatigue
- Nausea or sickness
- Sore mouth or throat
- Diarrhoea (if the bowel is included in the radiotherapy)

Chemotherapy

Chemotherapy is the general term used for anti-cancer drugs given to destroy cancer cells and to control or shrink a tumour. The drugs work by damaging cancer cells so that they are unable to divide and grow.

Unlike surgery and radiotherapy, which are local treatments, chemotherapy drugs are systemic, because they enter the bloodstream and therefore, in the short term, also damage normal cells and can cause side effects. A course of chemotherapy can affect the lining of the mouth and digestive tract, making it difficult to eat. It can influence the immune system, leaving you susceptible to infection, and eating can also be affected by its other side effects, including:

- Sore mouth
- Nausea and vomiting
- Diarrhoea
- Fatigue
- Taste changes
- Infections

Immunotherapy

Immunotherapy is a term used to describe treatments using substances that help the immune system recognise cancer cells and supporting the body to kill them. They may include vaccines, bacteria or antibodies, all of which are used to treat the cancer. They may be used in combination with other treatments such as chemotherapy, and may affect your eating habits because of:

- Reduced appetite
- Taste changes
- Flu-like symptoms
- Side effects such as diarrhoea or colitis (inflammation of the bowel)

Hormone therapy

Hormone therapy tends to be used for cancers whose growth is influenced by hormones, for example, some types of breast and prostate cancers. These treatments may be given alongside other treatments and are often used for long periods of time. Their side effects impact in various ways on health and diet as they can result in:

- Weight gain
- Fat stored around the waist
- Decreased muscle bulk
- Other conditions, such as heart disease and osteoporosis, being affected

How does diet affect cancer treatment?

Your diet has a strong bearing on your overall health and your ability to withstand cancer treatment: there is much truth in the saying 'You are what you eat'. The food you consume affects whether you lose or gain weight and can influence your muscle strength and how you feel. The overall balance of your nutrient intake can also affect how well your body responds. People who lose a lot of weight before or during cancer treatment may find it more difficult to cope with the treatment and side effects may be more common or harder to withstand. Increasingly there is a focus on preparing people for treatment in the time between diagnosis and when treatment commences. This is called 'prehabilitation' and focuses on eating well, being active or increasing exercise and having a good approach with mental health. It is hoped that this approach helps improve fitness and enables people to cope with planned treatment.

Eating well during cancer treatment is a question of ensuring you have a balanced, healthy diet that provides enough energy from protein and nutrients to maintain your weight, your muscle mass and strength and allow your body to recover from the side effects caused by the treatment.

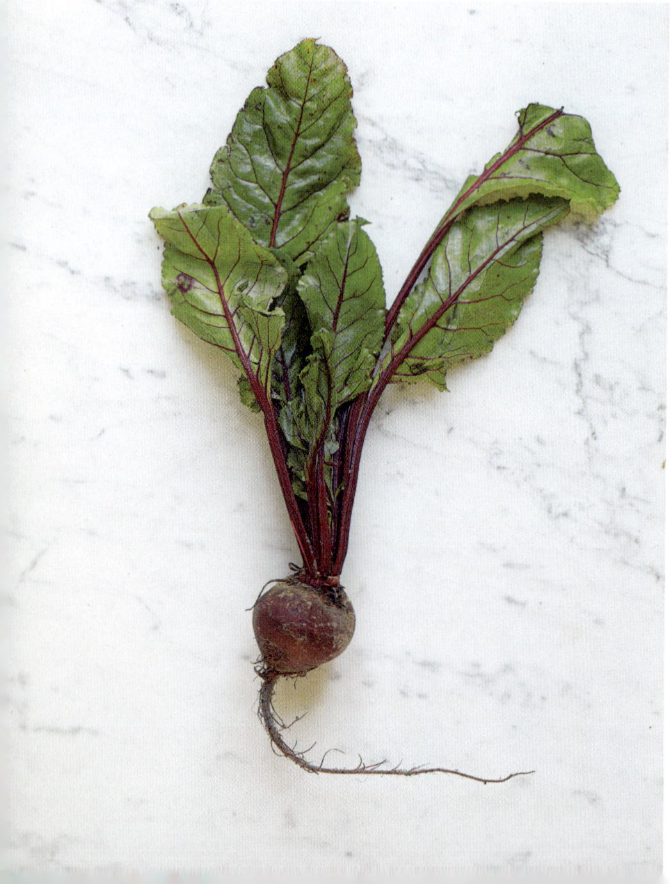

Not everyone experiences difficulty with eating – you may find that your treatment does not give you many side effects and that you are able to eat well. If that is the case, your main focus can be to get the correct balance of nutritious foods in your diet.

The first part of this book will help you decide which balance of foods suits you. What you need may change over time according to how you feel, changes in your weight and your taste or other factors that influence your food choices. The second part, the recipe section, is divided into two sections. It begins with recipes for the period when eating is more difficult. The dishes here are designed to be high in protein and energy (calories) and provide plenty of vitamins and minerals. They may be built around particular flavours to tempt your palate or give ideas for times when cooking is a chore. The recipes are designed for all the family so there is no need to cook separate meals. However, for times when you need more energy or protein, if you are struggling to eat or recovering from treatment, there are hints and tips on how to fortify your foods as necessary or choose high-energy foods. The remainder of the recipe section contains healthy recipes for those who are eating well or may even wish to lose weight, or watch that they don't gain any extra! Again, these recipes are not just for those who have cancer: good, healthy eating applies to everyone.

Does diet directly influence the growth of cancer?

Many people diagnosed with cancer change their diet, by eating or avoiding certain foods to try to prevent their cancer growing or spreading. There's a wealth of information on the internet and in books on how diet can affect the growth of cancer, although the ideas on what people should and should not eat are often not tested by rigorous research. Where there is evidence that particular foods or the overall balance of your diet can improve certain types of cancer, the information is included later on to ensure you make a good choice.

There is no 'special diet' for people with cancer. What is essential is that your diet provides all the nutrients that you need to function well, which is where this book will help.

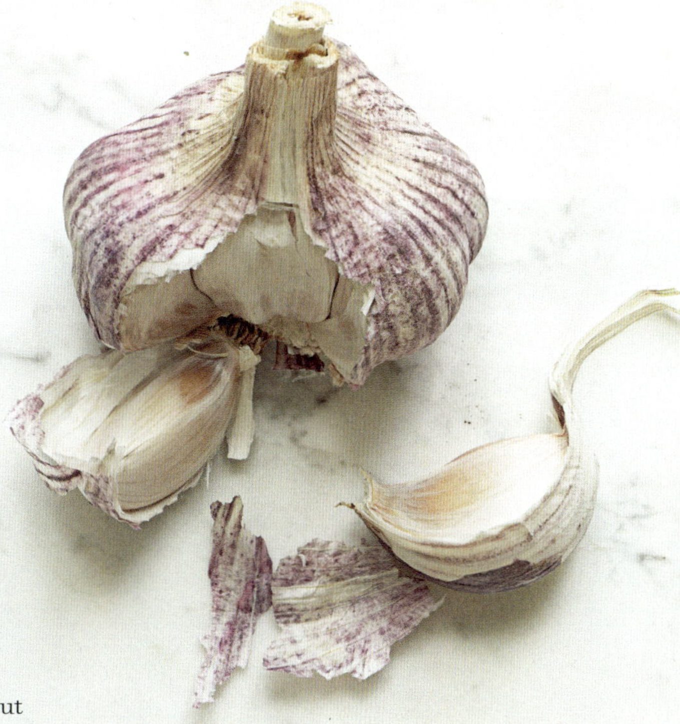

What is healthy eating?

Healthy eating is about the overall balance of your diet throughout the days, weeks, months and years. It is about choosing foods that taste good but also are packed with the nutrients you need to ensure the body works well. It is about having enough food, but not too much of anything, and, importantly, it is about enjoying good food. The essential points for your health are:

- Aim to have a healthy body weight in the normal range for your height. (If you are unsure of what weight you should be, then you can check your weight on a Body Mass Index [BMI] Chart). If you have lost weight, then try to gradually increase it; if you have gained weight, follow the healthy eating ideas to avoid further weight gain and eventually you should lose some weight. Don't be discouraged if you are unable to achieve your ideal body weight straight away – even some weight loss is beneficial for your health.
- Eat some protein-containing foods each day, such as chicken, fish, eggs, cheese, nuts, beans and pulses. Limit consumption of red meat such as beef, pork and lamb to about 500g (18oz) cooked red meat per week. This would be about 700–750g (25–26oz) of raw red meat.
- Eat more plant foods and aim to eat these with each meal, for example:
  - Wholegrains such as cereals, including bread, rice, oats and pasta
  - Pulses such as beans, lentils and chickpeas
  - Vegetables and fruit
  - Starchy foods such as potatoes, sweet potatoes and yams
- Choose a wide range of colourful fruit and vegetables to help ensure there is a good variety of nutrients in your diet.
- Keep processed meat that has been cured, smoked or salted to a minimum.
- Take care with sugar in your diet, especially if you are overweight, but if you are losing weight sugar may be a useful way to increase your energy intake.
- Take care with salt in your diet, but if you lack appetite and struggle to eat, or have taste changes, then it may help make food palatable.
- Take care with the amount of fat, particularly saturated fat, in your diet, but, again, if you are losing weight then it is a useful way to increase your energy intake.
- Drink alcohol in moderation or avoid it altogether.
- Whenever possible, try to take some exercise.

Eating well during cancer treatment

While it is easy to outline a healthy diet, when you are undergoing cancer treatment the balance of foods may need to change to ensure that you are able to eat enough and obtain sufficient nourishment.

Protein-containing foods

Protein is the building block of all cells and tissues, most visibly in our muscles, skin and hair, and, more difficult to see, in our blood. Your diet can include protein from animal and vegetable sources. Where protein comes from affects the quality or biological value, with sources from meat, fish and poultry tending to be of a higher quality than vegetable sources. Protein of a higher biological value is used more efficiently by the body. This is generally not a problem when eating a varied diet, as most people eat sufficient protein without any difficulty. However, this can be harder to do if appetite is poor or if the diet is already restricted, for example if following a vegan diet.

Sometimes people with cancer are told that the protein in their bloodstream, called albumin, is low. This is often the result of the cancer, an infection or a trauma, such as surgery. While it is important to eat enough protein, eating more may not increase these low levels as they are dependent on many factors. For example, whether there is continued stress on the body, owing to infection, when recovering after surgery or due to a course of chemo- or radiotherapy. These and other treatments for cancer may also increase the body's need for protein during recovery. Good sources of protein include:

- Meat, including offal such as liver and kidney
- Chicken
- Fish and shellfish
- Dairy products, including milk, yogurt and hard and soft cheeses
- Eggs
- Beans and pulses
- Nuts and seeds
- Vegetable protein, for example, soya products such as tofu (see page 40)
- Manufactured protein sources such as meat substitutes made from mycoprotein (e.g. Quorn™)

Protein-containing foods also contain other key nutrients such as fat, vitamins and minerals. Be aware that manufactured sources of protein in the diet may have added fat and salt, for example meat products such as pies, bacon, sausages, salami and kebabs. Any symptoms of cancer or problems with eating can make it more difficult to eat enough protein. Some foods and recipes can easily be fortified with protein foods to boost their protein content if you are really struggling to eat. Examples include dried skimmed milk powder, eggs and ground nuts.

Carbohydrate foods

There are two groups of carbohydrates: starches and sugars. The starchy carbohydrates include cereals, grains and starchy vegetables such as potatoes, sweet potatoes, yam, corn, cassava, beans and peas. Eaten in their natural form with little processing, for example wholegrain cereals, these foods contain the maximum amount of nutrients, such as vitamins and minerals. They are also higher in dietary fibre, which is essential for the normal functioning of the digestive tract. Starchy carbohydrates take longer for the body to absorb than those that are high in sugars, and therefore slowly release energy over a longer period of time, making you feel fuller. The term glycaemic index (GI) is used to describe the rate of absorption of carbohydrate from different foods. Foods with a low GI, such as some fruits and vegetables, pulses and wholegrain cereals, deliver sugar glucose into the bloodstream slowly. This is especially helpful if you are trying to lose weight, because you don't feel the need to eat more than necessary or snack between meals. Not all foods with a low GI are necessarily 'healthy foods' as the presence of fat can slow down the rate of absorption of sugars. However, it is really useful to include low-GI foods to help maintain that full feeling.

Sucrose is the type of sugar we commonly know as cane or beet sugar, which may be added to recipes, but there are other forms of sugar present naturally in foods: glucose, fructose (mainly in fruit and honey), lactose (in milk and yogurt) and maltose (in sweet potato and malted grain). If you are experiencing problems with eating, such as weight loss or poor appetite, then adding these sugars to your diet will provide extra energy.

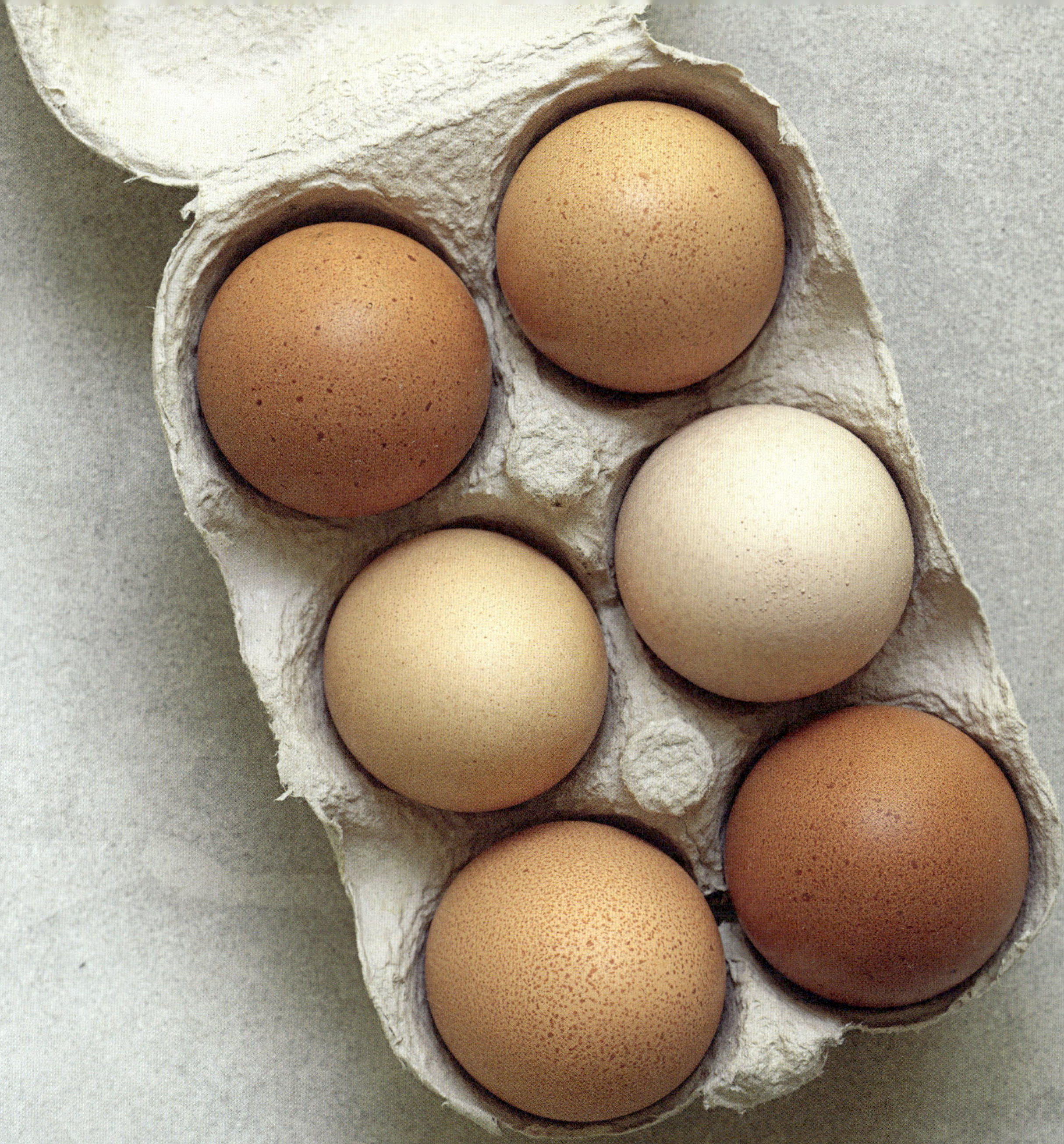

It is best to have carbohydrates in their natural form by eating fruit, some vegetables and milk, but adding sugar for its sweetness and flavour also gives you extra energy and helps your appetite. However, because sugar provides energy in an easily usable form, an excess of sugar causes weight gain. So, if you are eating well or want to watch your weight, then added sugars in your diet should be limited to small amounts. The World Health Organisation recommends no more than 10 per cent of our daily intake of energy should come from sugar, although other experts consider this is too high.

Fat

Like protein, fat is present in both animal and vegetable foods, or can be added to meals in the form of butter and oil. All fat has a high-energy density, meaning it provides lots of energy (calories), so the amount of fat in your diet should depend on whether you are under- or overweight. Fat also helps make food palatable, so you may wish to choose foods that are slightly higher in fat if you need to be tempted to eat. Fat is a source of fat-soluble vitamins such as vitamins A, D and E, which are essential for good health. There are different types of fat, healthy and otherwise.

Saturated fat

This is generally from animal sources or vegetable fats that have been processed (hydrogenated). They include:

- Meat (some lean meat, such as lean beef, pork or game has little fat, but some fatty cuts of meat, where the fat marbling can be seen or the meat is processed, contain considerably more).
- Dairy including cheese, cream, butter and ghee.
- Manufactured foods that have added fat, including crisps and savoury snacks, biscuits, cakes, pastries and chocolate.
- Hydrogenated vegetable and seed oils, including spreads, which are unsaturated fats that are artificially converted to saturated fats in the hydrogenation process. Most margarines or spreads made in this way will be a mixture of both saturated and unsaturated fat. The harder the margarine at room temperature, the more saturated fat present.
- Coconut oil, but it includes medium-chain triglycerides. It is a saturated fat that can be absorbed directly into the body without the usual digestion required for fat. It does not appear to have the same effect on blood cholesterol as other saturated fats. As it can withstand high temperatures it is suitable for cooking, but still needs to be taken in moderation.

Concern has been expressed regarding saturated fat in the diet as it may contribute to raised blood cholesterol levels. This, coupled with other health-related concerns, such as excess weight, high blood pressure, smoking and lack of exercise, can be linked to the risk of heart disease. For anyone who has been diagnosed with cancer and is undergoing treatment that may affect their weight and food intake, the risk of heart disease may, temporarily, become less of a priority. Some people even find their cholesterol levels drop if they lose weight as a symptom of their cancer or during treatment. However, post treatment, part of the return to a normal lifestyle is to consider the effect of diet on overall health.

Unsaturated fat: This type of fat tends to be found in oily fish, nuts and some fruit and vegetables. These oils are chemically slightly different and are often liquid rather than solid at room temperature. They include both monounsaturated fats, such as olive oil, and polyunsaturated fats, such as sunflower and sesame oils. This group of fats includes essential fatty acids that need to be eaten as they cannot be produced by the body. The two main types are omega-3 and omega-6 fatty acids. Omega-3 fatty acids are present in oily fish and flax oil. They have been shown to reduce the body's inflammatory response and there is interest in their use for inflammatory conditions such as rheumatoid arthritis and in the inflammation that can occur due to cancer. Omega-6 fatty acids are present in poultry, nuts, cereals and oils made from soybean, sunflower seeds and corn. Over the last few decades, the balance of omega-6 and omega-3 fats in the diet has changed. There is concern that this affects our health, particularly in terms of heart disease, but the full picture is not yet clear. Unsaturated fats may help lower blood cholesterol. If you need to gain weight these fats are excellent sources of energy, but if you need to lose weight be careful how much you eat. Examples are:

- Oily fish such as salmon, trout, mackerel, sardines and pilchards
- Nuts, including Brazil nuts, walnuts, hazelnuts and macadamia nuts
- Seeds such as pumpkin, sunflower and sesame seeds
- Vegetable oils from nuts, seeds and fruit, including olive, walnut, sunflower, sesame and avocado oils
- Some fruits and vegetables like avocados and olives

Trans fats

These have generated much interest as they have been shown to raise blood cholesterol. They are present in small quantities in meat and dairy produce and in manufactured foods containing hydrogenated vegetable fats. Many manufacturers have removed these types of fat from their products. If you wish to avoid trans fats there are ways to limit your intake:

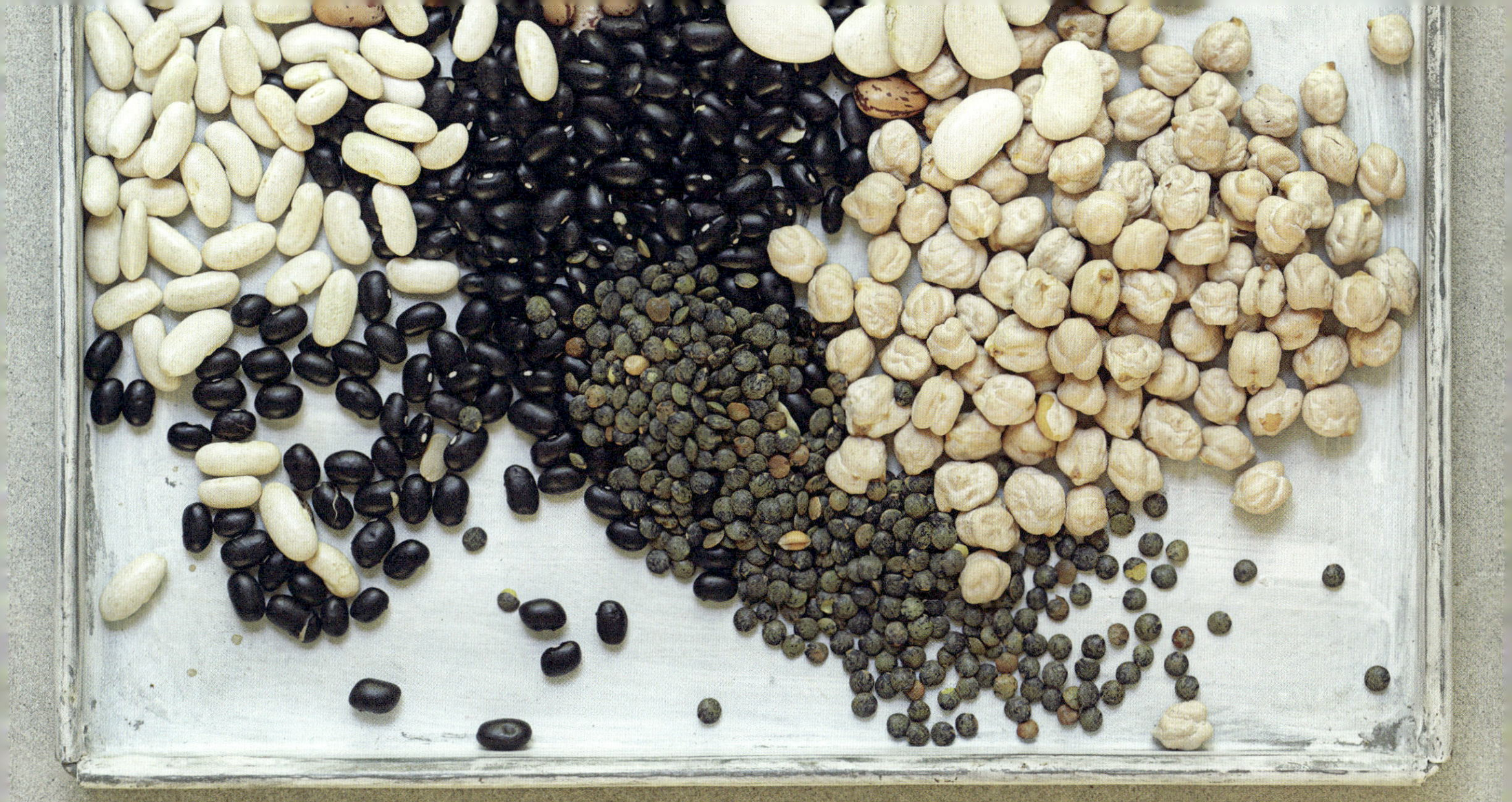

- Do not buy products that list partially hydrogenated fat or oil on the label
- Use liquid vegetable oil for frying food at home and try to eat fewer fried foods when eating out
- Eat fewer shop-bought biscuits, cakes and pastries

Dietary fibre

Dietary fibre is the part of fruit, vegetables and cereal foods that is not broken down in the digestive tract. It is described as either soluble or insoluble depending on its properties and the action it takes in the gut. It can help the digestive system work properly, keeping bowels regular, can reduce blood cholesterol levels and can help prevent digestive problems. Most people don't eat sufficient dietary fibre.

Foods that are a good source of dietary fibre are often an important source of vitamins and minerals. These include wholegrain cereals, fruit and vegetables, including pulses. Most foods are a combination of both insoluble and soluble fibres so, again, variety is key to ensure a balance of different types of fibre in the diet.

Soluble fibre

This is present in foods such as oats, beans and pulses, some vegetables and fruit. The soluble fibre can help thicken foods such as porridge, made from oats, which slows the digestion and absorption of glucose. These slow-release foods can make you feel full for longer – very helpful if you are trying to eat less.

Soluble fibre is fermented in the large bowel and can help both constipation and diarrhoea. This fermentation process adds bulk to the contents of the bowel and produces gas and short-chain fatty acids which are used by the cells lining the bowel and are also absorbed, providing a small amount of the overall energy we obtain from food.

Insoluble fibre

This type of fibre is not broken down by the digestive system and adds bulk to the contents of the bowel. Including insoluble fibre in your diet keeps the bowel regular and avoids constipation. Foods that have a high insoluble fibre content include wholegrain cereals, oats and other high-fibre breakfast cereals, wholemeal bread, brown rice and pulses.

Vitamins

Vitamins are essential for good health. They have many different functions in the body and, as they cannot be manufactured by the body, our diet is the main source of them. There is much interest in whether vitamins and certain minerals can protect the body against cancer. Often vitamins, particularly antioxidants, are singled out as helping the body to protect itself against the disease. Once cancer has been diagnosed it becomes much less clear whether these vitamins, particularly if taken as supplements, are of benefit, especially during treatments such as radiotherapy. Concern has been raised over whether the protection some vitamins may provide to tissues could reduce the effectiveness of cancer treatment. One study of supplements of beta-carotene and vitamin A given to people diagnosed with lung cancer was stopped early when it was shown that taking these supplements increased the risk of cancer returning. However, these undesirable outcomes have not been observed when vitamins are eaten in their natural form in everyday food, so this must be the best way to get the vitamins you need. Choosing a wide variety of foods that provide many different nutrients will ensure that your diet includes all the vitamins and minerals you need.

Which foods should you eat to get your vitamins? All fruits and vegetables, fresh, frozen and canned, can be an important source of vitamins, as are eggs, milk, cheese, fish, pulses, red meat and liver. Some vitamins deteriorate the longer they are exposed to oxygen, which is why you need to buy and use food while it is fresh. Others will also deteriorate when exposed to heat, so quick-cooking methods using minimal water, such as steaming or stir-frying, will help preserve the vitamin content. These methods also help preserve other nutrients including electrolytes such as potassium. And although raw, fresh ingredients are excellent for providing many micronutrients, this does not mean that raw is always better! There is some advantage to certain foods – carrots and tomatoes, for instance – being cooked, as the cooking process helps to make some vitamins more available to the body and easier to absorb. Using as many different types of vegetables and fruit as possible is the way to ensure you are getting all the essential vitamins and minerals you need.

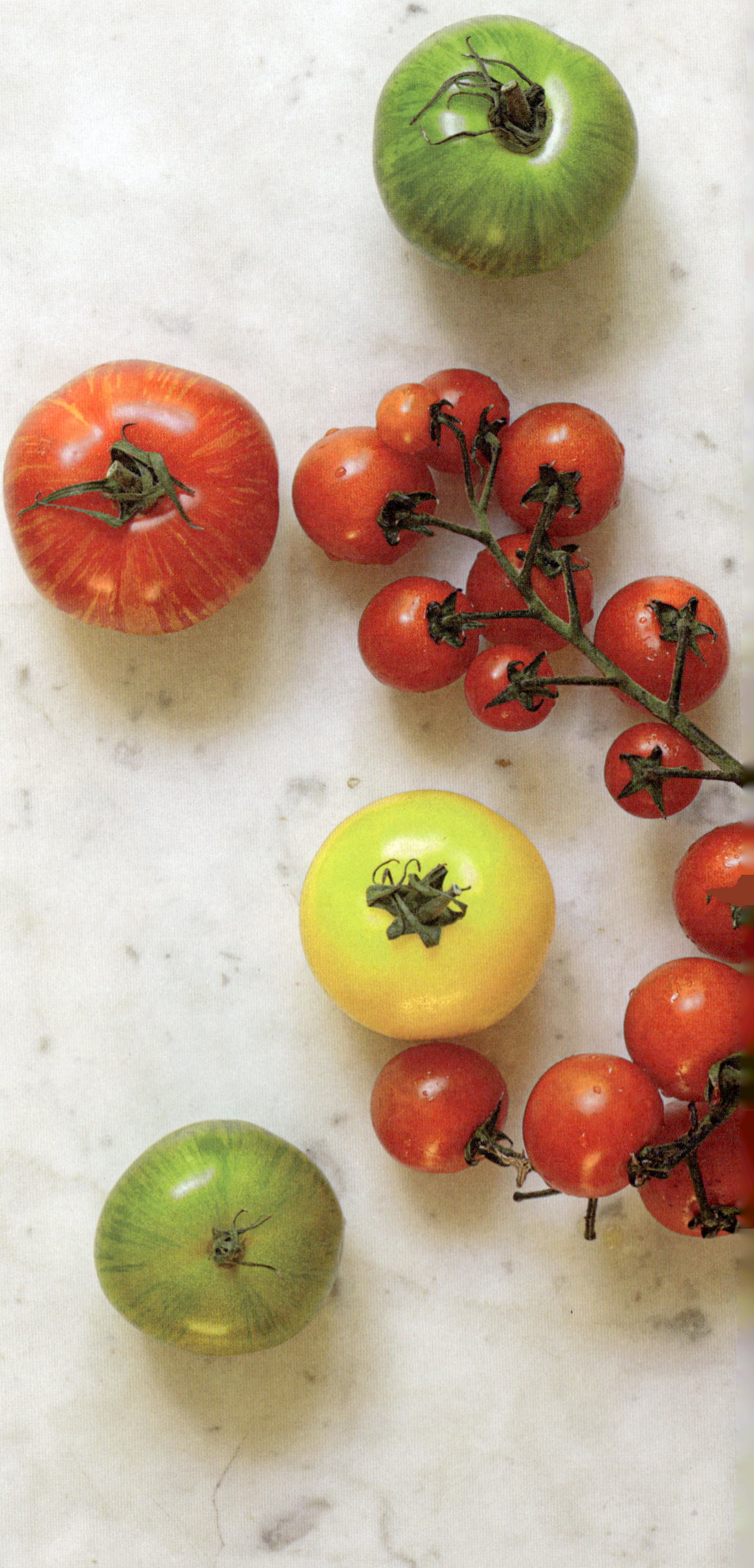

Vitamin A (Retinol)

Vitamin A is important for healthy skin and hair, and has antioxidant properties, protecting cells and tissues. It is a fat-soluble vitamin (retinol) found in oily fish such as mackerel, trout and sardines, and in eggs and cheese. It is also present in full-fat dairy products such as milk, butter and yogurt. However, if you are being careful about fat intake, you can also obtain vitamin A from your diet as beta-carotene (see below). Because the body cannot get rid of surplus vitamin A it is important not to have very high doses in the form of supplements on a regular basis. High intake of vitamin A are associated with an increased risk of bone fracture; your diet should provide the recommended daily amounts.

Beta-carotene

Beta-carotene is one of the family of carotenoids. They are a group of pigments that contribute the yellow and orange colours to a variety of fruit and vegetables. Beta-carotene is converted to vitamin A in the body and is therefore a very useful vitamin to include in your diet as it can provide a significant amount of the body's daily vitamin A needs. Extra beta-carotene, if absorbed by the body and not used, is deposited in fat stores – which explains why the skin develops an orange hue if larger than required doses of beta-carotene are consumed.

There has been much interest in beta-carotene from food and its possible role in helping prevent cancer through its actions as an antioxidant. However, once cancer has been diagnosed, it is not clear whether higher amounts of beta-carotene in the diet continue to have this protective effect against the cancer recurring or new cancer developing. However, it is an essential nutrient and can be found in a variety of fruits and vegetables. Good sources include yellow, green, orange and red vegetables such as carrots, pumpkins, sweet potatoes, spinach, tomatoes, broccoli and red peppers. Fruits that contain beta-carotene include mangoes, apricots and orange-fleshed melon.

B Vitamins

The B vitamins include thiamine (B1), riboflavin (B2), niacin (B3), pantothenic acid (B5), pyridoxine (B6), biotin (B7), folic acid and cyanocobalamin (B12). This water-soluble group of vitamins serves many different functions in the body, including helping it obtain energy from the food you eat. Some are particularly important for the formation of red blood cells and for nerve function. Foods that provide a good source of B vitamins include:

- Wholegrain cereals, yeast and yeast extract containing thiamin and riboflavin. These B vitamins are often added to grains and breakfast cereals.
- Meat such as pork and liver, seafood, potatoes and kidney beans, which are all sources of thiamin.
- Dairy products, eggs, liver, yeast extract and fortified breakfast cereals, which contain riboflavin.
- Meat, fish, wheat and maize flours, milk and eggs, which all contain niacin.

Pyridoxine is found in a wide variety of foods, especially pork, chicken, turkey, fish, eggs, vegetables and wholegrain cereals such as wholemeal bread and oats.

Folic acid works with vitamin B12 to form red blood cells. It is found in liver, broccoli, spinach, Brussels sprouts, peas, brown rice and fortified breakfast cereals.

Vitamin B12, important for nerves and red blood cells, is found in meat, fish, milk and eggs. The absorption of vitamin B12 from food depends on both the stomach and the intestine working effectively. In cases where treatment has involved surgery or radiotherapy to the stomach or intestine, vitamin B12 may need to be given as an injection.

Vitamin C

Vitamin C, or ascorbic acid, has received much attention with respect to cancer. This water-soluble vitamin has a key role as an antioxidant, helps with the absorption of iron from the diet and the production of collagen, a protein essential for the growth and repair of soft tissue. Collagen is essential for wound healing and so is especially important after surgery. Vitamin C received particular attention from nutritionists and dietitians when suggestions were made that in high doses it could be a treatment for cancer. A number of studies were carried out that administered vitamin C as a supplement rather than in food, directly into the blood stream (intravenously) and by mouth, but the results failed to endorse it as a treatment for cancer.Vitamin C is an essential water-soluble nutrient that cannot be stored in the body and therefore ideally needs to be taken on a daily basis. Vitamin C eaten in food is very important for the body and has been shown to be particularly so for people who are recovering from cancer. If you are eating well and including plenty of fruit and vegetables it is easy to take sufficient vitamin C. Excellent sources include citrus fruits such as oranges, grapefruit, lemon and limes and their juice, blackcurrants, kiwi fruit, guava and mango. Other particularly good sources are strawberries, red and green peppers, broccoli, Brussels sprouts and potatoes. If you cannot eat much fruit and veg, drinking fruit juices or fruit smoothies is an easy way to ensure you get your daily requirement. All fruit and vegetables need to be fresh for maximum value because vitamin C is destroyed by oxygen in the atmosphere and by heat. If you are cooking the food, choose a method that cooks quickly to preserve the vitamin C content.

Vitamin D

There is real interest in vitamin D because of its possible links with cancer development as well as its importance for those who have been diagnosed with cancer. Vitamin D is a fat-soluble vitamin present in food as calciferol and cholecalciferol. The latter can also be produced by the body when exposed to sunlight meaning that vitamin D levels are dependent both on diet and exposure to sunlight. It has a number of functions in the body, including the regulation of the amount of calcium and phosphorus absorbed from food and deposited in bones. It also affects other organs in the body, including the intestines, kidneys and the parathyroid gland.

The vitamin D produced after exposure to sunlight is determined by a number of factors, including a person's age, skin colour, how much skin is exposed, where the person lives, the time of day and the use of sunscreen products. It is also affected by the time of year, particularly for people who live further away from the equator, whose vitamin D levels often drop during the winter months.

Many people have low levels of vitamin D in their bloodstream and this has been shown to be more common in some people with cancer. The significance of this may vary according to the type of cancer, but low levels may affect the likelihood of cancer returning and other aspects of health such as the risk of bone fractures. Vitamin D is a very important nutrient whether it is sourced from food or sunlight. For those with cancer it is particularly valuable, as some treatments may impact on bone health, weakening the bones and increasing the chance of fractures. If you are concerned about vitamin D then do talk to your medical team. They can discuss with you the most appropriate ways to investigate your bone density, vitamin D levels and, if required, what type of supplement is best for you. Both calcium and vitamin D are required to help with bone density (see the section on calcium on page 21).

Vitamin D occurs naturally in egg yolks, butter and oily fish, including mackerel, sardines and salmon. It is also added to manufactured foods such as margarine and some cereals.

Vitamin E

Vitamin E, also known as alpha-tocopherol and gamma-tocopherol, is another essential antioxidant. It works to protect the body's tissues from damage by free radicals and supports the working of the immune system to protect the body against bacteria and viruses. Like vitamin B12, it helps with the formation of red blood cells. Fat-soluble vitamin E is present in vegetable oils, including sunflower, safflower, corn, rapeseed and soybean oils, as well as in wheatgerm, almonds, hazelnuts, peanuts and seeds such as sunflower seeds. Green leafy vegetables, such as spinach and broccoli, contain vitamin E, which is added to some fortified cereals, margarines and spreads.

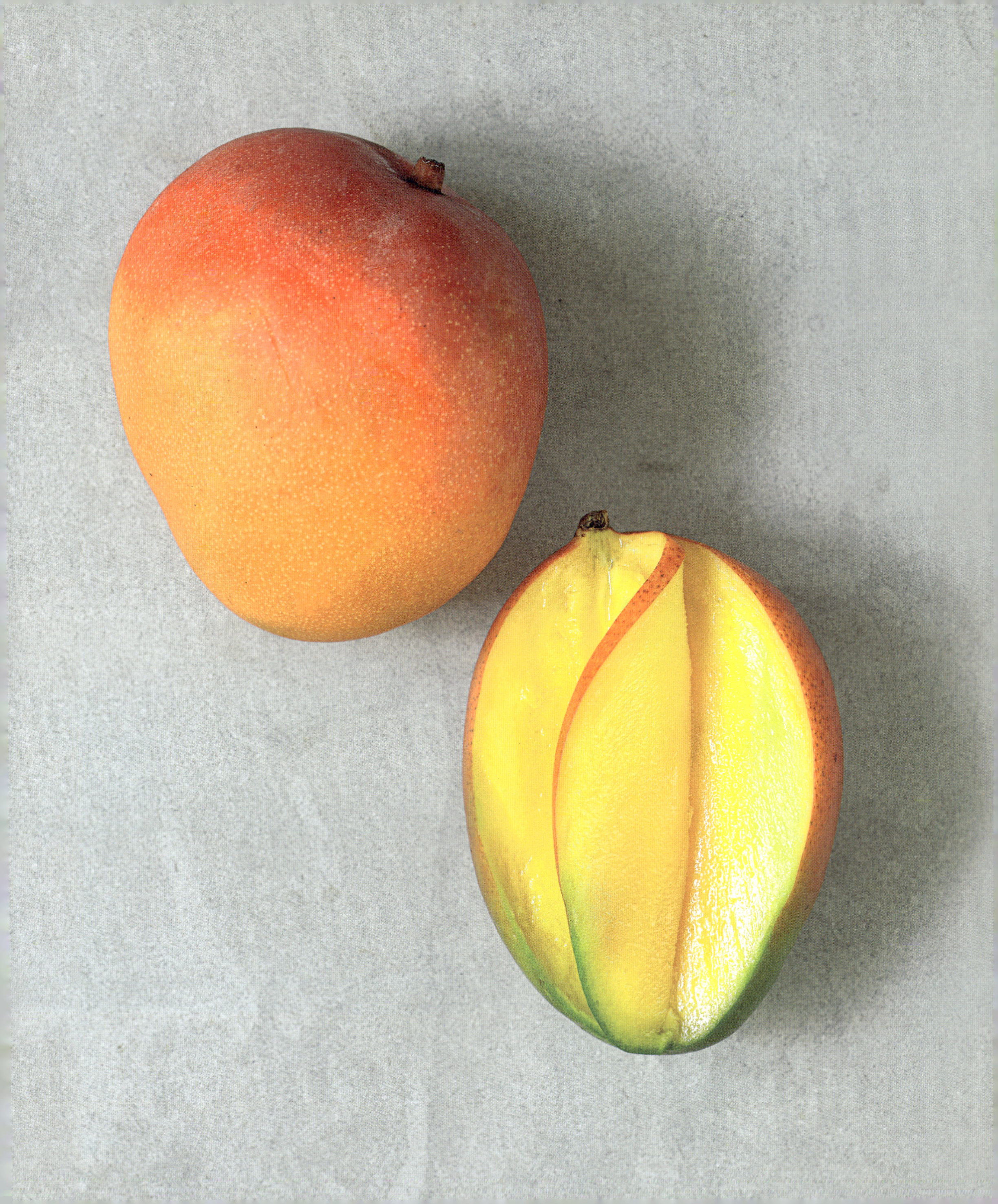

Electrolytes

The salts, or electrolytes, that are present in the bloodstream are particularly important for health. Levels of these salts, which include sodium, potassium, chloride and bicarbonate, are usually controlled by precise mechanisms within the body. However, they can be affected by many factors, including illness, drugs and losses from the body, for example, from sickness or diarrhoea or as a result of certain medications. They are important for the composition of the blood and support the way that muscles, nerves and tissues function.

Sodium

Most of the sodium in our diet is sodium chloride – salt. The salt used in cooking or added to food at the table is only part of our daily intake; the majority is obtained from other foods, including: many preserved or processed foods, such as ham, bacon, salami and salt fish; pickled foods such as vegetables and olives; salted snacks including nuts, pretzels and crisps; and seasonings such as soy sauce, stock cubes and yeast extract. Most of us eat far more salt than we actually need. For healthy eating it makes sense to limit the amount of salt you consume as high intakes of salt may be associated with increased blood pressure.

Potassium

Potassium is an especially important electrolyte, vital for the functioning of nerves and muscles, including the heart. It also helps the transfer of nutrients, such as glucose, into the cells. It can be lost from the body by the action of some drugs, such as diuretics (water tablets), and from diarrhoea, a common side effect of cancer treatment.

It's not difficult to include potassium in your diet because it is present in many fruit and vegetables – particularly bananas, dried apricots, potatoes and sweet potatoes – and in pulses, nuts and seeds, fruit juice and smoothies, coffee, milk and protein foods such as meat, chicken and fish.

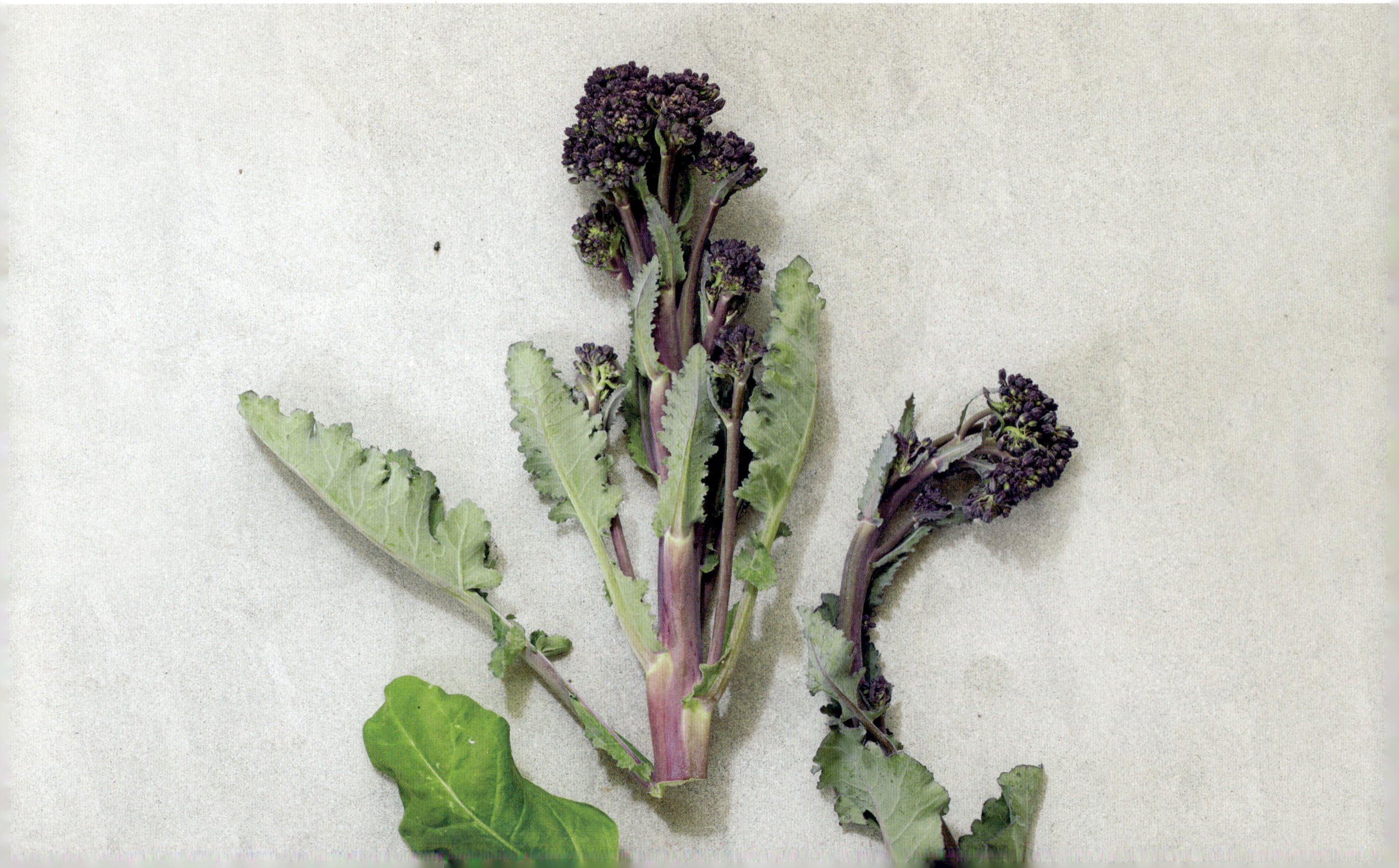

Minerals

Calcium

Calcium is a very abundant mineral in the body. It forms the structure of bones and teeth, helps muscles contract and enables normal blood clotting. There is much interest in whether calcium is important in protecting us from some forms of cancer, although little evidence of its protective power once cancer has been confirmed. Nonetheless, calcium has a vital role in bone health (see vitamin D on page 18), making it a key mineral for anyone with a cancer diagnosis. That said, there is some concern about those people with prostate cancer taking large amounts of calcium, as some studies suggest that high doses are associated with more advanced or aggressive prostate cancer. This may be a risk when calcium intakes are particularly high – 1,500–2,000mg per day – which is more than double the recommended intake.

Good sources of calcium include milk, cheese, yogurt and other dairy foods, plus green leafy vegetables such as cabbage and broccoli. Soya beans, soya drinks with added calcium and types of fish where the bones are eaten, such as pilchards and sardines, all provide calcium.

Iron

Iron has a number of roles in the body. It forms part of haemoglobin, the pigment in our red blood cells, which is essential for transporting oxygen from the lungs around the body in the bloodstream. Anaemia, the lack of red blood cells, is common in people diagnosed with cancer. It can occur due to a lack of iron or other nutrients in the diet or for a number of causes that result in blood loss, for example, following surgery or due to ongoing bleeding.

Dietary sources of iron include animal protein (haem iron) and foods of vegetable origin (non-haem iron). Haem iron is best absorbed from food sources and absorption can be optimised by taking vitamin C at the same meal, for example, as fruit juice. Excellent sources of iron include red meat, liver and eggs. Good vegetable sources include wholegrains, such as wholemeal bread and brown rice, fortified breakfast cereals, beans and pulses, dried fruit, such as apricots, nuts and dark green leafy vegetables, including spinach and kale.

Selenium

Selenium is important in helping to prevent damage to cells and tissues where it works with complex antioxidant systems in the body (see FAQ What are antioxidants? on page 34). It is also important to ensure the immune system and thyroid function well. Selenium is present in many foods, including Brazil nuts, fish, meat and eggs. Although the amounts of the mineral we consume in our food are perfectly safe, in high doses it can be toxic, so taking selenium supplements should be done with care.

Selenium levels in the body may fall during times of stress, illness and during treatments such as chemotherapy and radiotherapy, although this change is not universal. Throughout the recovery period your diet should include suitable sources of this trace element to replenish any shortfall.

Zinc

Zinc is a trace element that is essential for making new cells, supporting the immune system to work well, and processing nutrients, including protein, fat and carbohydrate. Its key roles are healing wounds and helping the body to repair itself.

There is much interest in whether zinc can affect taste changes. Studies of older people have shown that it may be linked with some taste changes and this has led some people to speculate that it is also responsible for taste changes during chemotherapy. However, there is no clear link between zinc deficiency and the taste changes associated with cancer. These changes are complex and are likely to be caused by various drugs and other medication. Similarly, it is not clear whether low zinc levels occur before the onset of cancer or as a result of it. As with selenium, the amount of zinc in the bloodstream may decrease with stress, illness and treatment. It can be unclear if this is happening in the tissues and organs of the body. What is certain, though, is the need to include enough zinc in your diet to ensure all the systems are functioning properly.

Good dietary sources of zinc are: red meat, poultry, beans, nuts, some types of seafood such as lobster and crab, wholegrains, fortified breakfast cereals and dairy products.

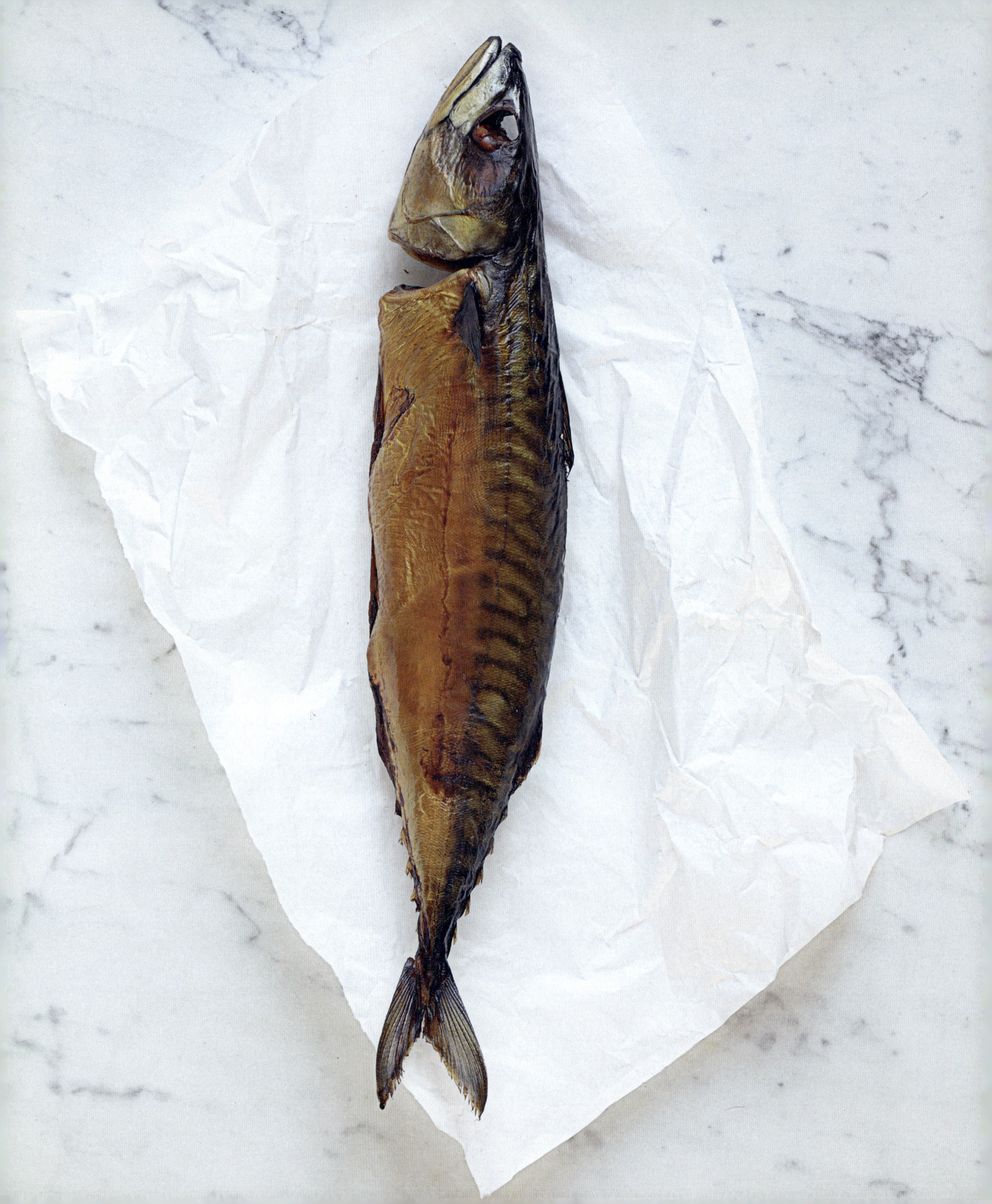

Alcohol

Drinking is part of social life for some of us. It is well known that alcohol can affect our mood and that excessive drinking impacts on many aspects of our physical health, contributing to heart disease, cancer, high blood pressure and liver problems, and can encourage weight gain. Anyone trying to eat healthily needs to either drink alcohol in moderation or avoid it altogether.

Many people who are undergoing cancer treatment find that their desire for alcohol decreases. Alcohol is an irritant to the tissues in the mouth and can aggravate symptoms of a sore mouth or throat. However, for people with a poor appetite, a small glass of alcohol before a meal may increase their desire for food. Not everyone will find this works, but sometimes just the social aspect of having a drink with others can help.

How important is body weight?

Weight loss may be a symptom of cancer and some people find they have lost weight by the time they are diagnosed. This may be due to loss of appetite or difficulty eating or swallowing, or it may be caused by the worry of knowing you are unwell and undergoing a number of tests. Your weight may be important to you both during and after treatment.

When you step on the scales the reading is total body weight: bones, muscles, internal organs and body fat. If someone loses weight then it is not just body fat that is lost but also some of the muscles that are needed for movement and for crucial functions such as breathing. Although people often focus on total body weight, it is actually the weight of the various components of the body that are more critical. The individual components can be measured using specialised equipment, but often hospitals use the simple measure of body weight.

Loss of body fat and muscle can arise as a result of changes in food intake, but are often in combination with the metabolic effects of the cancer and treatment. An inflammatory process can occur, which accelerates the loss of skeletal muscle, depresses albumin (protein) levels in the bloodstream and can make people feel weak and tired. Some studies have tested whether foods, particularly omega-3 fatty acids found in fish oils, can reduce this inflammatory response and help the body to utilise nutrients to replenish body stores. While it is not clear how much they help, they are certainly useful as part of a balanced diet, along with physical activity.

This book is full of ideas to help you eat well and try to avoid weight loss. At the beginning of any treatment, even if you are overweight, it is often still advisable to try to minimise weight loss unless your doctor has specifically advised you otherwise. Research has supported the idea that if people manage to stay well-nourished during treatment they are better able to cope with the treatment itself and make a better recovery. Maintaining muscle mass is particularly important and this is reliant on good nutrition and physical activity.

Physical activity during cancer treatment

The side effects of cancer treatment, such as tiredness and fatigue, can make it difficult to maintain the lifestyle you enjoy. The advice used to be to rest during treatment. However, the latest research suggests that it's beneficial to maintain a balance between good-quality rest and some physical activity during treatment. Where possible, try to plan your day so that there are periods of both rest and activity. Exercise doesn't necessarily mean going to the gym but could involve activities such as going for a walk or even doing some housework. It has been shown that aerobic exercise along with relaxation can help lessen both the severity and the duration of fatigue. Strengthening exercises are also important as they help maintain the size and strength of muscles. There is still a lot to learn about which exercise is best, but the important thing is to try to do some physical activity during treatment rather than rest all the time.

The challenges to healthy eating during cancer treatment

Eating well during cancer treatment is an essential part of keeping well, and the aim of this book is to help you with that goal by providing appetising ideas for tasty meals that will ensure you are eating a good range of nutrients. The guidance on healthy eating in the book is for when you are able to eat well and do not have any problems with appetite or symptoms as a result of treatment.

Symptoms

If you are experiencing symptoms that are affecting how much you eat, then speak to someone from the team of specialists caring for you. It is important to make them aware of your symptoms such as nausea, sickness, pain, sore mouth, poor appetite and alterations in bowel habits, any of which can have a profound effect on the amount and type of food you can eat and may make it harder to stick to a good balanced diet. Proper management of these symptoms can make a huge difference to how you feel and how well you eat.

If you find it difficult to eat and feel you are not managing to have a balanced diet, ask your GP to refer you to a registered dietitian. Dietitians are expert at using nutritional science to devise a realistic eating plan that meets your individual needs during treatment. They will provide specific advice and information on how you can improve your food intake, and whether vitamin and mineral supplements might be beneficial.

Poor appetite

Anorexia, which just means loss of appetite (not to be confused with *anorexia nervosa*), is perhaps one of the most common factors that may affect your food intake. Stress and anxiety over future investigations or treatment can contribute to your not wanting to eat. You may try to continue with your usual meal pattern but with a reduced portion size, or you don't finish meals and you don't eat snacks either, so overall your food intake decreases – and your weight may too. Some people lose interest in food altogether and mealtimes become a chore. Family and carers are likely to try to encourage you to eat more. This is well-meant, of course, but it can become a source of tension if you already find it harder to eat now that your appetite is low. If you have days when your appetite is better, then write down meal and snack ideas that appeal to you. Thinking of what you like to eat can be difficult when your appetite is poor. When possible, write down meal and snack ideas to help you later.

Ideas to help address the problem of poor appetite:

- Serve yourself smaller portions of food. Too much on your plate is likely to put you off and make you feel overwhelmed with how much you are expected to eat.
- Select a smaller plate, which will reduce how much food can be put on it and may help family and carers to judge how much you are able to eat.
- Consider changing your meal pattern during the day to 'little and often'. By eating small meals and snacks frequently during the day, overall you are likely to eat more food and therefore more nutrients.
- Avoid filling up on low-energy foods such as low-energy soups, tea, coffee and water. While fluids are important, these drinks tend to make you feel full without providing the necessary nutrition. So try to eat high-energy soups and drinks that will give you both fluid and nourishment.
- If you are losing weight, then choose high-energy meals and snacks, which allow you to manage with smaller portions.
- Choose foods that you fancy. You may worry that they are not the most nutritious foods but it is important to eat what you are able.
- Be flexible in your meal pattern. It is important to eat when you are hungry, so have lots of snacks available and take advantage of these.

The emotional aspects of eating

Not wanting to eat can cause friction with family and friends who are concerned for you and spend time and energy trying to persuade you to eat. Eating well is synonymous with good health so it is understandable that everyone who loves you feels they can help in this way. Such persuasion, though, can create an atmosphere of tension around mealtimes and eating.

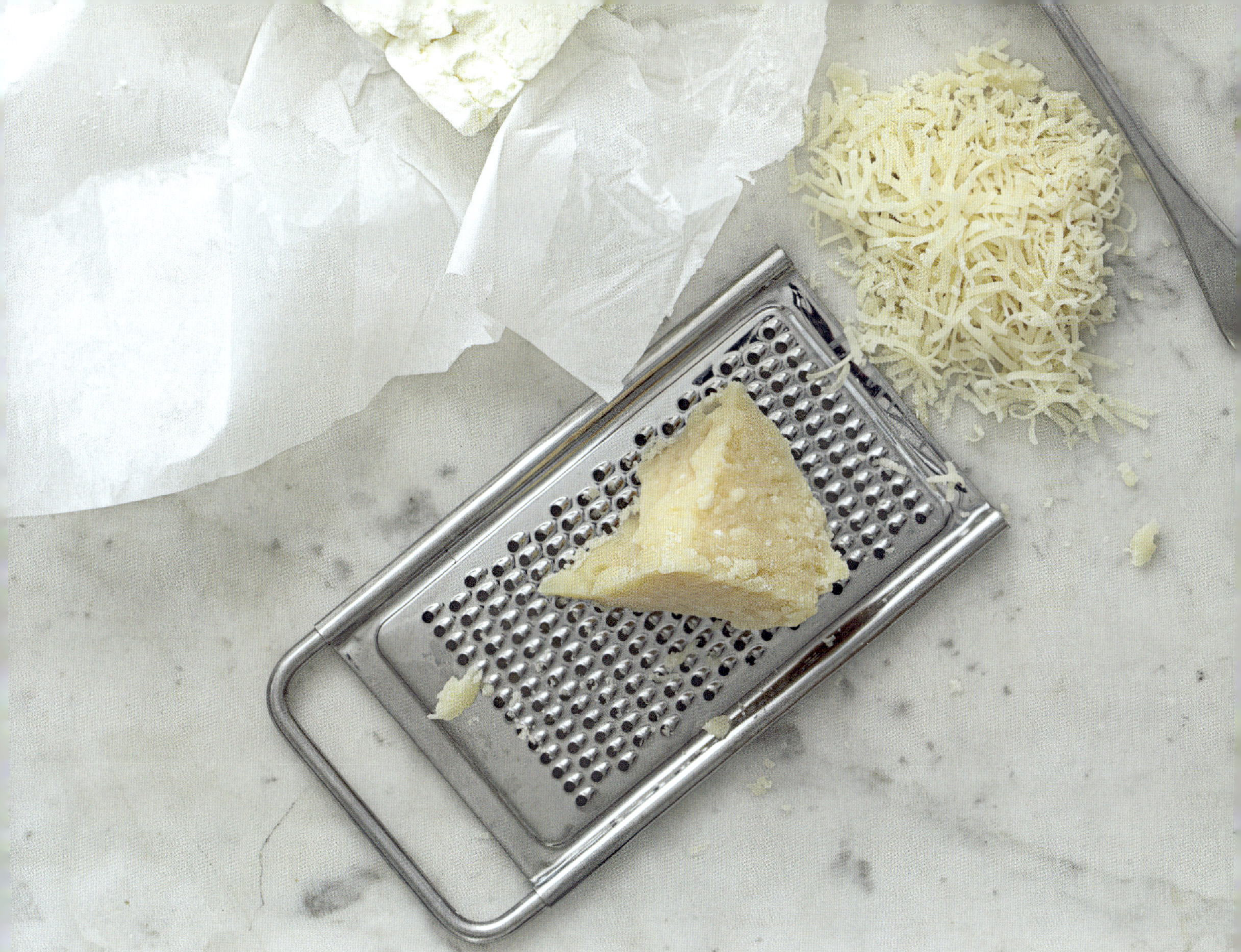

Strategies to avoid mealtimes becoming stressful:

- Speak to your family and friends about eating and how you feel about mealtimes.
- Discuss what time of day you find it easier to eat – it may help to change mealtimes to suit when you most feel like eating.

How to avoid feeling full

At times, the problem can be that you do want to eat but feel full having eaten only a small amount. The advice here is similar to managing a poor appetite, but there are specific strategies you can adopt.

- Try to avoid foods that are high in dietary fibre, as these may make you feel full before you have eaten enough.
- Avoid filling up on liquids before eating – this includes water, tea, coffee and soup. The gas content in fizzy drinks may also make you feel full, so they too are best avoided.
- Try small, frequent meals and snacks throughout the day rather than three meals.
- Go for high-energy drinks, such as milk-based drinks, fruit smoothies and fruit juice-based drinks, rather than water-based ones.
- If soup is easy to eat, enrich it with extra cheese, cream or crème fraîche.

Managing weight loss

One of the reasons people go to their doctor before cancer is diagnosed is because they find they have lost weight. If you have been overweight you may have struggled with keeping your weight down in the past then suddenly you find you are losing weight without trying. Losing weight in this way can result in a number of unwelcome outcomes:

- You feel weak and tired and find you have lost muscle bulk
- Your body is physically less able to withstand cancer treatment such as surgery or chemotherapy
- You start to feel uncomfortable or self-conscious about your body, particularly if you lose weight quickly

It is advisable to try to avoid weight loss during treatment. Often losing weight is the result of loss of appetite, nausea or being too tired to prepare food. Wherever possible, you need to increase the energy in your diet to try to prevent further weight loss.

Many people comment that the high-energy foods suggested are not necessarily 'healthy choices' but it is important to remember that they are being recommended for a particular reason and often for a limited period of time. The overall balance of your diet is still important and eating sufficient energy and protein is a priority. If you are concerned that you are not able to eat a good variety of foods to ensure you are getting a balanced diet you should seek advice from a health care professional such as a dietitian.

Tips to make eating easier:

- Opt for foods that are soft and easy to eat. Use sauces and gravies to make food moist and appetising.
- Make a batch of sauce and freeze in small portions to use at a later date.
- Try to have a dessert after meals. If you are too full to eat it straight away, then try an hour or so later. Keep high-energy ice cream in the freezer so preparation is simple and quick.
- Make desserts that will last so that they are easy to serve as a snack or at mealtimes.

Ways to increase the energy of food

- Choose energy-dense foods when you can. These include full-fat versions of everyday items including milk, yogurt, crème fraîche and cream, spreads and oils.
- Increase the energy content of everyday foods by adding a little olive oil, butter, milk, cheese or sauce, for example, to mashed potato, or drizzle some flavoured oil on pasta or into couscous.
- Look for the recipes here that are higher in energy – you can eat a small portion but still get lots of essential nutrients.
- Avoid low-fat or low-energy foods, for example, low-fat versions of salad dressings, desserts, dairy products or savoury snacks.
- Snack between meals choosing high-energy foods such as nuts, dried fruits or treats such as chocolate or homemade cookies.
- Add a swirl of cream to porridge or desserts for a deliciously creamy texture and taste.
- Avoid relying on soup alone as your meal as this can often be low in nourishment. Fortify soup by blending in protein sources including chicken, milk and milk powder, or pulses such as lentils. Serve with grated cheese.

Recipe ideas

- Reconstitute skimmed milk powder with ordinary full-fat milk rather than water. Use this fortified milk for cereal, sauces, drinks and milk puddings.
- Plant-based milks can be low in energy and protein. Add protein powder (for example pea, brown rice, soya or flaxseed protein powder) to plant-based milks. Use this fortified plant-based milk for cereals, sauces, drinks and puddings.
- Add an egg to mashed potato or rice before serving. Make sure that it is hot enough to cook the egg properly.
- Add extra cheese to mashed potato and sauces, and use extra as a topping on cooked dishes such as shepherd's pie, cottage pie and fish pie. Crumble feta cheese into side salads and serve extra Parmesan on soup and pasta dishes.

- Make high-protein shakes by adding milk, yogurt, peanut butter, powdered peanut butter, ground nuts eg. almonds or cashews or tofu to fresh fruit and blend until smooth.
- Use nuts and seeds in stir-fries, desserts, breakfast cereals or just enjoy as snacks.

Ideas for snacks

- For savoury snacks to eat between meals choose biscuits with cheese, cheese spread, cold meats, fish or vegetable pâté, avocado or hummus. Use butter on savoury cheese biscuits, crispbreads, pitta bread, toast or bread.
- Olives, sun-dried tomatoes in oil, potato crisps, rice crackers and vegetable chips are all easy snacks that are high in energy.
- Oatcakes, wheat or rye crackers, bread or toast – spread with butter and serve with a topping such as: nut butter (peanut, almond or hazelnut); cheese or full-fat cream cheese topped with tomato, cucumber, fruit or chutney; cold meats, such as ham or salami. Serve with salad vegetables (tomatoes, carrots, celery or cucumber sticks).
- Toasted teacake with butter and jam, honey or lemon curd.
- Small sausages or sausage rolls.
- Samosas or spring rolls.
- Popcorn with added butter or syrup.
- Nuts (plain, roasted, salted or unsalted) – try cashews, Brazil nuts, walnuts, hazelnuts and almonds.
- Seeds, including pumpkin, sunflower or sesame.
- Dried fruit (apricots, pear, mango, dates, sultanas and raisins).
- Trail mix – a mixture of dried fruit, nuts and chocolate.
- Individual pots of full-fat yogurt, custard, mousse, crème caramel, rice pudding and fruit fool. These can be bought or made beforehand and stored in the fridge as easy and nutritious snacks. If using plant-based yogurt choose those with a higher energy content. Serve with fresh or canned fruit or fruit coulis to add flavour and variety. Add granola or chopped nuts and honey to Greek yogurt.
- Homemade flapjack or cookies (freeze ready-rolled biscuit mix to bake when needed).
- Plain biscuits such as shortbread.
- Cake or muffins.
- Muesli or yogurt-coated fruit and nut bars.
- Scotch pancakes with butter and jam, or a topping such as fruit, honey or maple syrup.
- Toasted crumpets or English muffins with butter, cheese or jam.
- Fruit smoothies made from fresh or frozen fruit blended with yogurt or bought ready prepared.
- Drinking yogurt.
- Hot milky drinks such as hot chocolate or malted milk.
- Milkshake – add ice cream or fruit for extra flavour.

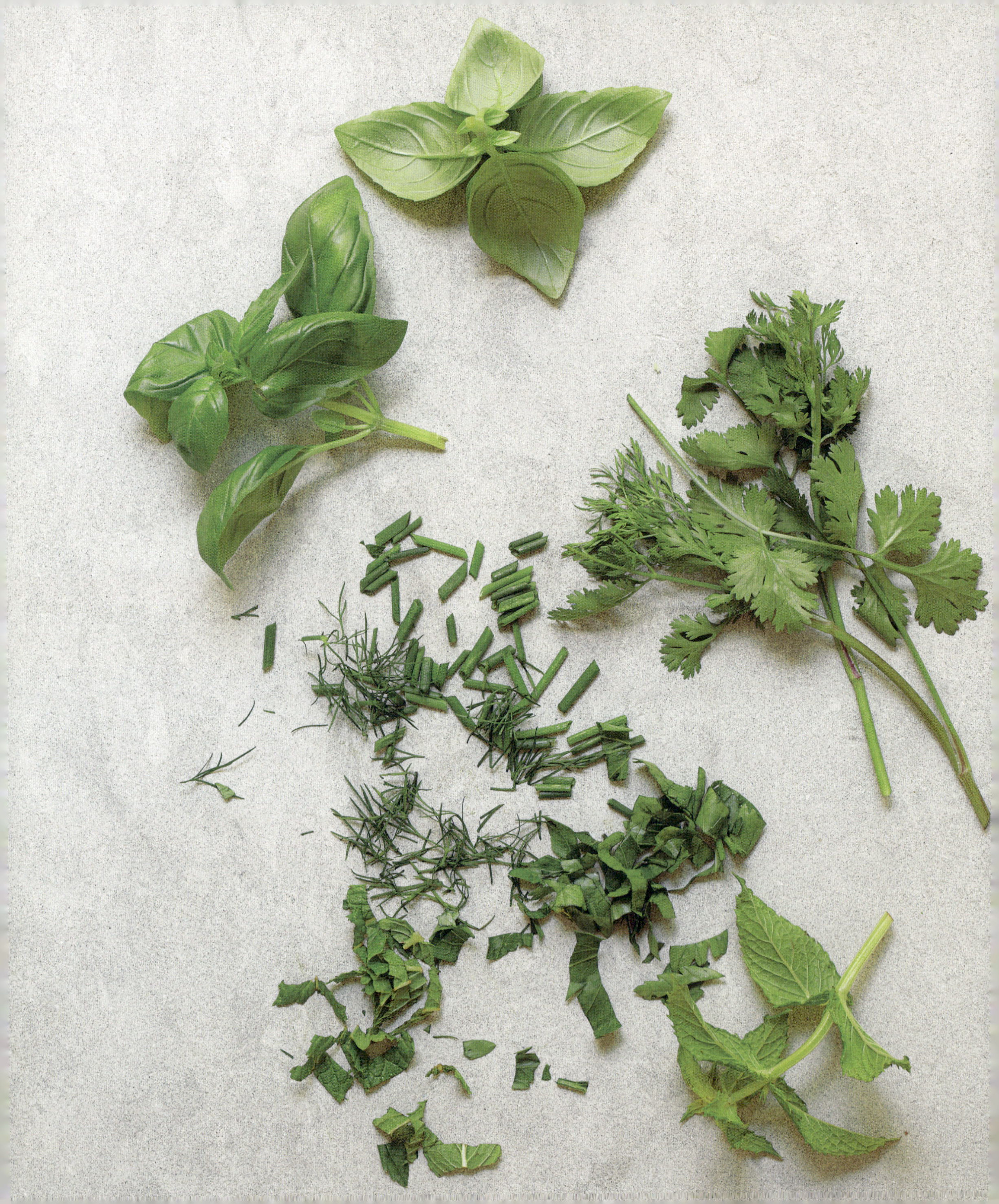

Taste changes

Taste changes can be difficult to deal with. It is thought that the cells in the oral cavity are damaged or desensitised by cancer drugs or therapy. Most people experience taste changes, particularly if they are undergoing chemotherapy, although such changes can occur during or after any type of cancer treatment. The effect, which makes usually delicious foods taste bland, tasteless, unusual or even unpleasant, removes much of the pleasure of eating. Dealing with taste changes requires patience and a willingness to try new flavours or combinations of foods.

Changes to smell perception may also be altered during cancer treatment. This can affect a person in many ways and can significantly affect their quality of life. Firstly, as smell and taste are inextricably linked, changes to the sense of smell may affect how foods taste. It may make identifying flavours more difficult. Secondly, it may contribute to feelings of nausea or aversions to food if smells seem unpleasant or overpowering. Trying to avoid such smells is crucial to managing these aversions, although that is not always easy. Aiming to stay away from cooking smells, keeping the home well ventilated and choosing cold foods with little odour may help some people.

Tastes and smells can change over time and those experienced early in treatment may not persist, although new ones may develop. The good news is that this side effect often diminishes with time, but while the changes persist try to ensure that they do not cause you to reduce your food intake or alter the balance of your diet. Eating is about how your food looks and smells as well as tastes, so choose and prepare dishes that appeal to all the senses. Hopefully the ideas in this book will help identify flavours to stimulate the taste buds. Trialling regular and new flavours is thought to be a useful way of managing taste changes and stimulating the taste buds. Below are the most common taste changes that have been identified, with suggestions of ways to deal with them:

Food does not taste of anything

Tastes and smells may be harder to identify. This means that the principal flavours – sweet, sour, salty and bitter – are trickier to detect. Here are some tips and tricks to help the flavour along:

- Use herbs (fresh or dried) and spices.
- Choose foods that are moist and served with sauces.
- Add a little more salt to food – best to do this at the table, particularly if others are eating the same dish.
- Try hot or warm foods – our taste buds more readily detect flavours when food is warm.
- Add a little more sugar, or use honey or syrup – this adds more energy as well as flavour to recipes and meals, and some people tolerate sweet foods well.
- Try fruit coulis on desserts to give a pleasingly sharp tang to the dish. These could be made from red berry or citrus fruits, provided your mouth isn't sore.
- Try adding sauces or dressings, such as soy sauce or balsamic vinegar, at the table or during cooking.
- Unless your mouth is sore, try citrus flavours such as a squeeze of lemon and lime on your food, or sip lime cordial with sparkling water and ice.
- Add slices of lemon or lime to a jug of iced water or a glass of iced green tea.
- Crush fresh mint leaves into a cup and pour over boiling water for a refreshing drink.

Food tastes bitter or metallic

People with cancer commonly cite foods such as meat, citrus fruit, chocolate, tea and coffee as becoming less palatable or experience particular aversions to some foods, which may be worse if they are associated with feeling sick or if there are strong smells around, particularly food or cooking smells. Some people find that they have a bitter taste in their mouth, which may occur at meal times or between meals and snacks, or that certain foods themselves, such as meat, taste bitter. Medication may be an influence in these taste changes.

- Consider alternative foods – meat, for example, can be replaced by eggs, yogurt and cheese, which may be more palatable.
- Try some of the ideas on page 169 and drink fruit or herbal teas, cordials or smoothies.
- Try hot chocolate or malted milk drinks as an alternative to tea or coffee – milky drinks will also give you protein and energy.
- Try to eat foods that are cold or at room temperature.
- Soak meat in fruit juice or a fruity marinade to help counteract a bitter taste.
- Suck sweets between meals and snacks to offset a bad taste in your mouth.

Cravings

You may experience a craving for sweet or salty foods which would not be your typical choice. Keep an open mind and try these new flavours that you would not normally have while keeping a good balance overall with as much variety as you can.

Sore mouth or throat

There can be many reasons why your mouth or throat is sore during treatment. The tissues lining the mouth are particularly susceptible to damage during chemotherapy, you may have had radiotherapy to the mouth or throat, or you may have an infection in the mouth. If you find eating or swallowing painful, seek advice on the best way to manage this. Below are ways to make swallowing less difficult or painful:

- Continue to drink plenty of fluids and, if your lips are sore, try using a straw.
- Choose foods that are bland, soft, moist and easy to eat.
- If you are only able to eat small amounts, fortify your food to increase the protein and energy by adding milk powder, full-fat milk or cream. Grate cheese on top of soup or add some to sauces.
- Avoid food that is dry, rough and takes a lot of chewing, for example, bread, muesli and nuts.
- Avoid foods such as citrus fruits, tomatoes or tomato-based sauces – these are acidic or tart and will inflame the lining of the mouth.
- Reduce the amount of salt and seasoning in savoury dishes as this can irritate the lining of the mouth. Similarly, spiced dishes such as chilli, chutney or curry should be avoided.
- Use homemade stock to make soup, as ready-made stock can be rather salty. Add milk or cream to increase the energy and protein content.
- If chewing is difficult mash vegetables such as potatoes, sweet potatoes, carrots, swedes and yam, and stir in extra butter, margarine or oil to soften them.
- Cook cereals until they are soft, for example, porridge, also for rice pudding.
- Choose easy-to-swallow desserts such as custard, crème caramel, crème brûlée, mousse, full-fat yogurt and ice cream.
- Suck ice cubes or freeze fruits such as pineapple, grapes, blueberries and raspberries, and eat straight from the freezer, provided your teeth are not too sensitive to the cold. Try drinking the juice from canned pineapple.
- Choose sorbet for dessert made from fruits that are not too acidic, such as mango, apple or pear.

Dry mouth and difficulty swallowing

Eating and speaking can be very difficult if your mouth is dry. This can result from a number of reasons, but radiotherapy to the mouth or throat or the drugs you have been given are especially likely to cause a dry mouth. These are some ways that will make it less difficult:

- Choose foods that are very moist and easy to eat. Many of the recipes in this book are designed to be soft or have plenty of sauce or gravy.
- Avoid foods that are dry or difficult to chew, such as meat, especially cold meat, pastry, bread and crackers – these will only make your mouth even drier.
- Choose moist fish, eggs and cheese dishes. Well-cooked pulses in dahl or stew can also be easy to eat.
- Make extra sauce or gravy and freeze in small portions. That way you'll always have some ready to serve with other meals.
- Consider puréeing your meals, for example, stews and casseroles, if eating is very difficult. Or you can blend parts of a meal separately so that you have more colour, flavour and interest on your plate, which will look more appetising.
- Have extra nourishing drinks or desserts between meals to increase your intake.

Combating nausea

There are many different drugs that can be used to help alleviate nausea and sickness, so do let your doctor or nurse know if this is a problem as feeling sick can make it very hard to eat and drink, particularly if you have other side effects too, such as taste changes or having a bad taste in your mouth. Getting the medication right can make a huge difference to how much you can eat and it can restore the enjoyment of eating.

Other triggers for feeling sick include certain smells and brushing your teeth. It may help if you are able to relax or use the television or hobbies as a distraction. Here are some tips to help choose foods and drinks for when you feel especially sick:

- Try bland foods with little seasoning or strong flavours.
- Choose carbohydrate-based foods such as crackers, savoury or plain biscuits, cookies, bread or toast.
- Combine protein foods if possible with carbohydrate foods, for example cheese with mashed or baked potato or pasta.
- Try yogurt or cold desserts such as crème caramel, custard or mousse.
- Ginger is an old remedy for nausea – try as ginger biscuits, ginger beer or ginger ale or the syrup from perserved ginger. Try ginger tea as an alternative to black tea or coffee.
- Sip drinks containing sugar such as fruit juices – try apple, grape, cranberry, red berry, orange or grapefruit juices.

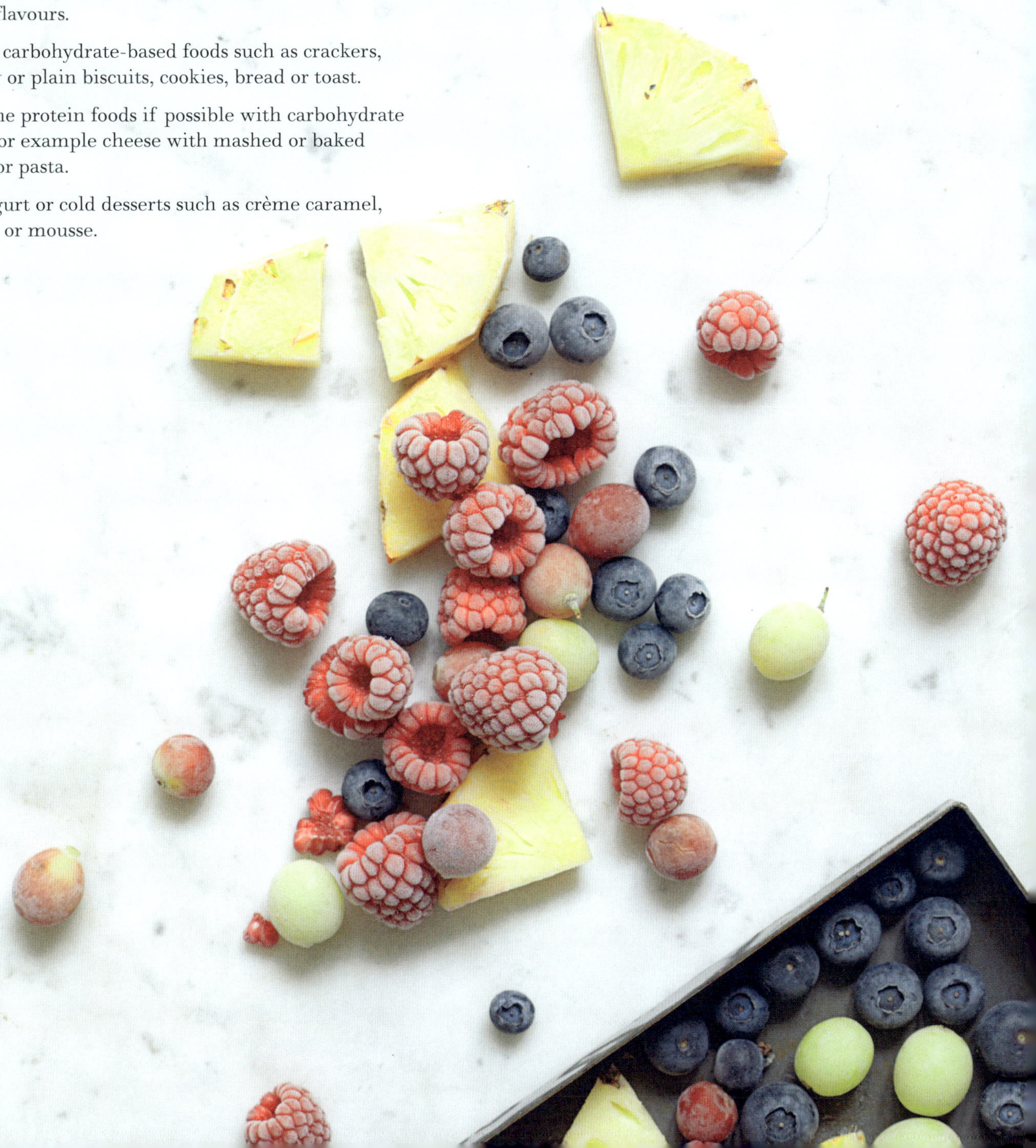

Managing the digestive system

The digestive system is very sensitive to changes in diet, medication and treatments. There are some simple measures which may be helpful for reflux and bloating:

- Eat small, frequent meals and snacks
- Try not to eat immediately before lying down
- Take care with fizzy/carbonated drinks as they can make you feel bloated
- Avoid drinking with a straw as it may encourage air to be swallowed

All forms of cancer treatment can affect how your digestive system works. Problems with digestion can be a side effect of chemotherapy, radiotherapy or medication you are prescribed for pain. All of these can alter how much you can eat, how quickly or slowly food travels through your system and possibly how efficiently nutrients are absorbed from your food. During chemotherapy a small proportion of people may develop an intolerance to lactose (milk sugar). This is often short-lived and can be managed by using alternatives to milk such as soya, rice, almond, hazelnut or oat milk with a return to cow's milk when symptoms of diarrhoea have settled. Many people are not sensitive to lactose so it is worth discussing this with your doctor before changing your diet. Remember that some alternatives to milk may be lower in essential nutrients, such as energy and protein, so always check the nutritional information.

Any changes in your bowel habits should always be discussed with your specialist team. Diarrhoea may be a sign of infection or result of chemotherapy and therefore need specific measures to manage. Similarly, with radiotherapy to the abdomen such changes in bowel habits need to be managed by your team. It can be tempting to change your diet to try to control bowel habits in these circumstances, but there is an ongoing debate as to whether changes in types of diet or quantities of foods, such as fruits, vegetables and wholegrain cereals, actually make enough of a difference when treatment is the cause.

In the case of radiotherapy to the abdomen or pelvis, changes in bowel habits may occur months or years after treatment and are known as pelvic radiation disease (PRD). The problems experienced are very individual and can vary greatly but they are common to a great many people who have been treated for cancer. It is very important that you talk to your medical team about the problems you have and how they affect you. Often people worry that their symptoms mean that the cancer has returned, but this is not necessarily the case. You may need some further investigation to find out what is causing the symptoms but the outcome may mean you are better able to manage in the future. Sometimes medication or changes to your diet will improve things but any remedial action should always be undertaken with the help of health care professionals.

If you have finished radiotherapy treatment to the abdomen but continue to have loose stools or urgency to get to the toilet or are woken at night to open your bowels, then this should always be discussed with your GP. You would benefit from referral to a gastroenterologist for specialist advice and management. See the contact details for the Pelvic Radiation Disease Association for advice and support on page 47.

Restricted diet

Many people find that their diet becomes more restricted during cancer treatment. There may be foods that they are unable to tolerate due to a sore mouth, nausea or taste changes, or they may develop aversions to certain foods. There may be foods that they would normally eat without any problem but suddenly they feel unable to cope with, such as coffee, tea, chocolate, citrus fruits, meat or milk. Diet may already be limited prior to treatment due to problems with swallowing or feeling full. In addition, many people already make choices about their food intake for medical, religious or cultural reasons, avoiding foods such as meat and animal products, high-fat foods, salt or sugar.

Ideally, try to find alternatives to usual foods to keep variety in the diet both for taste and nutrition. Often, it may feel easier just to manage on a limited number of foods but this is neither interesting nor nutritious. If you really struggle to find alternatives or follow a medically prescribed diet, then always ask for advice from a registered dietitian. There are many food and recipe ideas in this book to help guide you to make good and varied choices.

Frequently Asked Questions

What can I eat to help my nails and hair?

This is probably the most commonly asked question of all, since treatments for cancer affect many tissues in the body and you will be especially aware of the damage to your skin, hair and nails. Many people will lose their hair or experience thinning, and changes to nails are also very common as they may become fragile, develop ridges and grow slowly. Hair loss and nail changes that result from chemotherapy will improve when the drugs are stopped, although it may take time to resume normal growth. It is not known to what extent the quality of your diet can influence this regrowth but certainly a good balanced intake with all the necessary nutrients will do much to support the body during its post-treatment recovery. Our tissues are made of protein, and their composition and health reflect our diet and blood levels of minerals such as zinc and selenium. Look to include foods in your diet that contain a variety of vitamins and trace elements to really support nail and hair growth following cancer treatment. Good sources of minerals are outlined on page 21.

Is there anything I can eat to help my immune system?

Being able to fight infection is important, especially for people with cancer. Cancer itself, particularly leukaemia and lymphomas, and cancer treatments can lower the immune system and make people more susceptible to infection from bacteria, viruses or fungal infections. It is important to try to avoid losing weight, as this can make it difficult for the immune system to recover, particularly between courses of chemotherapy. Having a good balanced diet and following the principles outlined in this book are also helpful, although there are no specific nutrients or foods that can be eaten to actually boost the immune system.

It is very important that food does not become a source of infection, so follow guidance to reduce the chance of food-borne organisms. You may receive specific advice from your medical team about foods to avoid during treatment. Always discuss these with your doctor so you are clear on why you need to avoid them and for how long. If these restrictions make it difficult for you to follow a good varied diet, then ask to speak to a dietitian who can help you plan a good intake.

Some foods may pose a high risk of food-borne organisms. Good food hygiene is essential for everyone, but particularly for those who are undergoing cancer treatment. There are some foods that should be avoided as they carry a high risk of being a source of food-borne pathogens, or germs. These include raw eggs (a source of salmonella), liver pâté (a source of listeria), cheese made from unpasteurised milk and sushi.

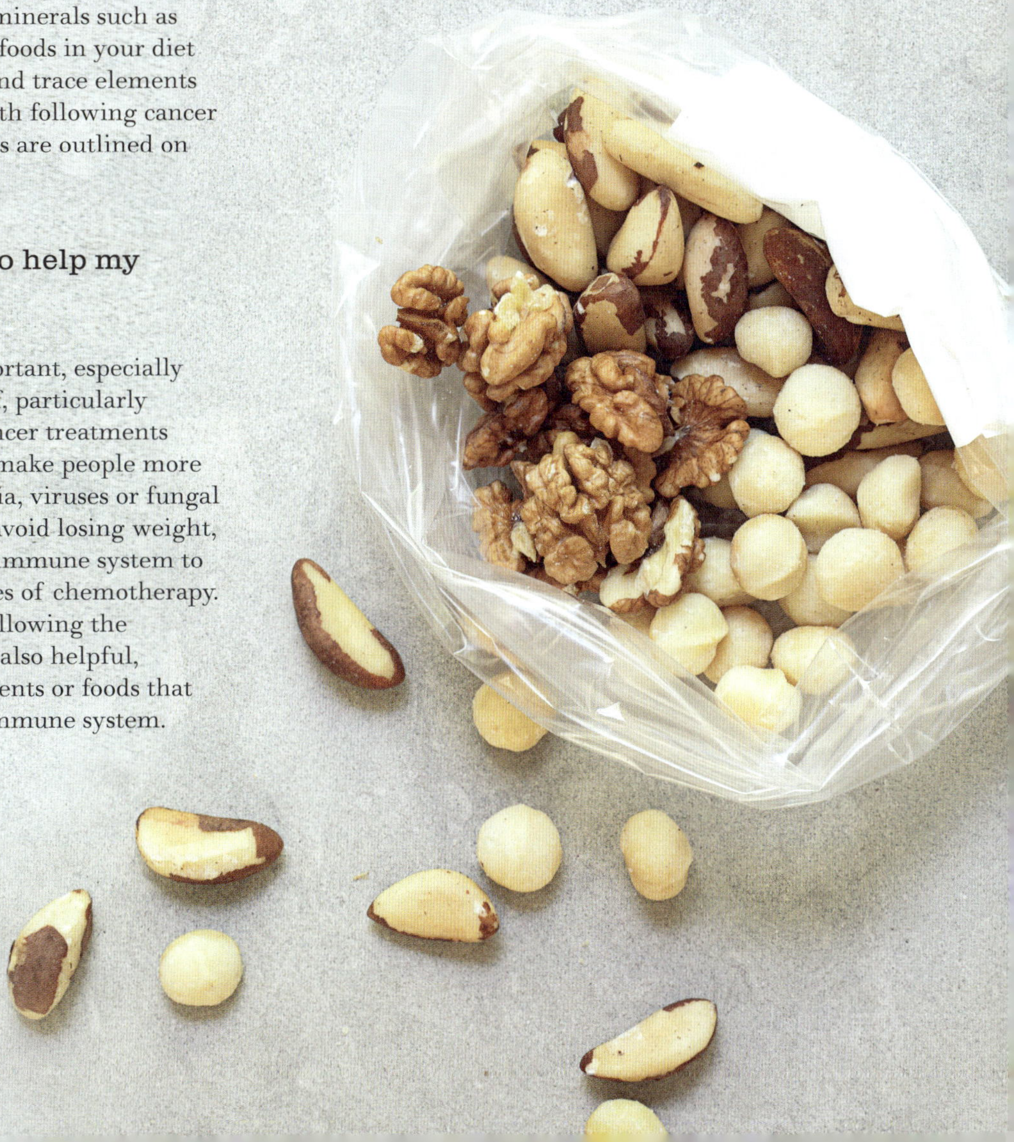

Tips for good food hygiene include:

- Always wash your hands before preparing food. This is especially important and should be done thoroughly, using soap and hot water, and a clean towel to dry them.
- Wash all worktops and preparation surfaces before and after food preparation using hot soapy water.
- Keep dishcloths and tea towels clean by washing them regularly and letting them dry before using.
- Keep separate chopping boards for raw and ready-to-eat foods and use a separate board for meat. Wash and dry well between uses.
- Keep raw meat, chicken and fish separate from either cooked or ready-to-eat foods such as fruit, salad, cheese and bread. Ensure that raw meat is stored at the bottom of the fridge so it cannot drip on any other foods. This is particularly important if these foods do not undergo cooking before being eaten.
- Cook food thoroughly and ensure it is piping hot before serving. Cook meat thoroughly until the flesh is no longer pink.
- Keep your fridge below 5°C to reduce the growth of bacteria. Always put chilled food in the fridge as soon as you return home after shopping. Check with a fridge thermometer if you are unsure how well your fridge works.
- Cool any cooked food that you are not going to eat straight away as quickly as possible (within 90 minutes) and store it in the fridge or freezer. Some of the recipes in this book can be reheated so make sure you use them within a couple of days or store in the freezer if you are not sure when you will eat them. Defrost in the fridge before reheating and check that they are heated through properly before eating.
- Cooked rice is a particularly high-risk food if it is cooled and reheated. Rice left at room temperature is susceptible to growing the spores of a bacterium, *Bacillus cereus*, which causes food poisoning.
- If you buy ready-prepared foods always eat before the 'use by' date.

Is there a connection between sugar in the diet and cancer?

Both healthy cells and cancerous cells use glucose (a simple sugar) for energy. This is sourced from sugars and starchy carbohydrates in the diet. Some people have suggested that by avoiding sugar you can alter the growth of cancer cells. However, restricting sugar in the diet has not been proved to be effective in controlling the growth of cancer cells. Sugar occurs naturally in many foods. It's a source of energy (calories) and makes food palatable, which helps if your appetite is poor and you have lost weight, but should be eaten in moderation if you are trying to lose weight after treatment. It should be balanced with foods that provide nutrients such as protein, fat, vitamins and minerals.

What are antioxidants?

Oxidation is a term for the chemical reaction that takes place when oxygen interacts with molecules. This is a common occurrence and involves reactions such as obtaining energy from our food. The process of oxidation occurs throughout the body and it is during this process that free radicals are produced. Free radicals are often thought of as bad, but this is not always the case. They have a number of jobs in the body, including protecting it against bacteria, and some types of cancer treatment, such as chemotherapy and radiotherapy, may work by producing free radicals. However, free radicals can also damage healthy tissues in the body and this is why there is much interest in antioxidants such as vitamin C, selenium and lycopene. These nutrients may work directly on the free radicals themselves or via the body's own chemical reactions, resulting in the free radicals being inactivated. The body needs antioxidants from food we eat, but there is concern that taking higher doses in supplements may not be helpful.

What should I do about my weight at the end of my treatment?

Once your treatment is over, or you begin maintenance treatment or surveillance, it may be a good time to think about your body weight. If you lost weight during treatment you may need to continue with a high-energy and protein diet to help you regain your weight and strength. On the other hand, if you are overweight, think about reducing your weight to within the normal range by following a healthy diet and taking suitable exercise. Always speak to your doctor and agree when is the right time before you deliberately try to lose weight.

Why is it important to not be overweight?

We know that being overweight is associated with the development of some types of cancer, such as breast and prostate cancer. Treatment, particularly some chemotherapy and hormone treatments, can encourage weight gain. Steroids, which may be used in conjunction with chemotherapy or given in low doses as anti-sickness drugs, may increase appetite and body weight, and make it harder to lose weight. It can be particularly frustrating and upsetting to find you are heavier at the end of treatment than you were at the beginning and that your clothes no longer fit. Some people develop negative feelings about their body image, and find it more difficult to exercise, which, ultimately, is bad for their overall health and recovery.

There is also concern that additional weight after treatment may actually influence the risk of some types of cancer recurring. Increasingly, studies suggest that weight gain and being overweight are not good for women with post-menopausal breast cancer and this may be the case for those with colorectal cancer and men with prostate cancer. This is a complex subject and varies greatly according to the type of cancer, so it is crucial that the issues are discussed fully with your medical team before you aim to change your weight.

How do I know if I am overweight?

The Body Mass Index (BMI) is one of a number of ways to judge if you are overweight. It is calculated by dividing your weight in kilograms by the square of your height in metres. Charts and programmes to calculate your BMI using your height and weight measurements are easy to find on the internet. For most adults the ideal range for BMI is 18.5–24.9kg/m^2. If your BMI is above 25kg/m^2 this is an indication that you are heavier than the ideal for your height.

A simpler method to check whether you are carrying too much weight is to take a simple measurement of the size of your waist. Carrying too much weight around your middle can increase your risk of a number of conditions including heart disease and type 2 diabetes.

If your waist measurement is greater than the following, then your risk of health problems is higher:

Men – more than 94cm (37 inches)
Men (African Caribbean, South Asian, Chinese and Japanese origin) – more than 90 cm (35.4 inches)
Women – more than 80cm (31.5 inches)

Remember, if you are overweight and not struggling to eat, then any weight loss is beneficial to your health.

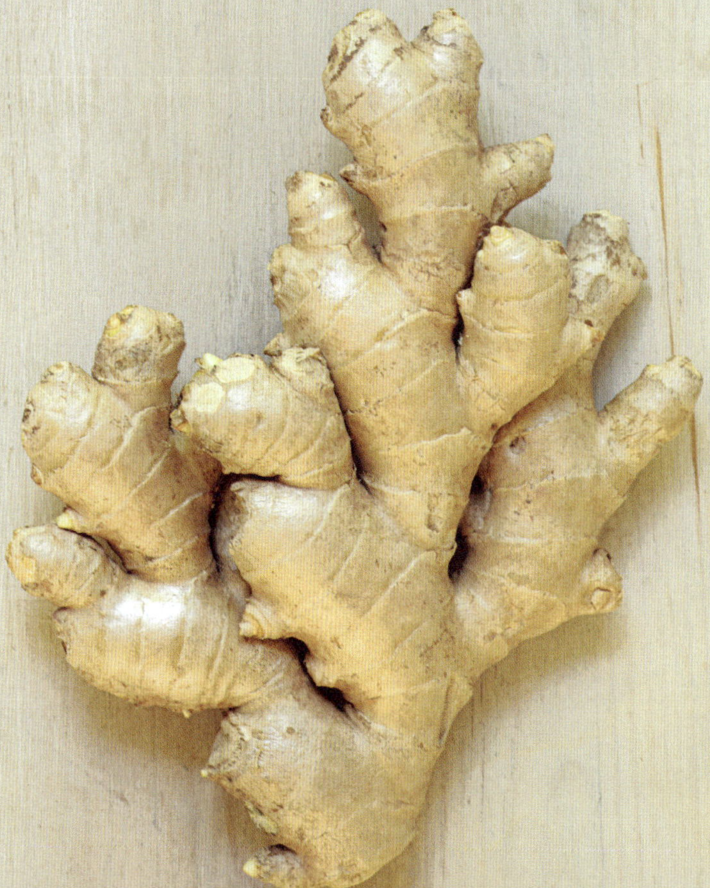

What is the best way to lose weight?

Any dietary changes should aim to reduce overall energy (calorie) intake while maintaining good food choices and therefore sufficient nutrients in the diet. This may include changing foods you choose to eat but also reducing the quantity or portion sizes you eat on a regular basis. There are many opinions on losing weight and there are hundreds of books on dieting. Not all of them give good, balanced advice so it can be difficult to know what is right for you. Many of these diets will work in the short term but it is important that they are not extreme, avoid many foods and give you a regime that is difficult to continue. A truly healthy diet must be adequate in all the nutrients and lower in energy so that you burn your own body fat stores.

If you are overweight, then losing even a small amount of weight can improve your chances of not developing cancer, heart disease, high blood pressure and the risk of diabetes. It may have particular benefits for those diagnosed with hormone-dependent cancer, such as breast and prostate cancer. Don't be put off if you feel you have too much to lose; losing weight may be a long process but is worth it in the end. You will feel better, have more energy and feel more comfortable in your clothes.

There is endless discussion over which types of diet are best for weight loss. However, there is broad agreement that a healthy weight-reducing diet should be low in fat and sugar and high in plant-based foods (vegetables, fruit, grains and pulses) and that lean protein foods are important because they help you to feel full after a meal.

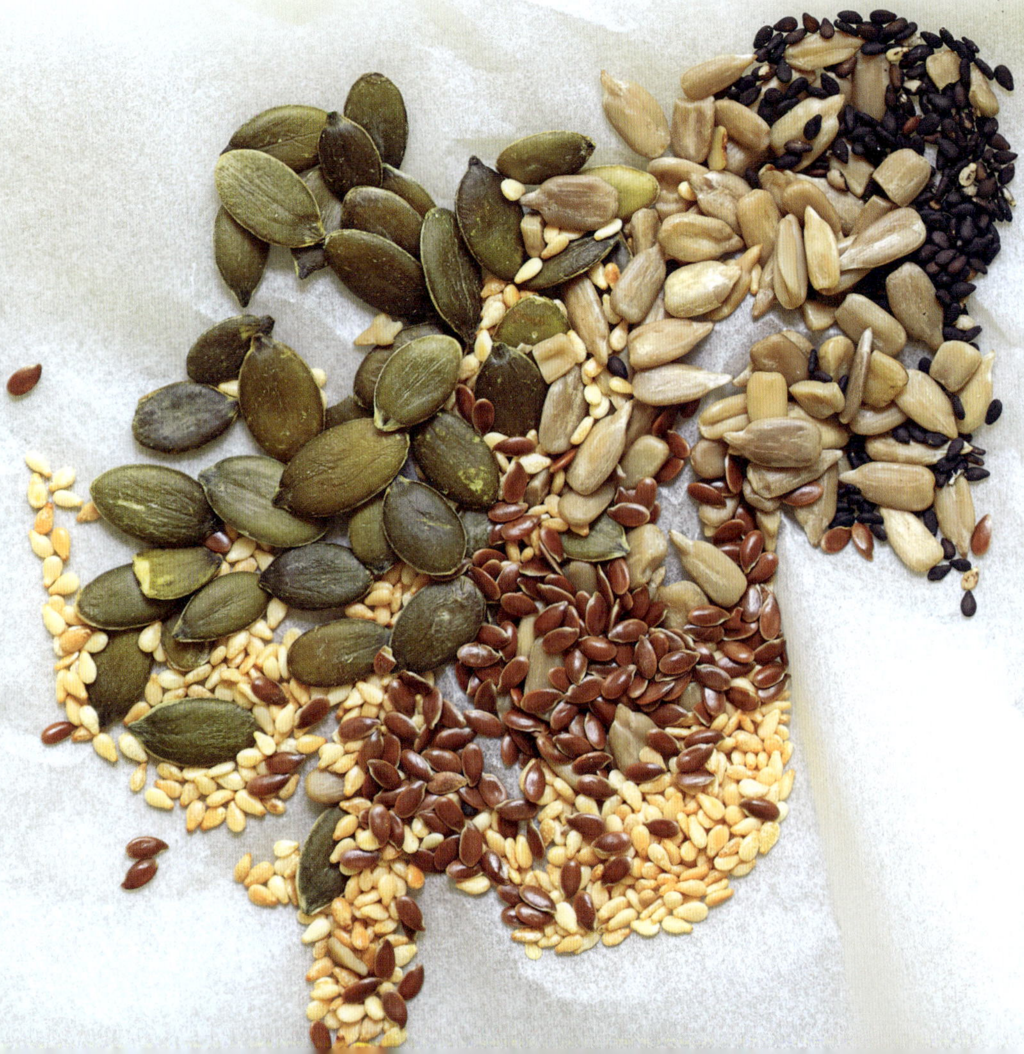

There is currently much interest in the use of 'intermittent' diets, such as the 5:2 principle, which is eating a balanced Mediterranean-style diet for five days, then restricting your food intake to a low-carbohydrate diet providing 600–650 kilocalories, or kcal, (2,500–2,700 kilojoules) per day for the remaining two days. Some studies of women with breast cancer found that this compared well with trying to restrict intake every day. More studies are needed to determine the safety and effectiveness of these diets, but the early results are encouraging.

Perhaps the most important part of losing weight is changing your behaviour. A diagnosis of cancer can be a motivating factor to change aspects of your life, of which diet and exercise may be a part. You may need help to do this, so do ask your healthcare team for advice. Weight-loss support groups or the encouragement of friends and family can make a big difference in helping you to achieve your goal.

Mindfulness in eating may be an important part of making these changes in the long term. This involves the person considering the links between external influences on food choices, such as habit, enjoyment, lifestyle, peer pressure, portion size, and triggers for overeating. This may be particularly helpful in managing your food choices when hungry, and really understanding why you make some food choices at certain times. Understanding these influences is often the first step to making effective changes to your food intake.

Increasing exercise when you are trying to lose weight can also make a real difference to your health. It helps to maintain your muscle strength and burns energy, so that you lose weight.

If you are overweight and have finished treatment, then always speak to your medical team to check whether it is a good time to try to reduce your weight to a healthy level. Some treatments, such as steroids or hormone treatments, may make losing weight more difficult but this does not mean it is not possible. You may benefit from some support, either from the hospital, from community health care or via online weight-support groups. Always check that these are reputable and do not give strict advice that results in you eating an unbalanced diet. If the advice is very different from the principles outlined here, then it may not be the best diet for you.

Here are some tips to help you lose weight:

- Plan ahead so you have the right foods in the fridge and cupboard to avoid the temptation to eat snacks or make poor choices.
- Eat regularly throughout the day and always eat breakfast, making sure it's healthy.
- Choose meals that include starchy carbohydrate foods that are also high in dietary fibre – porridge, sugar-free muesli, wholegrain bread, baked potato, brown rice, pulses.
- Include protein foods in your meals – fish, chicken, lean meat, egg, cheese, pulses (beans and lentils) and tofu – as these will make you feel full.
- Watch portion sizes and eat a little less than usual at mealtimes – using a smaller plate may be helpful.
- Take care to restrict intake of fats, including oils and spreads.
- Avoid sugary foods and drinks.
- Don't be too strict on yourself – you will find it much harder to keep to such a diet.
- Aim to lose 0.5–1kg (1–2lb) per week.
- Following the meal ideas and recipes in this book will give you high-nutrient meals to ensure you get all the vitamins and minerals you need.
- Take time with meals – slow down your eating, giving your body time to tell you when you have had enough.
- If you are hungry and want a snack, swap high-fat and high-sugar foods for ones that are lower in fat and sugar. For example, choose fresh or dried fruit if you are looking for a quick sweet taste. Choose kale chips, baked crisps, vegetable sticks, unsalted nuts and seeds, popcorn and unsalted rice cakes and oatcakes when looking for a savoury snack.
- Choose foods with a low glycaemic index – they are absorbed into the bloodstream more slowly and therefore reduce the insulin response produced by the body. They take longer to digest and may help reduce feelings of hunger. Foods with a low glycaemic index include vegetables, pulses, wholegrain foods (including porridge), unsweetened muesli and some fruits. The glycaemic index is not the only important consideration when choosing a healthy diet, so it is important not to focus on this alone.

- Drink plenty of water – aim for a total of 1.5–2 litres (50–68fl oz) of fluid daily. This can include tea, coffee, water and other drinks. Remember that you need more fluid if it is hot or you take exercise.
- Cut down on alcohol.
- Have a treat on an occasional basis – this may help you keep to healthy eating changes in the long term.

What are the best physical activities after treatment?

There has been a great deal of research to assess whether adopting a healthy lifestyle after cancer treatment brings benefits both in terms of managing side effects and reducing the risk of recurrence. Although as yet unproven for all cancer types, there are positive indications that the combination of a healthy diet and regular exercise can make a significant difference to your recovery and wellbeing, and will help you maintain normal body weight.

Currently, the guidance recommends that everyone should be exercising five times a week for 30 minutes. This may sound a lot but each 30 minutes can be broken down into three 10-minute episodes. Generally, these recommendations also apply for all people with cancer after treatment, although research varies depending on different tumour types.

Exactly what form of exercise is best still needs to be established, but generally the advice is to engage in moderate exertion which increases your heart rate and makes you slightly breathless, but still able to talk and finish a sentence.

Ideas on different forms of exercise:

- Gardening such as digging and raking up leaves
- Housework such as changing bed linen, cleaning windows and vacuuming
- Walking briskly
- Cycling
- Dancing
- Yoga
- Swimming
- Bowling
- Racquet sports such as tennis and badminton

How much fruit and vegetables should I eat?

It is often confusing to know how much is 'enough' when it comes to fruit and vegetables. If you are eating well, then aim to include vegetables or fruit in each meal, with some extra as snacks between. By doing this you should find it easy to eat at least five portions each a day – which is a great starting point. Extra fruit and vegetables, in addition to your five portions, will give you more of those essential vitamins and minerals as well as the phytochemicals that are also present in them. Both vegetables and fruit also give you water and fibre and can make you feel full, which is helpful when you are trying to lose weight. If you are finding it difficult to eat, they can be included in soups, stews, casseroles, baked dishes, desserts and smoothies. You'll find plenty of great ideas in this book for incorporating fruit and vegetables in your diet.

What is a 'portion' of fruit or vegetables?

The term 'portion' is often used to describe fruit or vegetables. A portion is used to describe a weight of about 80g (3oz) of either vegetables or fruit and is based on the recommendation from the World Health Organisation that we should be eating at least 400g (14oz) per day. Some health organisations consider that our daily intake should be higher than this, so consider this amount as a basic regular intake.

Fruit and vegetables can be fresh, frozen, canned or dried. At least 150ml (5fl oz) of fruit juice can also contribute to this daily target, although it should only count as up to one portion, because it lacks the dietary fibre that you get from eating the whole fruit. Beans and pulses also only count as one portion, no matter how much is consumed (the minimum portion is 3 heaped tablespoons). This is because they contain fewer nutrients than other fruit and vegetables.

Starchy plant-based foods, such as potatoes, yams, plantain and cassava, should not be included in the daily portions as they contain mainly starch. Try to get a good range of fruit and vegetables, because their nutritional value varies.

Should I eat a plant-based diet?

A plant-based diet is based on foods with few or no foods that come from animals. People choose plant-based diets for different reasons and these include concerns about animal welfare, health benefits or environmental concerns. A plant-based diet is recommended for cancer prevention but it does not necessarily need to exclude all foods that come from animals such as chicken, turkey, fish, eggs and limited red meat. After a diagnosis of cancer some people may choose to change to a more plant-based diet, however, it is important to ensure that such a diet continues to provide adequate nutrition. If you are vegan and used to eating this type of diet you may find it easy to continue to do so. However, if you are making changes to your usual diet this may require more planning to ensure that you eat sufficient protein (from beans, pulses, tofu, nuts, seeds, meat substitutes made from soya), enough energy (calories) to ensure that you do not lose weight during treatment and a variety to provide sufficient vitamins and minerals. A vegan diet will need to include foods fortified with vitamin B12 as this is not present in a plant only diet. One option may be to take a daily supplement of vitamin B12 to ensure that you receive sufficient. The vitamin and mineral content of a plant-based diet will depend on the types of foods eaten. Some nutrients are more difficult to absorb from plant foods, for example, iron but this can be boosted by including good sources of vitamin C in the same meal eg. citrus fruits, blackcurrants and vegetables such as broccoli, peppers, potatoes and salad.

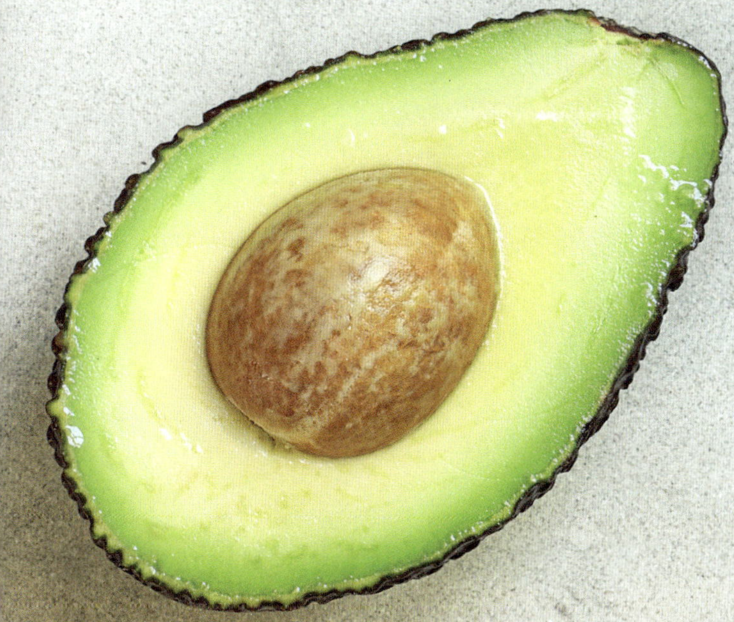

If appetite is low then it can be a challenge to eat sufficient to get all the vitamins and minerals that are required. Look at the ideas on page 26 for adding extra energy and protein to foods.

Sources of protein in a plant-based diet

- Beans and pulses eg. chickpeas, cannellini beans, kidney beans, baked beans
- Nuts and seeds including almonds, hazelnuts, Brazil nuts, linseeds, or sunflower seeds
- Peanuts, powdered peanut butter
- Soya beans and foods made from them ie. edamame beans, soya milk, tofu, tempeh
- Meat free mince or sausages (made from soya, pea and rice protein)
- Quinoa or freekah

Are there any vegetables or fruits that I should include in my diet'?

We often read about 'superfoods' in the media but what does the label mean, and should they be included in your diet? A superfood is one that claims to have special health-giving properties, because it contains particularly beneficial vitamins, minerals or other substances. In relation to cancer, certain berries, pomegranate, wheatgrass, broccoli and green tea have all been called superfoods. However, closer inspection often reveals that these claims are based on limited research, research on animals or popular opinion. The evidence is not conclusive enough for us to be certain that they slow down the growth of cancer in humans. Marketing superfoods is illegal in Europe unless there is substantiated research to support the view that they make a difference to a particular medical condition. Of course, such foods are still a valuable part of the diet, as they are great sources of vitamins or minerals – and, importantly, they taste delicious. This section looks in more detail at some of the particular foods that have been suggested as good for people with cancer to include in their diet.

Pomegranate and berries

Interest in the pomegranate centres on its polyphenol content. Polyphenols are phytonutrients that act as antioxidants. They have been shown to limit the growth of cancer cells in laboratory and animal experiments. Pomegranate juice is of particular interest as it contains the polyphenol compounds from both the juice and skin of multiple fruits. Some Middle Eastern cooking uses pomegranate syrup, which also contains polyphenols.

The polyphenol compounds in pomegranate and berries such as raspberries and blueberries include ellagic acid and luteolin. Natural fruits will vary in their chemical composition, and it has not yet been established whether the benefit from eating such fruits is due to one or more of these substances, or, possibly, to the combination present in the fruit. Some studies have used pomegranate extract to produce a tablet, making it easier to include substantial quantities of these compounds as a supplement to your diet.

In cases of prostate cancer, the presence of a protein known as Prostate Specific Antigen (PSA) is used as a marker of prostate cancer activity. It is not a guarantee of the activity of cancer cells but acts as a guide and has often been used in studies looking at the effect of pomegranate extract. Pomegranate extract appeared to slow the rise in PSA in prostate cancer patients when compared to those taking a placebo (non-active) tablet. More trials are needed to establish whether pomegranate extract can slow the growth of cancer cells. While work continues in this specific area, it is clear that pomegranates and berries provide many nutrients and phytonutrients, which may influence overall health. They taste delicious, are a source of dietary fibre and add an appetising colour to salads, desserts or cereals and yogurt.

Soy foods

Soy foods are of particular interest in those who have been diagnosed with hormone-dependent cancers, particularly breast cancer. Isoflavones are present in soy products such as soya beans and nuts, soya milk and yogurt, tofu, tempeh, textured vegetable protein, miso paste, and, in smaller amounts, in other legumes. Isoflavones, or phytoestrogens, exert an effect that mimics, in a number of ways, the body's own oestrogens. Laboratory experiments indicated that these isoflavones may stimulate the growth of breast cancer cells, but such experiments do not mimic what happens in real life. Large studies of people in the early stages of breast cancer suggest that eating soy foods each day actually reduced the risk of their breast cancer returning.

Brassicas

Vegetables from the brassica family – for example, broccoli, cauliflower, cabbage, kale, Brussels sprouts and pak choi – have generated much interest. These leafy vegetables are good sources of many nutrients, including vitamin C and folate (as folic acid) in addition to vitamins A and K, beta-carotene, calcium and fibre. They also contain other antioxidants, such as isothiocyanates, which had an effect on cancer prevention in laboratory and animal experiments, although human trials have not shown quite the same benefit. Their high nutrient content means that brassicas are an ideal part of a varied diet. They are incredibly versatile and they don't have to be boiled! Try them raw, stir-fried, steamed or baked.

Garlic

Laboratory experiments into the properties of garlic have attracted much attention. The pungent bulb is valuable for its potential ability to reduce blood pressure and hardening of the arteries. Garlic has been used in herbal medicine for millennia. It has been shown to lower cholesterol levels and can make it more difficult for blood to clot, which is why it is good for people with circulation problems, although to date there is little evidence to suggest it is of special benefit to those with cancer. It does add its delicious flavour to sauces, casseroles and stews and may be especially helpful if taste sensation is poor following treatment.

Green tea

Green tea, like other so-called superfoods, has been linked to the prevention of cancer. It contains polyphenols, which are prized for their antioxidant effect. It makes an enjoyable alternative to other hot drinks, although you should limit your intake to no more than six cups a day because very high intakes of green tea may irritate your stomach, alter sleep patterns and possibly influence your heart rate, as some brands contains high levels of caffeine.

Tomatoes

Tomatoes are an excellent source of a number of natural carotenoids including lycopene, which gives tomatoes their distinctive red colour and which has generated a lot of interest because of its antioxidant properties. Lycopene is readily absorbed by the body, particularly when tomatoes are cooked and have oil added to them. This explains why lycopene is present in higher levels in processed products such as tomato purée, sundried tomatoes and tomato sauce.

Studies of lycopene have centred primarily on the apparent link between diets high in tomatoes and a reduced risk of prostate cancer. Whether men diagnosed with prostate cancer can benefit from a diet high in lycopene is unclear. Studies have tended to use lycopene as a dietary supplement and have monitored markers of prostate cancer (such as PSA – see opposite) and therefore there is no concensus so far on whether we should recommend high intakes of tomatoes or other foods containing lycopene, such as watermelon, guava and pink grapefruit. Even so, tomatoes are a high-nutrient food, a great source of vitamin C and potassium, and very easy to include in your diet, cooked or raw, for fantastic colour and flavour.

Turmeric

Curcuminoids are the active substances present in turmeric and mustard. The curcuminoids in turmeric have been taken as a supplement by people receiving radiotherapy. Although they are poorly absorbed by the digestive tract, there is interest in whether they work with treatments such as radiotherapy and chemotherapy to enhance their action of killing cancer cells. Studies have shown that it can reduce inflammation during treatment although it is not totally clear whether this is the most important action or how useful it is.

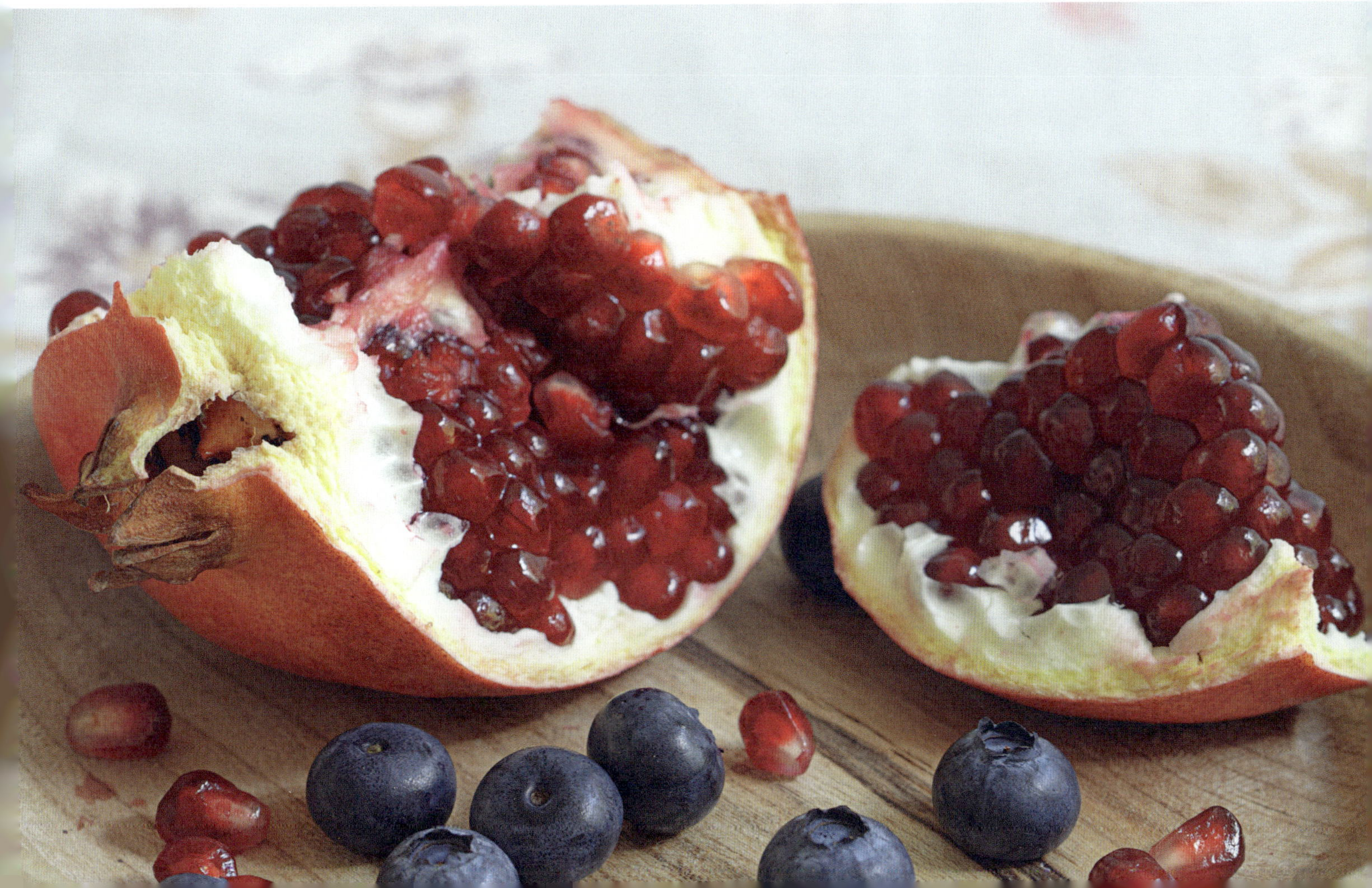

Do I need to take a vitamin and mineral supplement?

This book is filled with ideas for tasty and nutritious meals and snacks that are packed with vitamins and minerals. The best way to obtain all the nutrients you need is through good, healthy food, choosing variety on a daily basis. There are times when eating a balanced diet is not easy, particularly if you are experiencing side effects after treatment, and you may need to take a vitamin and mineral supplement. Always speak to your health care team before taking any supplements as they may adversely interact with medicines or other treatments.

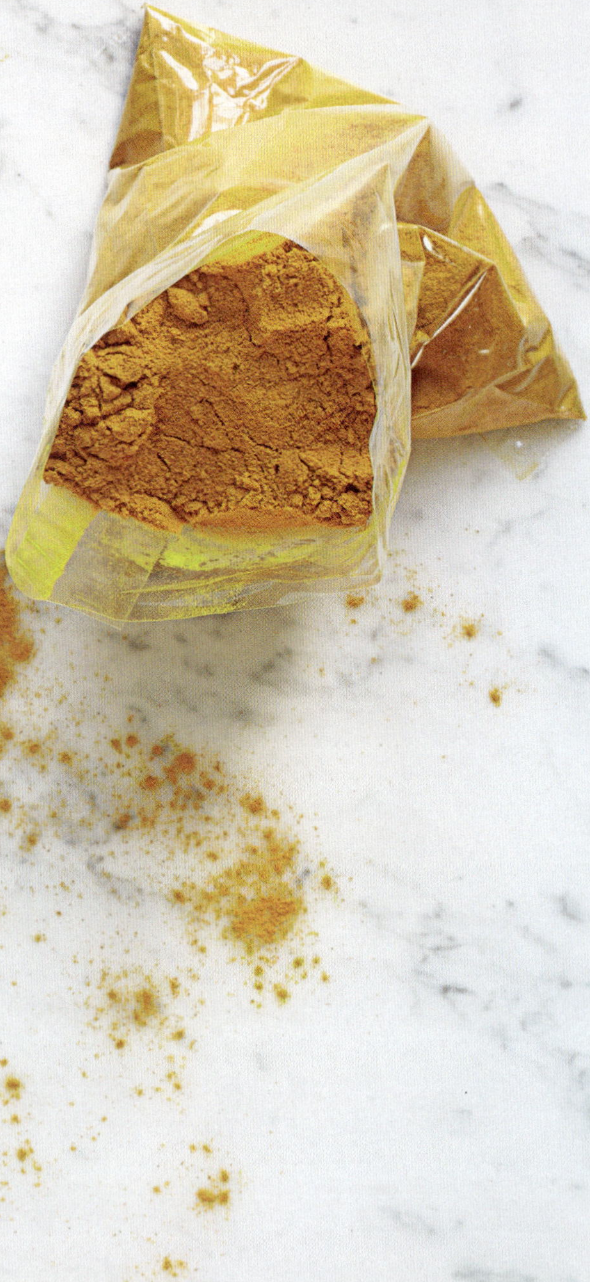

Will growth factors in food affect my cancer?

Artificial growth factors have been marketed to dairy farmers to increase milk yield in cows. Their use is permitted in some countries including the USA but not in Europe, Canada and some other countries. There has been concern about the effect on humans of using these substances as they increase milk production through the action of a hormone, the insulin-like growth factor known as IGF-1. Higher levels of IGF-1 have been detected in the bloodstream of some people but any link to diet is unproven because similarly high levels can be found in those who drink little or no dairy milk or use alternatives such as soya milk. It is not clear whether the IGF-1 in milk is absorbed, and the body is responsible for producing IGF-1, so the possible contribution to levels detected in our bloodstream is very small. On balance, it appears that growth factors in countries where their use is permitted do not appear to have an effect on the development of cancers.

Is raw food a better source of vitamins than cooked food?

Fresh raw fruit and vegetables have higher levels of vitamins and minerals than older fruit and vegetables of the same variety. This is why some people prefer to juice fresh fruit and vegetables so that we obtain vitamins and minerals, along with other phytonutrients, at their peak, as they are often lost during cooking. A balanced diet, one that is high in fruit and vegetables, is likely to contain all the necessary vitamins and minerals. Juicing is an easy means to contribute to your five daily portions and can really help if you have difficulty chewing or swallowing following treatment. However, eating the fruit or vegetable in its natural form also gives you the essential nutrients and dietary fibre your digestive system needs to work efficiently. Cooking fruit and veg, especially for long periods of time, can reduce the water-soluble vitamin content. This particularly applies to vitamins B and C but can also make some vitamins more readily available for absorption, as in the case of beta-carotene. For a good overall balance include both cooked and raw fruits and vegetables.

What about fermented foods and probiotics?

Our digestive system relies on many different types of bacteria. One of the functions they provide is to break down some of the dietary fibres in the diet that cannot be digested. Probiotics are particular strains of bacteria, such as Bifidobacteria and Lactobacillus, which are thought to be beneficial to our digestive system. Encouraging the growth of these microflora is thought to possibly reduce the presence in the gut of other bacteria that may be more harmful.

Probiotics, sold in the form of drinks or capsules, can be taken alongside a normal healthy diet. The full potential benefits of these bacteria are still being studied in trials of people without cancer and those undergoing cancer treatment. It is thought that probiotics may influence the way in which the digestive system works, interact with the body's immune system or alter the balance of bacteria after medication such as antibiotics. One concern is whether probiotics could be a source of infection in people who are undergoing intensive cancer treatment. As always it is advisable to discuss their use with your doctor before taking probiotics.

Fermented foods such as yoghurt, sauerkraut, kimchi and kefir have become an increasingly popular addition to the diet. Some of these foods rely on bacteria that are naturally present on the food, for example, kimchi, sauerkraut and pickled vegetables. Others have specific strains of bacteria added to them, for example, yoghurt, cheese, soy products, kombucha / fermented teas and wine. The resulting foods have a distinctive taste created by the by-products of fermentation products such as lactic acid. The bacteria present will depend on the food, how long it has been fermented and any other food processing that occurs after fermentation.

Some studies have suggested that if fermented foods are taken in on a regular basis that they can produce changes in the bacteria in the gut, however, they are too few studies to be definite about what these changes mean in terms of health.

How can I avoid wasting food?

No one wants to waste food, particularly as good food is expensive. Try to plan your meals before you shop and write a list. Choose recipes that will make more than one meal so that you can save the rest but do follow the guidance on good food hygiene (see page 34). Some of the ideas in the book are for a main meal or light meal with enough remaining to serve for lunch the following day, which saves on waste and requires less effort.

If you have a poor appetite it can be difficult to know what to buy. Choose ingredients that will store well without going to waste. Make use of some canned foods or those that can be stored at room temperature, so you have a choice without worrying about wasting food.

Freeze small portions of recipes to be defrosted and used later. Always defrost food in the refrigerator to ensure that it remains at the correct temperature. Reheat food until it is piping hot.

What if I am too tired to cook?

Fatigue during or after cancer treatment can be very debilitating. Keeping active is one way to help cope with this, but it can leave you too exhausted to prepare food. Don't be afraid to use shortcuts – it is more important that you have a good meal than worry about using ready-prepared foods at this time. Knowing a few shortcuts and using some ready-made items will make meal preparation easier.

Accept help from friends and family if it is offered. If they are able to prepare food and store it in the fridge or freezer, this can make a huge difference to your food intake. You may have to buy ready-made meals that can be reheated without any effort – just add some vegetables, salad or fruit to your meal or use these convenience foods as snacks between meals.

Ideas for the store cupboard, fridge and freezer

When you are tired or your appetite is poor, one of the hardest tasks is choosing what to buy and what to eat, either for meals or as quick snacks. Having the right foods to hand makes a huge difference to being able to prepare quick, easy and nutritious meals. If you have periods of time when you have a little more energy, then make the most of this to plan ahead for periods when you are particularly tired, especially immediately after a course of treatment. Shopping online can really help too. Here are some ideas for what to buy to store: Keep a good stock of canned foods in the cupboard, such as:

- Oily fish (tuna, sardines, pilchards, salmon, mackerel and anchovies).
- Plum tomatoes and tomato purée.
- Vegetables, such as sweetcorn and potatoes.
- Pulses, such as chickpeas, lentils, butter beans, cannellini beans and borlotti beans – they only need to be drained and rinsed thoroughly in cold water before using. (If you find canned beans too salty or are looking for a more economical alternative, buy dried pulses, which can be soaked, cooked and frozen in smaller portions ready to be used in soups, salads and casseroles.)
- Fruit, canned or frozen, which can be particularly useful – eat with ice cream, cream or full-fat yogurt. Most work well in cooked desserts such as crumbles, pies and cobblers.
- Vacuum-packs of rice, couscous, lentils, pearl barley and vegetables such as beetroot, which are useful for hot or cold meals – add to salads or blend vegetables with soured cream or crème fraîche to make a tasty dip.
- Cheese with a long use-by date, such as halloumi or feta, which is a quick source of protein. Store in the fridge and remember once the pack is open to keep it refrigerated and use within 3–5 days.
- Dried ingredients such as couscous, rice and noodles can form the basis of a quick and easy meal. Vacuum-packed pouches of 'ready-to-wok' noodles are also handy.

Frozen foods are a great standby when you are too tried to buy and prepare fresh:

- Vegetables are always frozen at their freshest and can be an excellent way to get variety into your diet without much effort. Good choices are peas, sweetcorn, broad beans, soya beans, spinach, green beans or mixed vegetables.
- Shortcrust pastry – just add fresh ingredients to make flans or quiches.
- Ready-to-bake bread rolls are a great standby if you are too tired to go out to buy a fresh loaf.
- Herbs and flavourings can really enhance the flavour of a dish, but it can be difficult to keep a stock of fresh ingredients ready for use. Look for frozen herbs or herb blends that cut down on waste. It makes adding delicious flavours both economical and easy.
- If you have sufficient room in your freezer, then freeze a plastic bottle of milk (semi-skimmed milk freezes better than whole milk). Always defrost it in the fridge, usually for 12–24 hours, depending on size.
- Jars of vegetables in oil or brine are useful ready-to-use ingredients, for example, artichoke hearts, sundried tomatoes, peppers and olives. Likewise, jars of pesto, passata or pasta sauces may be handy for stock. Some can be salty, though, so these may not suit all tastes during treatment, but they can take the strain out of meal preparation. Jars of peanut, almond or cashew butter are a delicious way to add protein and energy to snacks. Try them in dressings, marinades and desserts, or served on toast or crackers. They make excellent accompaniments to both sweet and savoury foods including cheese and jam.
- Other preserves, such as jam, honey and lemon curd, are not only delicious on bread, toast and crackers but can also be used as a topping on yogurt, porridge, rice pudding and custard, giving you extra flavour and energy. Honey can be a great alternative to sugar to sweeten drinks such as herbal teas.
- If you like yogurt, then keep a large tub of Greek or full-fat yogurt in the fridge. Adding honey, muesli, granola, fruit or fruit purée makes a delicious breakfast or dessert.
- Nuts (salted or unsalted) and dried fruit make a nutritious snack.

Should I eat organic food?

People make choices about the food they buy and eat for many different reasons – cultural influences, personal preferences and cost among them. The decision to eat organic food may be based on concern for the environment, particularly with regard to the chemicals or intensive farming methods used in non-organic farming, welfare of animals kept for dairy or meat, desire to support local farmers and producers, awareness of climate change and the effect of some large-scale farming practices regarding energy and water usage.

The term organic has different definitions in different countries. For some people the term is synonymous with health, and this extends beyond food production to toiletries, cosmetics and fabric. Recent studies have demonstrated that organically produced cereals, fruit and vegetables have higher levels of antioxidants and lower levels of pesticides compared to non-organic produce. This may be a major factor for some people in deciding to choose organically produced food.

However, to date, studies that have looked at organic-only diets and the risk of developing cancer are limited and inconclusive, and there have been none made with people diagnosed with cancer in order to try to establish whether changing to organic foods will make a difference to their cancer risk in the future. What is known is that a diet high in fruit and vegetables, whether organic or conventionally produced, can only be good for our health. If you are concerned about pesticide residue on food, then wash fruit and vegetables thoroughly before eating.

If you are concerned about how food is produced and where it comes from, then this influences your food choices. Choose fresh ingredients from producers and shops you trust to give you confidence that your food is providing the best range of nutrients and phytonutrients.

What about drinking tea or coffee?

Many people decrease their consumption of tea and coffee following a diagnosis of cancer. Taste changes of these beverages are often cited as being one of the main changes that people experience. Others alter their drinking habits, tending to drink more water and non-caffeinated drinks. This may be either because of concern about drinking too much caffeine or because these drinks don't taste the same as usual.

Caffeine is present in a number of drinks apart from coffee, including tea (both black and green), cola and other energy drinks. As caffeine is a stimulant it can have a number of effects in the body, usually when taken in larger amounts, including a temporary rise in heart rate and blood pressure in those who are sensitive to it. Some people find caffeine affects their sleep and so avoid these drinks before bedtime, but for other people it appears to make no difference to their quality or quantity of sleep.

Moderate amounts of caffeine should be quite safe for most people and there are certainly no studies to suggest that people who have cancer should avoid caffeine. Those who drink a large number of caffeinated drinks may experience some symptoms of withdrawal if they cut back suddenly. These include headaches, fatigue, anxiety and depressed mood. These symptoms are similar to some side effects of cancer treatment and therefore it may be difficult to identify their cause.

Perhaps the most notable fact is that people often find that tea and coffee taste different and are less palatable. If this is your experience, see the section on taste changes (page 29) for ideas for delicious alternative beverages to try.

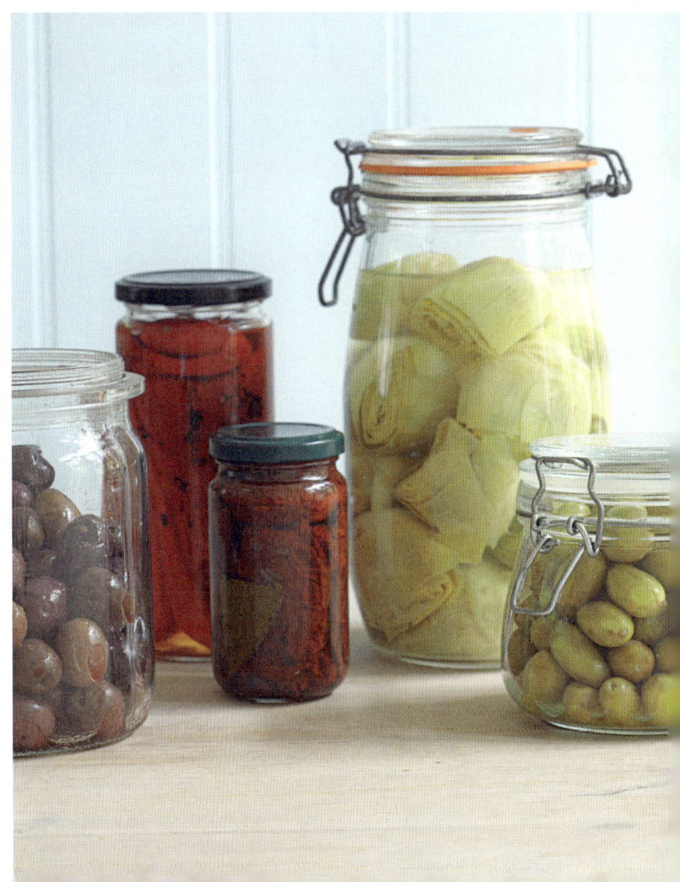

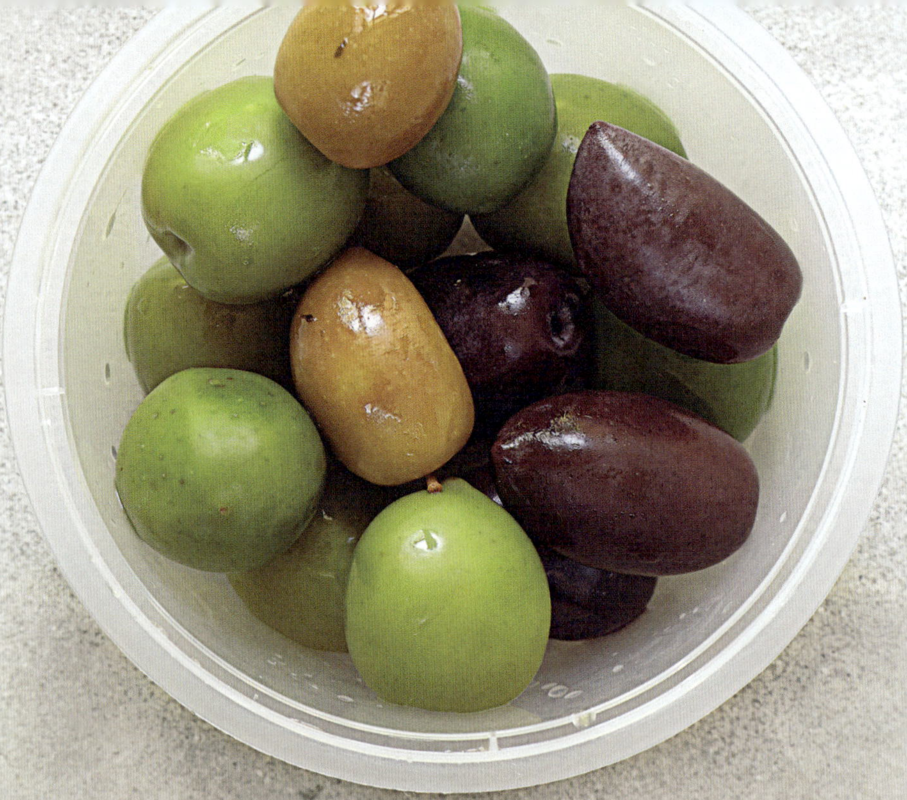

The emotional aspects of a cancer diagnosis

This cookbook looks mainly at the practical aspects of cooking, eating and how to eat well during cancer treatment. However, cancer has a huge psychological impact and for many this is more difficult to cope with than the physical symptoms that can arise due to cancer and its treatment. There are many things that people can do for themselves that may help with this aspect of having a cancer diagnosis. Some physical symptoms can influence how people feel and how they cope. For example, cancer fatigue and weight loss can profoundly affect people's resilience and mood. Strategies to help people manage these have changed over time. For example, it used to be commonplace for people who were fatigued as a result of treatment to be advised to rest whenever possible, but research has shown that activity and exercise actually help people cope with the fatigue of cancer and its treatment. Avoiding weight loss can also help people feel stronger, improve mood and better withstand cancer treatment.

Just as physical symptoms can affect how we feel, psychological techniques can affect how we experience and cope with physical symptoms. Relaxation, counselling, yoga or massage may help both psychologically and physically. Another popular psychological approach is 'mindfulness' – a form of meditation where you aim to accept the present circumstances, rather than avoid or suppress aspects of what is happening. These approaches can be instrumental in helping with pain, stress, anxiety, nausea and poor sleep patterns, enabling people to foster a positive attitude towards their treatment and recovery. Helping to improve your wellbeing and coping skills can be invaluable to deal with the emotions that having cancer creates.

These varied ways to provide support, along with positive healthy eating, can provide the best environment to help people be physically and mentally strong, to cope with whatever the future holds.

Cooking as therapy

During and after cancer treatment people often need to look for some normality in life. You may desire to return to routine tasks and carry out everyday activities. Food preparation and cooking can be an integral part of that. Many people love cooking and sharing dishes with family and friends. For some, this pleasure may be diminished or lost during cancer treatment, but it can be very therapeutic to reconnect with food, trying new recipes and cooking for health. Cooking may be physically challenging as you try to combat fatigue and poor stamina, a common occurrence following treatment. Preparation of even simple meals may be tiring, but they can contribute to improved strength and tolerance to activity. Returning to normal life can be difficult, especially when treatment comes to an end, but good food and nutrition have a strong part to play. Cooking can be a great mood enhancer. It is a creative activity that can be carried out with and for other people, and the benefits should not be underestimated. It brings people together and provides a strong sense of both purpose and achievement. Sharing food is one of life's most basic needs and is one of life's great pleasures.

Resources

Bowel Cancer UK

Bowel Cancer UK aims to save lives and improve the quality of life for all those affected by bowel cancer. It works to raise awareness of bowel cancer screening, as many people find it uncomfortable to discuss the symptoms. www.bowelcanceruk.org.uk

Breast Cancer Now

The research and care charity. https://breastcancernow.org/

Cancer Research UK

Cancer Research UK is a charity aimed at discovering new ways to prevent, diagnose and treat cancer. It provides good, reliable information on many aspects of cancer and its treatment. www.cancerresearchuk.org

Blood Cancers UK

Blood Cancer UK, is a UK-based charity dedicated to funding research into all blood cancers including leukaemia, lymphoma and myeloma, as well as offering information and support to blood cancer patients. https://bloodcancer.org.uk/

Macmillan Cancer Support

A charity providing advice and support for people following a cancer diagnosis. Provides good-quality information on all aspects of living with cancer including work, finances, cancer information and emotional support. www.macmillan.org.uk

Pelvic Radiation Disease Association

This is a charity aimed at developing a network of support groups throughout the United Kingdom for people who are affected by Pelvic Radiation Disease. www.prda.org.uk

Prostate UK

Provides a range of information and support for people concerned about prostate cancer or prostate problems. www.prostatecanceruk.org

The Royal Marsden

The Royal Marsden is a world-leading cancer centre specialising in diagnosis, treatment, care, education and research. www.royalmarsden.nhs.uk

The Soil Association

The Soil Association is a charity that campaigns for healthy, humane and sustainable food, farming and land use. It provides useful and interesting information for those who wish to find out more about food and the way it can be produced. www.soilassociation.org

World Cancer Research Fund

The World Cancer Research Fund is a charity that has a focus on cancer prevention, especially through lifestyle changes such as diet and exercise. The information they produce, *Cancer Prevention for Cancer Survivors*, is ideal for people who have had cancer and want to look at lifestyle changes to improve health. Information on eating well during cancer and taste changes are all supported by recipes and ideas for meals. www.wcrf-uk.org

EATING DIFFICULTIES DURING TREATMENT

Breakfast	Poor Appetite	Taste Changes	Nausea	Sore Mouth	Dry Mouth	High Energy	Low Energy
Cinnamon French Toast	•	•	•			•	
American-style Ricotta Pancakes	•	•	•	•			
Coconut Rice Pudding with Mango	•	•	•	•	•	•	
Clodagh McKenna's Poached Eggs	•	•			•	•	
James Ramsden's Courgette Muffins	•	•	•				
Blueberry and Avocado Smoothie	•	•	•	•	•	•	
Peach, Mint and Ginger Smoothie	•	•	•	•	•		
Lassi	•		•	•	•	•	
Sybil Kapoor's Pear and Blueberry Compôte	•	•	•				
Light Meals							
Celeriac Soup	•	•	•	•	•		
Nigella Lawson's Cauliflower Soup	•	•		•	•		
Ruth Rogers' Pappa al Pomodoro	•	•		•	•	•	
Chilled Avocado Soup	•	•	•	•	•		
Jo Pratt's Roast Pepper Soup		•	•		•	•	
Chicken Noodle Soup with Matzo Balls	•	•	•		•	•	
Thane Prince's Smoked Haddock Chowder	•	•		•	•	•	
Stanley Tucci's Cod Baked with Tomatoes	•	•			•		
Jane Baxter's Orecchiette						•	
Baked Eggs	•	•	•	•	•		
Creamed Spinach with Eggs	•	•	•	•	•		
Hugh Fearnley-Whittingstall's Pumpkin	•	•		•	•	•	
Stuffed Jacket Potatoes	•	•		•	•		•
Maggie Beer's Cavolo Nero							
Smoked Trout with Potato Salad	•	•					
Flatbread Pizzas	•	•	•				
Quick Tomato Sauce		•					•
Spinach and Egg Flatbreads	•	•					
'White' Pizza	•	•					
Spicy Lamb Flatbreads	•						
Divya Sharma's Roasted Chickpea Salad	•	•					
Salmon (or Tofu) with Soba Noodles	•	•				•	
Ways with Meatballs	•					•	
The Vegetarian Option	•	•				•	
Maria Elia's Watermelon, Black Bean Tacos	•	•	•			•	
Main Meals							
The Royal Marsden's Mongolian Stew	•	•			•	•	
Mary Contini's Spinach & Ricotta Crespelle	•				•	•	
Jack Monroe's Barley Risotto	•	•		•	•	•	
Jamie Deen's Butternut Squash Lasagne	•	•			•	•	
Mushroom and Swiss Chard Tart	•	•				•	
Poached Fish in Parsley Sauce	•	•		•	•		
Joe Woodhouse's Savoy Cabbage Gratin	•	•				•	
One-pot Roasted Fish with New Potatoes	•	•			•		
Paul Merrett's Mackerel Chermoula	•	•				•	
A Simple Fish Pie	•	•		•	•		

	Poor Appetite	Taste Changes	Nausea	Sore Mouth	Dry Mouth	High Energy	Low Energy
One-pot Chicken with Leeks	•						
Mindy Fox's Warm Chicken & Barley Salad	•	•				•	
Chicken and Pumpkin Curry	•	•			•		
Valerie Berry's Roasted Chicken	•	•				•	
David Tanis' Ham & Cheese Bread Pudding	•			•	•	•	
Nut Roast	•	•					
Angela Harnett's Pea & Pancetta Risotto	•			•	•	•	
Sausage and Puy lentil casserole	•				•	•	
Jeremy Lee's Warm Salad of Pork Belly	•					•	
Braised Lamb with Celeriac and feta bake	•				•	•	
Tim Hayward's Beef Cobbler	•				•	•	
Diana Henry's Breton Tuna Gratin	•						
Desserts							
Ching He Huang's Coconut Milk Puddings	•		•	•	•	•	
Prue Leith's Muscovado Heaven	•	•	•	•	•	•	
A Useful Apple Sauce	•		•		•		•
Soothing Fruit Salad	•		•		•		
Tom Aiken's Caramelised Plums	•	•			•		
Fennel Panna Cotta	•	•	•	•	•	•	
Plum and Star Anise Crumble	•	•	•			•	
Peach and Blueberry Cobbler	•		•			•	
Lucy Young's Summer Fruits Pavlova	•			•	•	•	
Chocolate Pots	•			•	•		
Green Tea (Matcha) and Peach Ice Lollies		•	•	•	•		•
Melon, Coconut and Mint Ice Lollies		•	•	•	•		•
Banana Ice Cream	•	•	•	•	•	•	
Mango Kulfi	•	•	•	•	•		
Divya Sharma's Strawberry Frozen Yogurt	•		•	•	•	•	
Elderflower Jelly	•	•	•	•	•		•
Pumpkin and Chocolate Chip Cookies	•					•	
Mary Berry's Sunday Orange Spice Cake	•	•				•	
Richard Bertinet's Gingerbread	•	•				•	
Snacks							
Bagna Cauda	•			•	•	•	
Radish tzatziki	•		•				
Peynir (or Feta) with Lemon and Olives	•		•				
Beetroot Hummus	•		•	•	•	•	
Grilled Peppers with Cumin and Chilli	•						
Fuchsia Dunlop's Tofu with Avocado	•		•	•	•		
Jekka McVicar's Panna	•	•				•	
Potted Cheese	•		•	•	•	•	
Date and Maple Syrup Flapjacks	•	•				•	
Malted Milkshake	•		•	•		•	
Banana and Maple Milkshake	•		•	•		•	
Chocolate and Peanut Butter Milkshake	•			•		•	
Traditional Iced Tea		•	•	•			•
Fruity Iced Tea		•	•	•			•
A Soporific Hot Drink		•	•	•			

AFTER TREATMENT

Breakfast	Poor Appetite	Taste Changes	Nausea	Sore Mouth	Dry Mouth	High Energy	Low Energy
Bircher Muesli	•		•		•	•	
Homemade Granola	•					•	
Multigrain Seeded Bread	•		•			•	
Turkish Eggs	•	•	•	•			
Masala Omelette		•					
Light Meals							
Cream of Tomato with Vegetable		•	•	•			•
Raymond Blanc's Vegetable & Chervil Soup			•	•		•	
Mary McCartney's Quinoa and Bean Soup							•
Sam Gates' Wontons in a Tasty Broth		•			•		
Ching He Huang's Hoisin Broccoli	•	•				•	
Shakshouka	•					•	
Watermelon Gazpacho with Feta Cream		•					•
Martin Morales' Quinoa & Avocado Salad			•				•
Lucas Hollweg's Goat's Cheese Salad	•		•			•	
Ming's Shiitake Brown Rice Pilaf	•		•				•
Felicity Cloake's Spinach and Tomato Dal		•	•				•
Pot Noodles		•	•				•
Gwyneth Paltrow's Chinese Chicken Salad		•				•	
Henry Dimbleby's Jackson Pollack Salad	•		•	•	•		
Mussels in Broth	•	•					•
Smoked Mackerel, Beetroot & Apple Salad	•	•	•			•	
Thomasina Miers' Spiced Lentils and Rice	•					•	
Spicy Beef Salad	•						•
Frittata	•	•					
Main Meals							
Stuffed Aubergines	•	•					•
Summer Vegetable Stir-Fry			•				•
Cauliflower, Chickpea and Spinach Curry		•					•
Theo Randall's Sea Bass	•	•				•	

	Poor Appetite	Taste Changes	Nausea	Sore Mouth	Dry Mouth	High Engery	Low Engery
Basil & Lime-Crusted Salmon	•	•					
Allegra McEvedy's Stuffed Trout						•	
Sam and Sam Clark's Bream	•	•					•
Rick Stein's Madras Fish Curry	•	•					•
Anjum Anand's Burmese Chicken Curry		•				•	
Yogurt-Marinated Chicken	•	•	•	•	•	•	•
Pot Roast Chicken	•	•				•	
Claudia Roden's Tagine of Chicken		•				•	
Shepherd's Pie					•		•
Desserts							
Blackberry and Apple Sorbet			•				•
Vanilla Poached pears & Chocolate Sauce	•	•			•		
Chocolate and Beetroot Cake	•	•		•		•	
Grilled Pineapple with Ginger & Mint		•		•			•
Baked Apples with Toasted Oats & Honey	•		•				•
Georgia Glynn Smith's Chocolate Drops	•	•				•	
Snacks							
Katie and Giancarlo Caldesi's Zhug	•	•					•
A Mediterranean Selection of Bruschetta	•		•				
Banana, Oat and Honey Smoothie	•		•	•	•	•	
A Green Smoothie				•			•
Falafel	•	•				•	
Liz Earle's Refreshing Green Juice		•	•	•			•
Fruit Leather	•		•				•
Power Balls	•		•			•	

Poor Appetite	These recipes can easily be adapted for small portions or snacks	**Dry Mouth and Difficulty Swallowing**	Foods that are moist and easy to eat
Taste Changes	Increased emphasis on chicken, fish and eggs rather than red meat	**High Energy**	For weight gain
Nausea	Increased emphasis on chicken, fish and eggs rather than red meat	**Low Energy**	For those who want to lose weight
Sore Mouth	Foods that are soft, easy to eat and not too spicy		

NUTRITION DURING TREATMENT

Breakfast	Beta-carotene	Thiamin	Riboflavin	Niacin	Folate	Vitamin C	Vitamin E	Calcium	Iron	Zinc	Selenium
Coconut Rice Pudding with Mango	•										
Blueberry and Avocado Smoothie							•				
Lassi								•			
Light Meals											
Chilled Avocado Soup							•				
Jo Pratt's Roast Pepper Soup	•						•		•	•	
Chicken Noodle Soup with Matzo Balls	•										
Jane Baxter's Orecchiette	•				•			•			
Baked Eggs								•	•	•	•
Creamed Spinach with Eggs	•						•	•	•	•	•
Hugh Fearnley-Whittingstall's Pumpkin	•	•	•				•	•			
Maggie Beer's Cavolo Nero	•				•				•		
Spinach and Egg Flatbreads	•						•				
Ways with Meatballs									•	•	
The Vegetarian Option									•		
Maria Elia's Watermelon, Black Bean Tacos						•					
Main Meals											
Jamie Deen's Butternut Squash Lasagne	•						•	•			
Mushroom and Swiss Chard Tart	•						•		•		
Poached Fish in Parsley Sauce								•			
One-pot Roasted Fish with New Potatoes							•				
A Simple Fish Pie								•			
One-pot Chicken with Leeks			•	•							
Mindy Fox's Warm Chicken & Barley Salad	•			•						•	
Chicken and Pumpkin Curry	•										
Valerie Berry's Roasted Chicken	•	•	•	•			•			•	

	Beta-carotene	Thiamin	Riboflavin	Niacin	Folate	Vitamin C	Vitamin E	Calcium	Iron	Zinc	Selenium
David Tanis' Ham & Cheese Bread Pudding	•	•	•	•			•	•	•		
Angela Harnett's Pea & Pancetta Risotto		•									
Sausage and Puy Lentil Casserole	•			•			•		•	•	
Jeremy Lee's Warm Salad of Pork Belly		•								•	•
Braised Lamb with Celeriac and Feta Bake	•	•						•	•		
Tim Hayward's Beef Cobbler	•	•	•	•				•	•	•	•
Desserts											
Prue Leith's Muscovado Heaven							•				
Soothing Fruit Salad						•					
Tom Aiken's Roast Plums	•								•		
Fennel Panna Cotta							•				
Plum and Star Anise Crumble	•						•				
Mango Kulfi	•										
Richard Bertinet's Gingerbread							•		•		
Snacks											
Beetroot Hummus							•		•		
Grilled Peppers with Cumin and Chilli	•						•				
Fuchsia Dunlop's Silken Tofu with Avocado							•				
Jekka's Panna	•						•				
Potted Cheese								•			
Malted Milkshake			•					•			
Banana and Maple Milkshake			•				•	•			
Chocolate and Peanut Butter Milkshake			•	•			•	•			
A Soporific Hot Drink								•			

The above recipes have been selected as they provide a significant amount of the nutrients identified. Many recipes provide a wide range of vitamins and minerals but some, for example the snacks, are eaten in small portions and therefore may not provide sufficient vitamins or minerals to appear on the list.

Many of the recipes contain vitamin C due to the use of vegetables and fruit. The amount of vitamin C present will depend on a number of factors, including freshness of the vegetables and fruit, cooking methods and time the dish may be kept hot. Because of these factors, only those containing raw fruit and vegetables are identified as providing a significant amount of vitamin C.

Iron

Total iron is included but iron from haem sources (meat) are better absorbed than from vegetable sources.

AFTER TREATMENT

Breakfast	Beta-carotene	Thiamin	Riboflavin	Niacin	Folate	Vitamin C	Vitamin E	Calcium	Iron	Zinc	Selenium
Bircher Muesli							●		●	●	●
Homemade Granola							●		●	●	●
Multigrain Seeded Bread							●		●	●	●
Turkish Eggs			●			●			●	●	●
Masala Omelette	●		●		●				●	●	●
Light Meals											
Cream of Tomato with Vegetable	●				●		●		●	●	●
Raymond Blanc's Vegetable & Chervil Soup	●				●				●		
Mary McCartney's Quinoa and Bean Soup	●						●				
Sam Gates' Wontons in a Tasty Broth							●				
Shakshouka	●	●	●	●	●		●		●	●	●
Watermelon Gazpacho with Feta Cream						●					
Martin Morales' Quinoa & Avocado Salad							●		●		
Lucas Hollweg's Goat's Cheese Salad	●				●				●	●	●
Ming's Shiitake Brown Rice Pilaf		●	●								
Pot Noodles	●			●	●	●					
Gwyneth Paltrow's Chinese Chicken Salad					●	●					
Mussels in Broth		●	●				●		●	●	●
Smoked Mackerel, Beetroot & Apple Salad				●		●			●	●	●
Thomasina Miers' Spiced Lentils and Rice	●	●	●	●	●		●		●	●	●
Spicy Beef Salad	●			●			●		●	●	
Frittata	●				●		●		●		

Main Meals	Beta-carotene	Thiamin	Riboflavin	Niacin	Folate	Vitamin C	Vitamin E	Calcium	Iron	Zinc	Selenium
Stuffed Aubergines	●				●		●	●	●		
Summer Vegetable Stir-Fry	●	●					●		●		
Cauliflower, Chickpea and Spinach Curry	●				●		●		●		
Theo Randall's Sea Bass									●		
Basil & lime-crusted Salmon	●			●			●		●	●	●
Sam and Sam Clark's Bream	●			●	●				●		
Rick Stein's Madras Fish Curry				●			●				●
Anjum Anand's Burmese Chicken Curry				●			●		●	●	●
Yogurt-Marinated Chicken										●	●
Pot Roast Chicken	●			●			●				
Claudia Roden's Tagine of Chicken				●					●	●	●
Shepherd's Pie	●								●	●	●
Desserts											
Vanilla Poached Pears & Chocolate Sauce							●				
Baked Apples with Toasted Oats & Honey							●				
Snacks											
Banana, Oat and Honey Smoothie							●	●	●	●	
A Green Smoothie	●					●	●				
Falafel	●						●		●		
Liz Earle's Refreshing Green Juice	●						●				

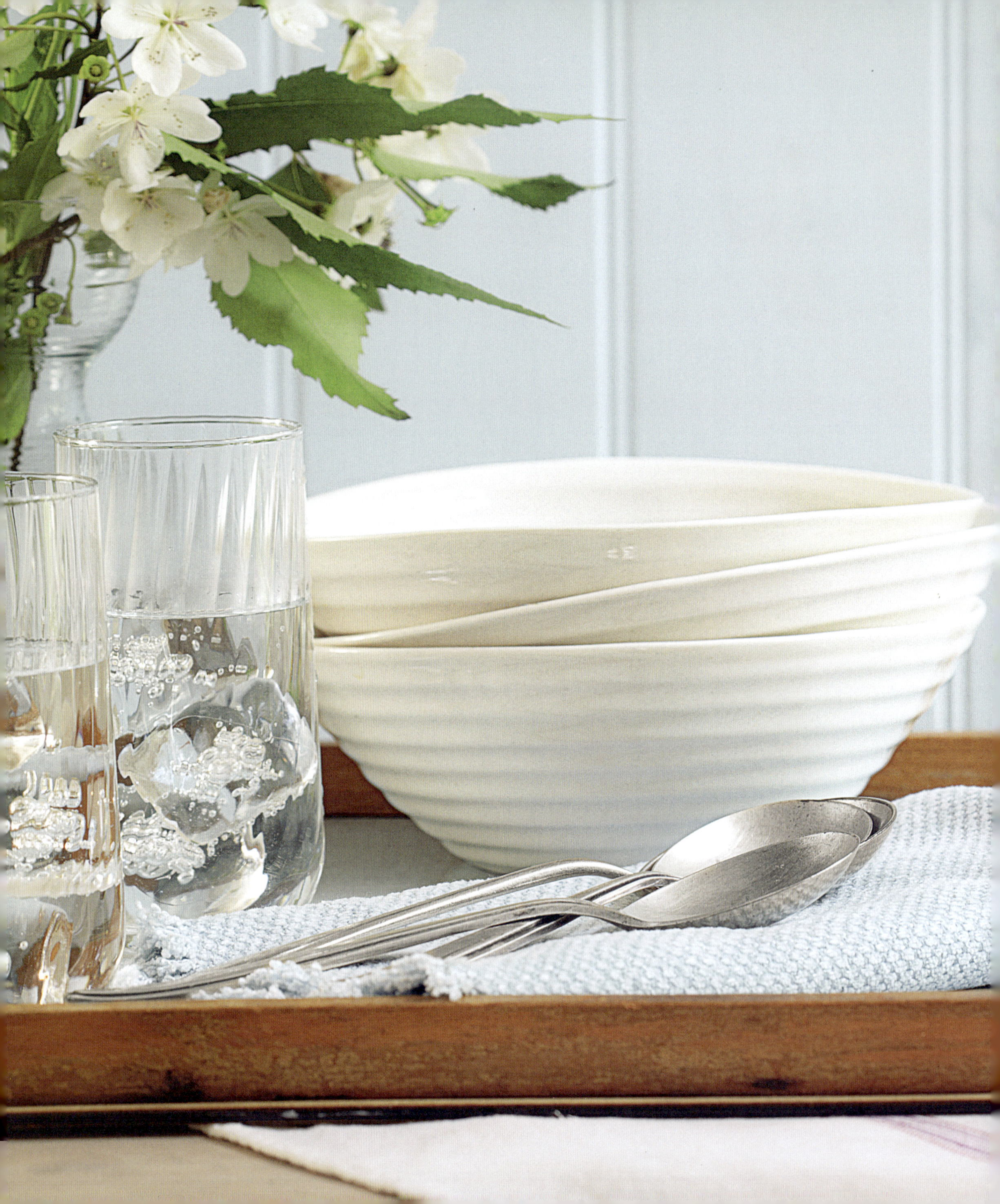

DURING TREATMENT RECIPES

These recipes are for the times when eating is more difficult. They are designed to be high in protein and energy while still providing plenty of vitamins and minerals. Remember, these recipes can be for all the family!

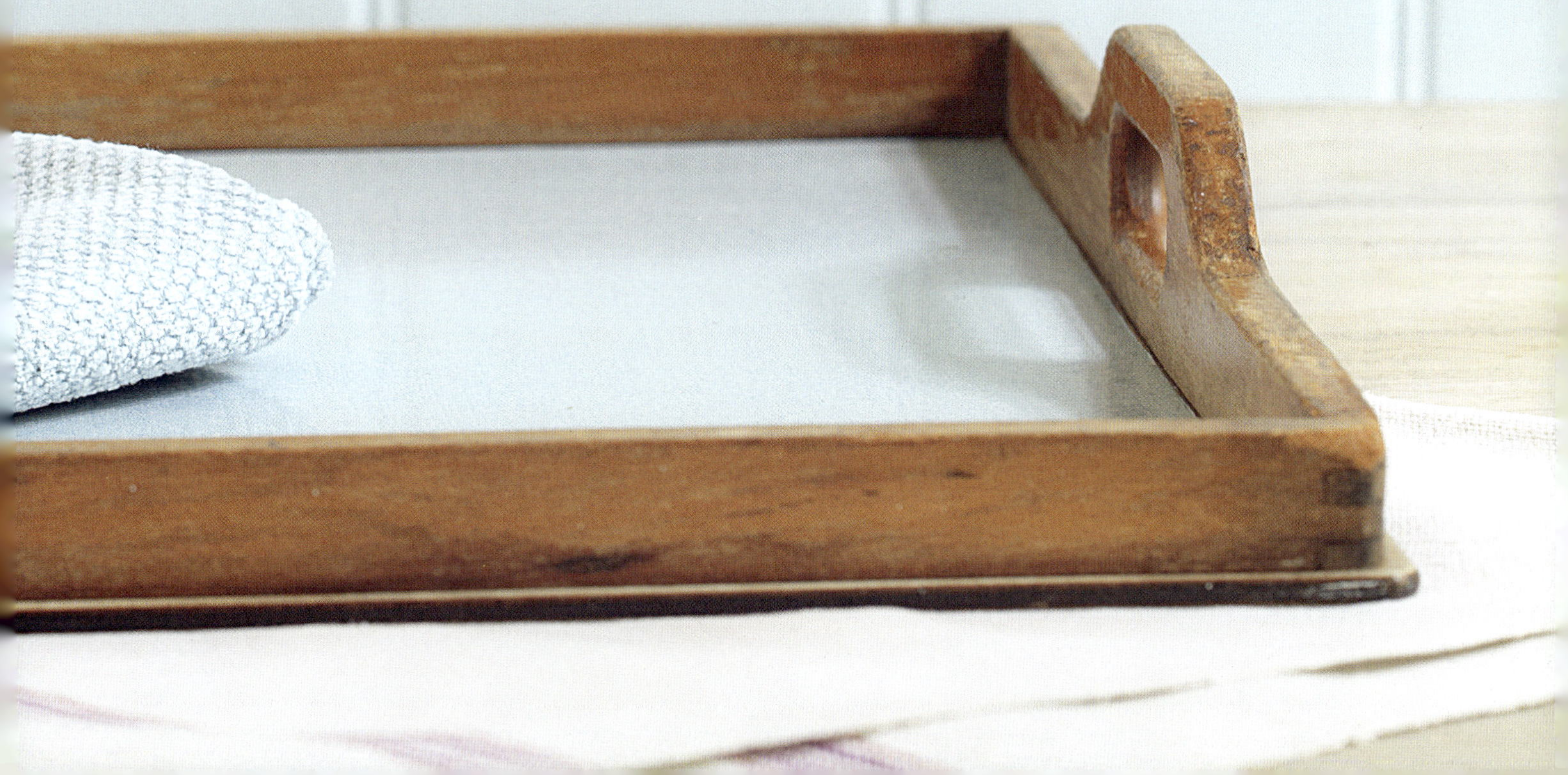

BREAKFASTS

Start the day with a good breakfast. Often this is one of the best times of the day, when appetite is better and energy levels are at their highest. If you cannot manage to eat as soon as you get up, then make the most of a late breakfast or brunch to eat well. Some of these recipes also work as snacks or light meals later in the day. A cooked breakfast can be an excellent and delicious way to set yourself up for the day ahead. Here are a few ideas:

Porridge made from oats, millet or rice (congee). Add topping of fruit compôte, fruit coulis or dried fruit. Stir in cream to increase energy.

Scrambled eggs with extra ingredients to boost the nutrition and add flavour:

- Smoked salmon or trout with herbs, such as dill or chives
- Grated cheese or cream cheese
- Cooked tomatoes, pepper or onions
- Good-quality bacon or ham
- Tofu

Hard-boiled eggs with buttered anchovy toast (use Gentleman's Relish).

Poached eggs with mushrooms, wilted spinach and cherry tomatoes on sourdough bread. Grilled bacon served with tomatoes or baked beans.

Pancakes with maple syrup, bananas and blueberries (see page 57).
Add strawberries or other fruits when in season.

Muffins made with dried fruit and nuts – make a batch that will last a number of days for breakfast or snacks. Serve on their own or with jam or cheese.

Toasted English muffins with butter, nut butter (for example peanut, almond or cashew) or cheese.

Toasted bagel with cream cheese. Smoked salmon or trout adds extra flavour and protein.

French toast and/or fruit compôte and Greek yogurt (see pages 55 and 64). Stir in cinnamon, maple syrup or honey for extra flavour.

If you really find it difficult to eat properly in the morning, there are some smoothie and lassi recipes at the end of this chapter to which you could add plenty of ice and just sip throughout the first part of the day.

CINNAMON FRENCH TOAST

with Apple and Blackberry Compôte

This is a very easy to eat alternative to toast, as it is soft and fluffy, with no sharp edges. I've included an apple and blackberry compôte here, but you can use whatever fruit you like or simply just use apples. I've given quite large quantities for the compôte – it's a very useful thing to keep in the fridge as it can be used in so many ways.

Serves 2 (with lots of compôte leftover to keep in the fridge or freezer)

For the compôte:
3 large Bramley apples, *peeled, cored and sliced*
2 tablespoons soft, light brown sugar (*or more to taste*)
Juice of **½** lemon
200g (7oz) blackberries

For the french toast:
4 thick slices of slightly stale white bread or brioche, *crusts removed*
2 free-range eggs, *beaten*
50ml (1⅗fl oz) full-fat milk
1 tablespoon caster sugar
½ teaspoon ground cinnamon
Grating of nutmeg (*optional*)
Large knob of unsalted butter

To serve:
Crème fraîche or Greek yogurt
Maple syrup

To make the compôte, put the apples in a large saucepan and sprinkle over the sugar. Add the lemon juice and 60ml (2 fl oz) cold water. Heat gently for 20–25 minutes or until the apples have softened but not disintegrated. Add the blackberries and simmer for another couple of minutes until they start releasing their juice. Taste for sweetness and add a little more sugar to taste.

Cut the bread in half. Put the eggs in a shallow bowl and pour in the milk. Add the sugar, cinnamon and nutmeg, if using. Dip the bread into this mixture, pushing it down and allowing it to rest there for a few moments so it is fully soaked.

Melt the butter in a large frying pan over a medium heat. Take the slices of bread out of the egg mix and brush off any excess. Fry the bread for about 2 minutes on each side until golden brown. Serve with the compôte and crème fraîche or Greek yogurt, and a drizzle of maple syrup, if you fancy it.

TIPS

- Maple syrup and crème fraîche or yogurt provide additional nutrients.
- This compôte freezes brilliantly.

Energy 486 kcal/2049 kJ
Protein 16.3g
Fat 11.8g
Sat. Fat 4.3g
Carbohydrate 84.9g
Fibre 7.0g

Nutritional information for 2 portions using half the compôte

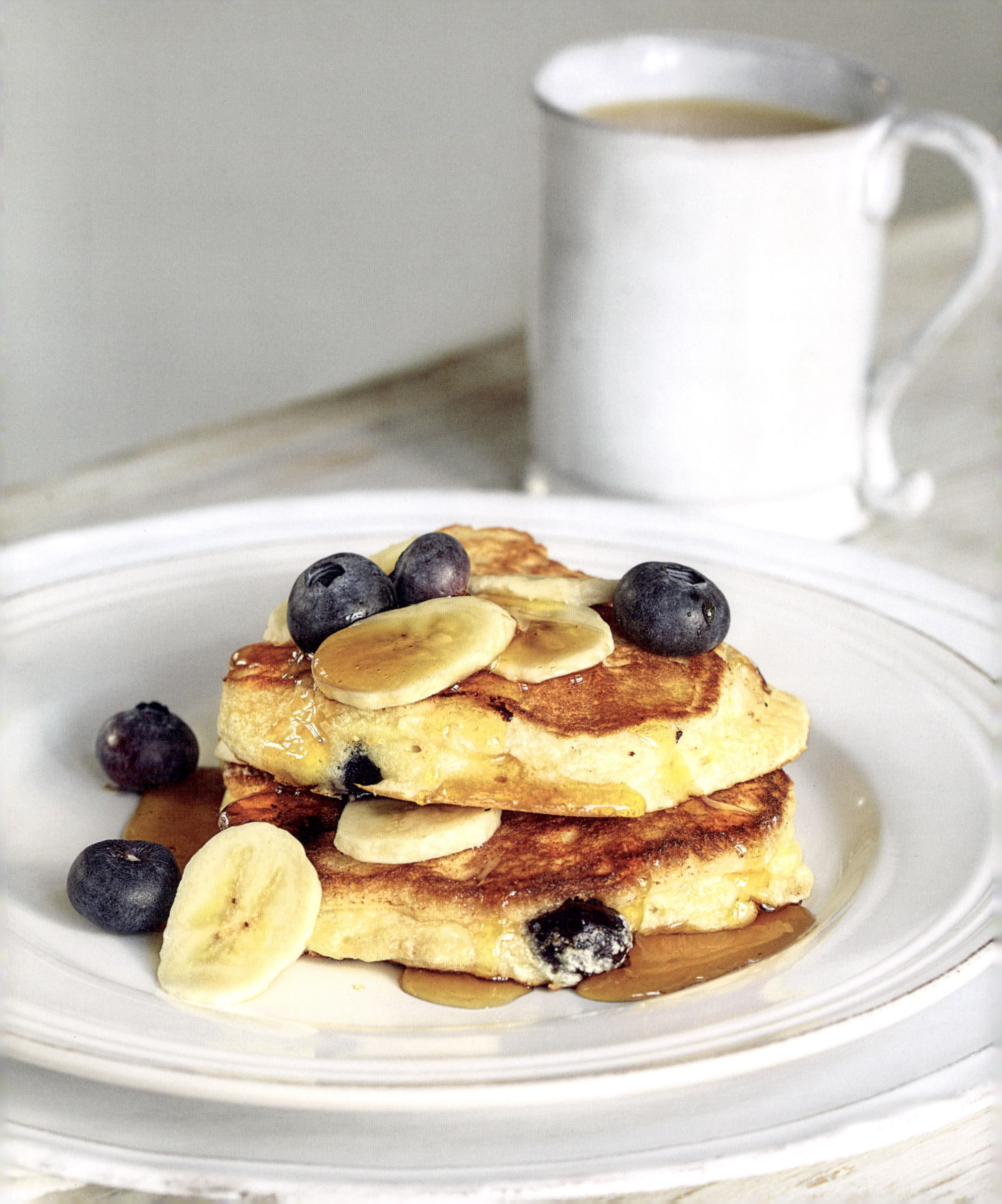

AMERICAN-STYLE RICOTTA PANCAKES

250g (8⁴⁄₅oz) ricotta cheese
125ml (4¼fl oz) whole milk
3 free-range eggs, *separated*
½ teaspoon vanilla extract
100g (3½oz) plain flour
1 teaspoon baking powder
Pinch of salt
1 tablespoon caster sugar
200g (7oz) punnet blueberries
25g (3/4oz) unsalted butter

To serve:
2 bananas, *sliced*
Maple syrup
Butter or crème fraîche

Energy 90 kcal/378 kJ
Protein 3.8g
Fat 4.7g
Sat. Fat 2.5g
Carbohydrate 8.9g
Fibre 0.6g

These American pancakes are much thicker than their British counterparts, but they are light and fluffy, which makes them very easy to eat. If you prefer them plain, don't add any blueberries to the batter, just have them on the side. Because of the addition of egg whites, this batter does need to be used up immediately, however, the pancakes will keep in the fridge or freezer – reheating them (best wrapped in foil and put in a warm oven) will restore their light texture.

Makes 16 pancakes

Mix together the ricotta, milk, egg yolks and vanilla extract in a large bowl until fairly smooth.

In a separate bowl, sift together the flour, baking powder and salt. Stir in the sugar. Using a fork, gradually whisk the dry ingredients into the wet, until your batter is lump-free.

Whisk the egg whites until they form stiff peaks. Using a metal spoon, stir a couple of tablespoons of the egg whites into the batter to loosen it, then fold in the rest as lightly as you can. Fold in half the blueberries.

Melt the butter in a frying pan over a medium heat. Pour it off into the pancake batter and stir it in. Wipe the frying pan, then ladle in rounds of the pancake batter. Make sure you do not try to make too many at once – they need room to spread. Cook the pancakes for about 3–4 minutes on each side until they are a deep golden-brown.

Serve the pancakes with the rest of the blueberries, sliced bananas and a generous drizzle of maple syrup.

TIPS

- Using the bananas, maple syrup and crème fraîche adds additional nutrients.
- For extra calories, you can also top with some melted butter or crème fraîche.

COCONUT RICE PUDDING WITH MANGO

100g (3½oz) pudding or risotto rice
400ml (13½fl oz) can coconut milk
400ml (13½fl oz) full-fat milk
½ vanilla pod, *split down the middle*
Zest of 1 unwaxed lime
Pinch of ground cinnamon *(optional)*
Pinch of ground cardamom *(optional)*
Pinch of ground ginger *(optional)*
Pinch of ground cloves *(optional)*
2 tablespoons golden unrefined caster sugar
100ml (3½fl oz) double cream *(optional)*

To serve:

Energy 367 kcal/1533 kJ
Protein 6.5g
Fat 18.3g
Sat. Fat 11.1g
Carbohydrate 45.1g
Fibre 1.9g

I know we tend to associate rice pudding with dessert, and you can eat this at any time of day – but, again, if you don't fancy oat porridge first thing this makes a great alternative. It's best made the night before, as it does take a while to cook, but it will reheat very well – you just might need to add a splash of extra liquid. I've given quantities enough for four servings, on the basis that it seems silly to go to this much effort for less. Just make sure that if you aren't eating it all straight away, you cool it down and put it in the fridge as soon as possible after cooking.

Pinches of spice work really nicely in this, but don't feel you have to include all or any of them. The addition of the lime gives an extra helping of vitamin C and the mango is a good source of beta-carotene.

Serves 4

Put the rice in a large saucepan or casserole and pour over the coconut milk and full-fat milk. Add the vanilla pod, lime zest and spices, if using, then sprinkle over the sugar. Slowly heat until it is almost boiling, then turn down the heat, cover, and leave to cook on the lowest heat for about 1 hour. Check regularly to make sure the rice isn't catching on the bottom of the pan.

Lightly whip the cream, if using, and fold into the pudding. This will add richness and lightness at the same time. If you are chilling the pudding or want to eat it cold, fold in the cream just before serving as it will help loosen it.

Dress the mango with the lime juice, if using, and serve on top of the rice pudding.

TIPS

- You can make larger batches of this and store in either the fridge or freezer. Just make sure that you transfer to one or the other as soon as the rice has cooled down.
- This also works very well as a dessert or as a snack between meals.

Clodagh McKenna's POACHED EGGS IN 'NDUJA TOMATO SAUCE WITH BUTTER BEANS

1 tablespoon olive oil
2 tablespoons 'nduja
1 garlic clove, crushed
½ teaspoon ground cumin
½ teaspoon smoked paprika, plus extra to serve
150g (5½oz) tomato passata
1 teaspoon balsamic vinegar
400g (14oz) can of butter beans, drained and rinsed
2 large eggs
1 tablespoon flat-leaf parsley, chopped
Sea salt and freshly ground black pepper

Energy 365 kcal/1521 kJ
Protein 19g
Fat 21g
Sat. Fat 5.7g
Carbohydrate 21g
Fibre 6.6g

If you haven't tasted 'nduja before, now is the time! It's a delicious, very spicy spreadable pork sausage from Calabria in Italy that you can buy in a jar and store in your fridge (once opened). Added to a rich tomato passata along with garlic, cumin and smoked paprika to create an amazing spicy, rich tomato sauce that you can make it just a few minutes. A cooked egg on top, with butter beans, makes it more a substantial supper.

Serves 2

Heat the olive oil in a medium saucepan over a medium heat. Add the 'nduja and fry for 1 minute, breaking it up with a spoon as it cooks. Add the garlic and fry for 30 seconds until fragrant. Add the spices and stir together for a further 30 seconds. Pour in the tomato passata and balsamic vinegar, stir well and simmer for 5 minutes.

In the meantime, poach the eggs in boiling water for 4 minutes.

Add the butter beans to the tomato sauce, stir through to warm and season to taste.

Spoon the beans into two bowls, top with a poached egg and finish with a sprinkle of smoked paprika, sea salt and scatter over the parsley.

TIP

- If you can't find 'nduja, then substitute diced cooking chorizo. For a vegetarian alternative, add ½ teaspoon of chilli flakes instead.
- If you are at increased risk of infection then cook the eggs thoroughly until both the white and yolk are solid.

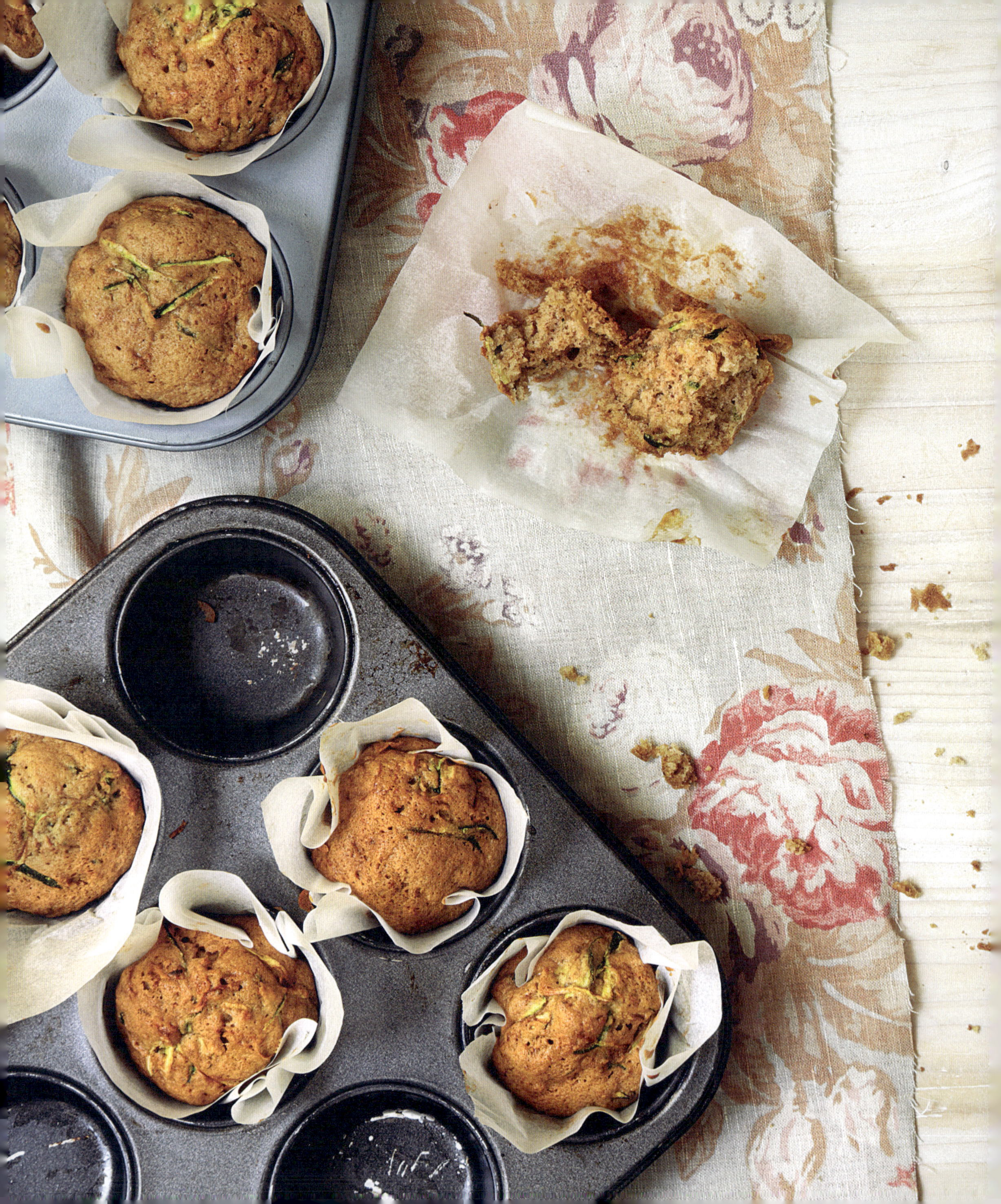

James Ramsden's
COURGETTE MUFFINS

'This recipe comes courtesy of my mum. Best enjoyed, in my opinion, with a cup of tea. It's dairy-free too, unless you're one of those who consider an egg to come from a cow.' *James Ramsden*

Makes 12 muffins

2 free-range eggs, *beaten*
200g (7oz) caster sugar
100ml (3½fl oz) sunflower oil
½ teaspoon vanilla extract
250g (8⅘oz) plain flour
1 teaspoon bicarbonate of soda
½ teaspoon ground cinnamon
Pinch of ground nutmeg
Pinch of mixed spice
Pinch of salt
200g (7oz) courgettes, *grated*

Preheat the oven to 180°C/gas mark 4/350°F. Line a muffin tin with 12 paper cases.

Whisk the eggs, sugar, oil and vanilla extract thoroughly together.

Sift the flour into a separate bowl and add the bicarbonate, spices and salt, then fold the wet ingredients through. Finally fold in the grated courgettes. Divide between the muffin cases and bake for 20–25 minutes, until a skewer comes out clean.

Turn out onto a cooling rack and store in an airtight tin (they will last 3–4 days).

Energy 230 kcal/965 kJ
Protein 3.5g
Fat 9.9g
Sat. Fat 1.4g
Carbohydrate 34g
Fibre 1.1g

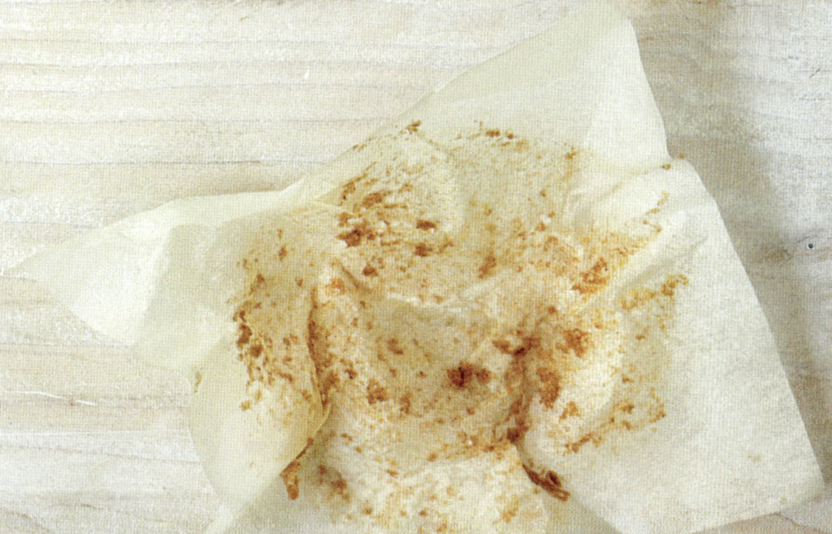

SMOOTHIES AND LASSI

Smoothies are a great way to increase your calorie intake when you just don't feel like eating. If you use fresh fruit, then you may even manage to have all your vitamin C for the day in just one glass. Smoothies tend to be quite thick, but you can always thin them down with a little more juice or water, if you prefer. To increase the sweetness of your smoothie – sometimes necessary if the fruit is on the sour side – you can add sugar, honey or maple syrup, but there's also a wonderful fruit from Peru called lucuma, which is sweet like maple syrup and you can buy in powder form either online or from health food shops. It makes a very good natural sweetener and can be sprinkled onto anything.

The method for all three recipes is exactly the same: blitz in the blender until smooth!

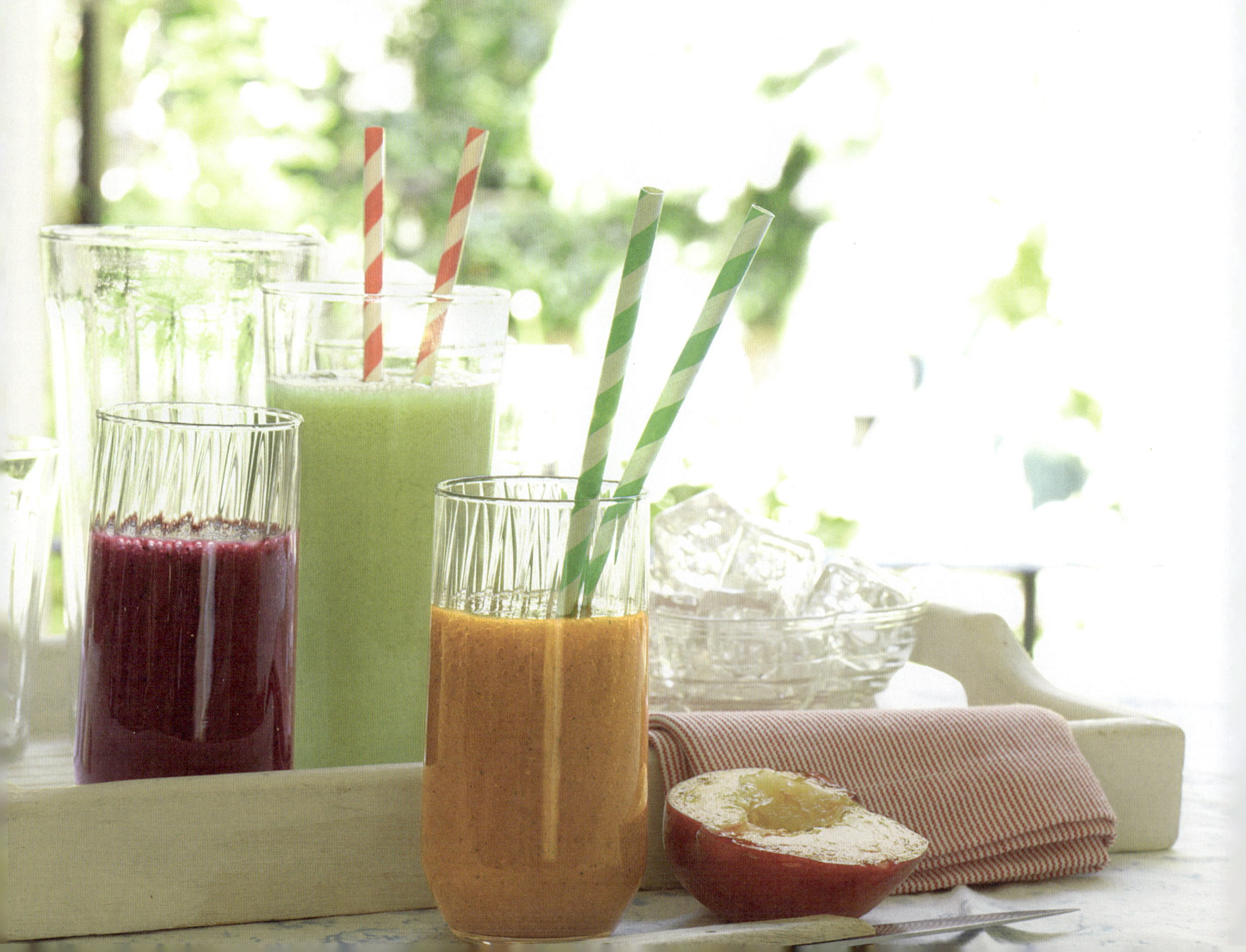

Blueberry and Avocado Smoothie

Serves 1
½ avocado, *peeled*
½ banana
150g (5½oz) blueberries
200ml (7fl oz) fruit juice – *cherry, blueberry or pomegranate are all good*
Handful of ice

We all know that avocados are highly calorific, but they are very nutritious, as they are an excellent source of vitamin E and dietary fibre. They work surprisingly well in smoothies. Use whatever kind of juice you like, but those richer in colour will make the smoothie look better.

Energy 300 kcal/1262 kJ **Protein** 2.8g **Fat** 10.3g
Sat. Fat 2.1g **Carbohydrate** 55.2g **Fibre** 6.3g

Peach, Mint and Ginger Smoothie

Serves 1
2 peaches, *halved and stoned*
150g (5½oz) grapes, *well washed*
Handful of mint leaves
Tiny grating of fresh ginger
Large handful of ice

This is a really refreshing, summery smoothie, good to make when peaches are at their ripest. If you feel like drinking this in the middle of winter, your best bet is to use canned peaches.

Energy 138 kcal /592 kJ **Protein** 2.1g **Fat** 0.3g
Sat. Fat 0g **Carbohydrate** 34.0g **Fibre** 4.2g

Lassi

Serves 2
250ml (8fl oz) plain yogurt *(not the thick or set version)*
125ml (4¼fl oz) full-fat milk
125ml (4¼fl oz) water
2 ice cubes

A lassi is basically just a yogurt smoothie. You can simply blitz yogurt with milk and ice, with perhaps a pinch of salt, for a very refreshing drink, or you can make it sweet with honey. This drink is a good source of protein and calcium. Add extra energy with sugar, honey or fruit (which will also add vitamins and fibre).

Traditional Savoury Lassi: Add a pinch of salt, and large pinches of cumin and turmeric.
Sweet Lassi: Add 1 tablespoon of sugar or honey. You could also add a few drops of rosewater and a pinch of cardamom.
Matcha Tea Lassi: Add 1 teaspoon of matcha powder and a squeeze of lime to the sweet lassi. You can also add these to regular yogurt and eat with fruit or granola.
Fruit Lassi: Add banana or ripe mango, or any soft fruit you like to the sweet lassi. It will be slightly thicker but you can thin it down with more water or milk if you like.

1 glass of basic lassi provides:
Energy 140 kcal/588 kJ **Protein** 9.2g **Fat** 6.2g
Sat. Fat 4.0g **Carbohydrate** 12.6g **Fibre** 0g

Sybil Kapoor's
PEAR, BLUEBERRY AND LEMONGRASS COMPÔTE

4 lemongrass stems
85g (3oz) granulated sugar
Juice of **1** lemon
4 ripe pears, *such as Comice or Concorde*
450g (16oz) blueberries

To serve:
Natural Greek yogurt or fromage frais

Energy 200 kcal/847 kJ
Protein 1.3g
Fat 0.3g
Sat. Fat 0g
Carbohydrate 53.2g
Fibre 6.7g

This delicate-flavoured compôte makes a lovely breakfast, especially if you serve it with a blob of natural Greek yogurt or some fromage frais.

Serves 4

Wash the lemongrass stems, trim and either halve lengthways or roughly bash with a rolling pin to release extra flavour. Put in a saucepan with the sugar and 300ml (10fl oz) cold water over a low heat and stir occasionally, until the sugar has dissolved. Then increase the heat slightly and simmer for 10 minutes. Set aside.

Meanwhile, pour the lemon juice into a small bowl. Peel one pear at a time, cut into quarters and remove the core. Cut each quarter into chunks slightly larger than the blueberries and mix them into the lemon juice, so that they don't discolour. Repeat with the remaining pears.

Strain the lemongrass liquid into a wide non-corrosive saucepan, pressing out any juices from the lemongrass. Tip the pears and their juice into the syrup. Simmer gently for 3–5 minutes or until the pears are just cooked. Add the blueberries, return to a simmer, then immediately remove from the heat and tip the fruit into a large strainer, reserving all the juice.

Transfer the fruit to a serving bowl and leave to cool. Return the syrup to the pan and boil vigorously for about 10 minutes or until it forms a sticky syrup. The time varies according to how much juice has been released by the fruit. Mix into the fruit and leave to cool. Cover and chill until needed.

To serve, spoon your desired amount of fruit compôte into a bowl and top with a few spoonfuls of yogurt or fromage frais, according to your taste.

TIPS

- It will keep for several days in the fridge, so can be made in advance and eaten as needed.
- Use yogurt or fromage frais to provide additional protein, energy and

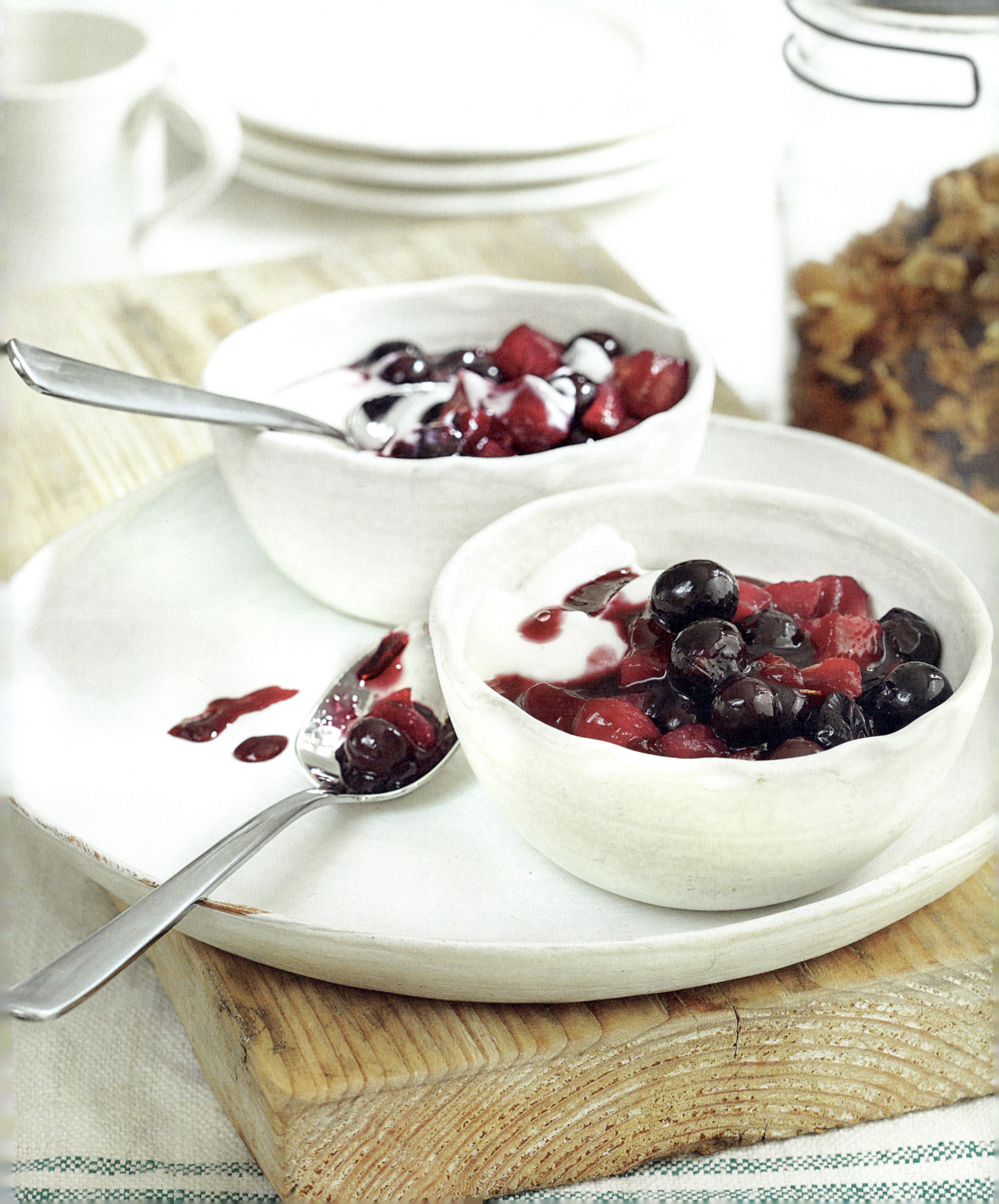

LIGHT MEALS

When appetite is poor or you just don't know what to eat, a light meal is the easiest way to eat as well as you can. During treatment the emphasis may be on eating higher energy foods, but if your weight is stable and in the normal range then increase the ratio of vegetables and salad and have smaller portions of higher fat, high protein foods (see page 180). These recipes work well as a meal or snack, or to graze on throughout the day. Don't worry too much about having meals at their usual times if you don't feel like it, but do try and eat small amounts regularly during the day.

Snacks on toast or pitta bread (also try sourdough or rye bread). Add salad vegetables for colour and flavour.

- Melted cheese served with tomato, chutney, pickle or toasted ham and cheese
- Full-fat cheese spread with cucumber, chives or pineapple
- Garlic mushrooms – try mushrooms and garlic in olive oil, add cream and chopped parsley and warm through
- Baked beans – add grated cheese
- Hummus or tzatziki with cucumber and tomato
- Sardines or pilchards – canned for a quick, easy meal
- Salmon pâté – blend smoked salmon together with mayonnaise, crème fraîche, pepper and lemon juice
- Taramasalata with cucumber, olives and tomatoes
- Smoked mackerel pâté – mix skinned smoked mackerel with crème fraîche or cream cheese, pepper and lemon
- Tuna mayonnaise on lightly toasted bread grilled until hot (add spring onions to the mix for extra flavour)
- Egg mayonnaise
- Mushroom or vegetable pâté, home-made, or buy ready-made if you are too tired to cook

Salads – serve with bread, a jacket potato or couscous. Use oil and vinegar or mayonnaise for extra flavour and energy.

- Prawns and avocado with mayonnaise (add tomato ketchup or lime for flavour)
- Chicken, avocado and bacon
- Feta cheese and olives
- Poached salmon or prawns with lime mayonnaise
- Quiche – buy shortcrust pastry or a pastry case then add beaten eggs, milk or cream and a filling of your choice

Baked potato or sweet potato with butter and a variety of easy toppings:

- Grated cheese or soft cream cheese and chives
- Baked beans with extra cheese or chopped cooked bacon
- Tuna mayonnaise and chopped chives or lime juice and coriander for extra zing
- Smoked mackerel mixed with cream cheese or crème fraîche and spring onions
- Coronation chicken (chicken in mayonnaise with some mild curry powder)
- Minced beef in a bolognaise or chilli sauce – top with grated cheese

Pasta with a sauce – make a large batch of sauce and freeze as individual portions or buy ready-made if you are too tired to cook. Serve with a salad or quick and easy vegetables. These ideas would also work with gnocchi:

- Cheese sauce – add oven-roasted tomatoes, cooked bacon, cauliflower or herb and garlic cream cheese
- Bolognaise
- Pesto, red or green
- Tomato and cream sauce with grated Parmesan
- Carbonara

CELERIAC SOUP

with Coconut, Lemongrass and Ginger

1 tablespoon vegetable or coconut oil
1 small celeriac, *peeled and cubed*
1 large potato, *peeled and cubed*
1 onion, *finely chopped*
3 garlic cloves, *finely chopped*
Small piece of fresh ginger, *grated*
¼ teaspoon turmeric
2 lemongrass stems, *outer leaves removed, very finely sliced*
2 tablespoons coriander leaf stems, *finely chopped*
1 teaspoon unwaxed lime zest
400ml (13½fl oz) can coconut milk
200ml (7fl oz) milk or water
Salt and freshly ground black pepper

For the herb oil:
Handful of fresh coriander
Handful of fresh basil
2 tablespoons olive oil
Squeeze of lime juice

Energy 217cals/905 kJ
Protein 6.1g
Fat 11.2g
Sat. Fat 2.6g
Carbohydrate 24.7g
Fibre 2.7g

Nutritional value for soup if made with milk

This very fragrant, lightly spiced soup is ideal to tempt jaded taste buds. If you can handle heat, you might want to add a chilli along with the garlic and ginger. And if you are eating this with someone who likes heat, serve some chilli oil at the table.

Serves 4

Heat the oil in a large saucepan. Add the celeriac, potato and onion, and sauté gently for about 10 minutes until everything has softened around the edges. Add the garlic and ginger, and cook for another couple of minutes, then add the remaining ingredients. Season with salt and pepper. Bring to the boil, then turn the heat down and simmer until the vegetables are completely tender – about a further 10 minutes.

Put the soup in a blender – you may have to do this in two batches – and blitz until smooth. If you feel it's not quite thin enough, add a little more milk or water. Return to the saucepan and reheat until piping hot.

For the herb oil, put the herbs and olive oil in a small blender and season with a pinch of salt. Add a squeeze of lime juice. Blitz everything together until fairly smooth. Serve the soup drizzled with the herb oil.

Nigella Lawson's CAULIFLOWER, GARLIC AND TURMERIC SOUP

1 head of garlic
3 tablespoons olive oil
1 medium onion, *chopped*
1 cauliflower, *broken into florets*
1 teaspoon turmeric
1 large potato, *peeled and diced*
1 litre (33⅘ fl oz) hot vegetable stock
(Marigold bouillon powder is fine)

Energy 187 kcal/780 kJ
Protein 6.9g
Fat 9.6g
Sat. Fat 1.4g
Carbohydrate 19.6g
Fibre 5.0g

'Packed full of vegetables and phytonutrients, it is undeniably true that this soup is both soothing and bolstering as well as easy and gratifying to eat. Baking the garlic gives a lot of depth while taking away any potential for bitter heat; strangely, the turmeric seems to assuage, if not remove, the school corridors smell of the cooking cauliflower. And the colour, an almost acid gold, is glorious.' *Nigella Lawson*

Serves 4

Preheat the oven to 200°C/gas mark 6/400°F. Cut the top off the head of the garlic so that you can just see the tops of the cloves. Sit the garlic on a generous square of tinfoil (shiny-side up) and drizzle a small amount of the olive oil over. Pull up the edges of the foil to form a tightly wrapped but baggy parcel and put in the preheated oven for 40 minutes. Remove and allow to cool a little while you get on with the soup.

Pour the rest of the oil into a wide saucepan and fry the onion gently for 10 minutes or so until softened but not browning. Add the cauliflower florets and turn in the oily onion. Add the turmeric and keep stirring, then stir in the potato. Cover and cook over a low to medium heat for about 10 minutes.

Squeeze in the pulpy, sweet, baked garlic cloves (just squish the head straight into the saucepan) and then add the stock. Bring to the boil, lower the heat to a simmer, then cover and cook for a further 15 minutes or so. Purée in a food-processor or blender or, if you like a soup with more texture, just stick a hand-held blender in the pan or bash about with an old-fashioned potato masher. Add freshly chopped parsley or coriander to the bowls as you eat.

TIPS

- Boost the protein and energy of this soup by adding a blob of crème fraiche or grated cheese just as you serve.
- Alternatively, eat with a light meal of bread and a selection of cold meats or cheeses, or hummus.

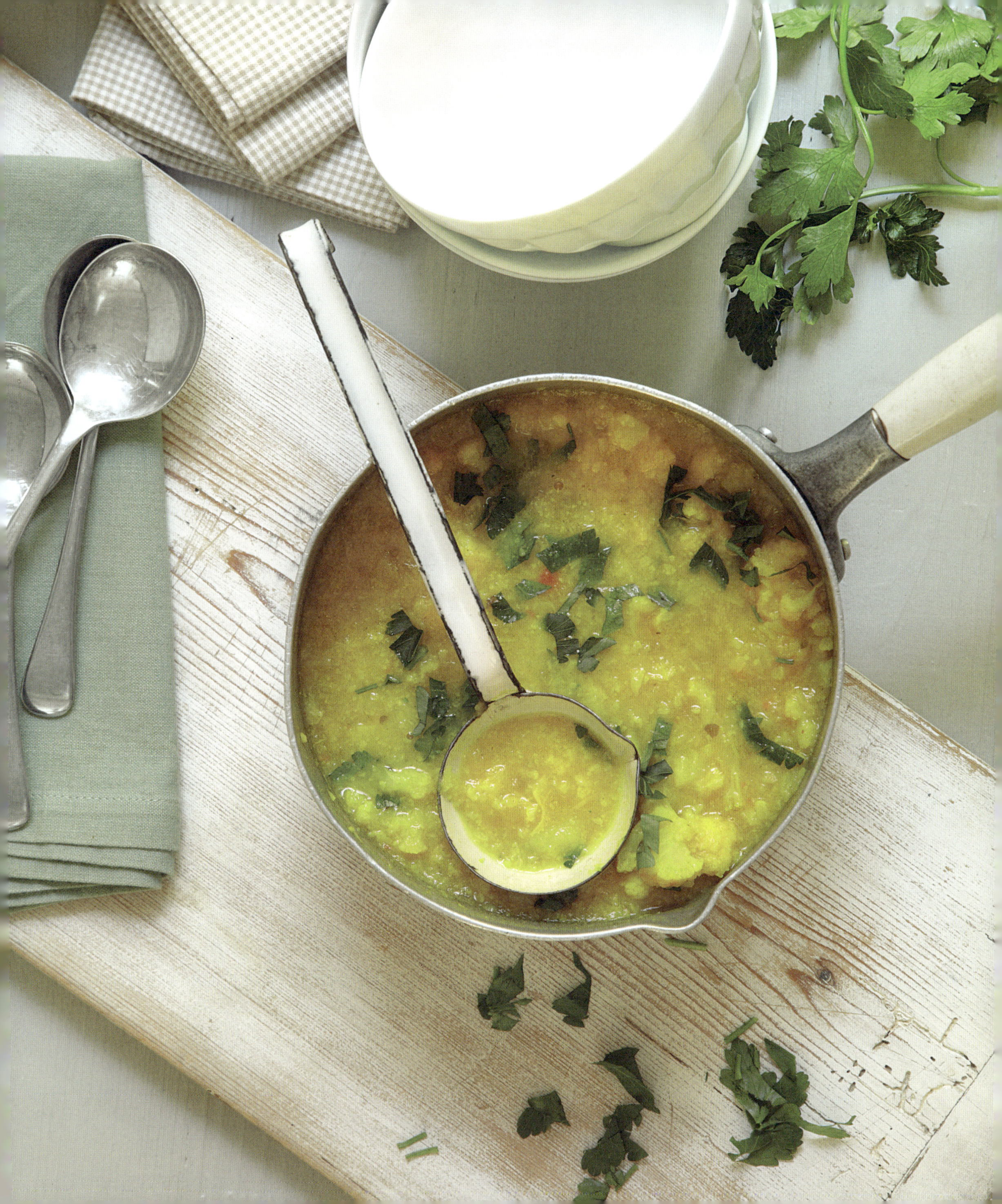

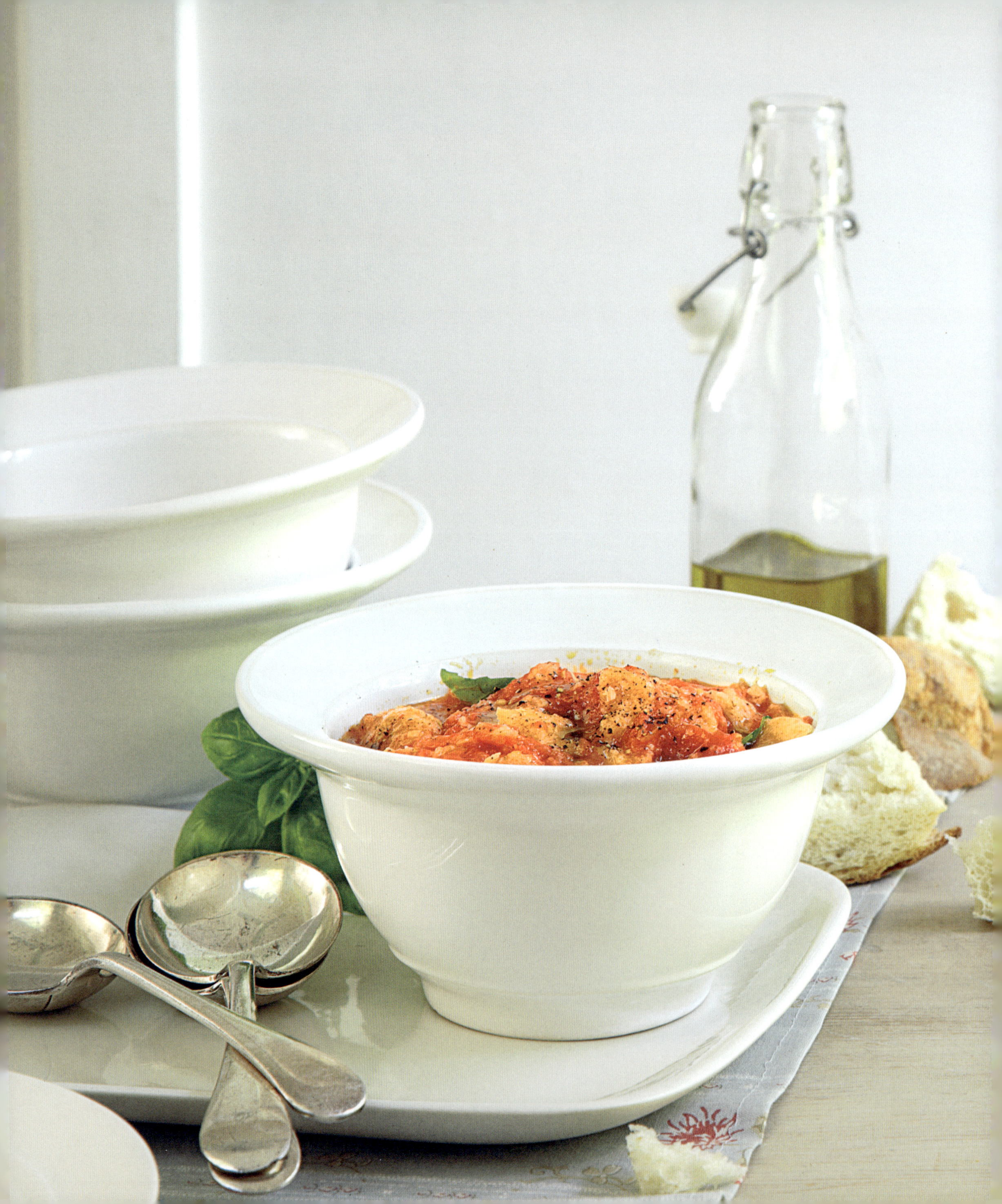

Ruth Rogers' PAPPA AL POMODORO

5 tablespoons olive oil
3 garlic cloves, *finely sliced*
2kg (70oz) sweet, ripe tomatoes, *skinned and seeded*,
or **1kg (35oz)** ($2\frac{1}{2}$ × 400g (14oz) cans) best-quality peeled plum tomatoes, *drained of most of their juice*
2 loaves of stale Pugliese bread
Large bunch of basil
Extra virgin olive oil
Salt and freshly ground

Energy 385 kcal/1625 kJ
Protein 11.5g
Fat 14.4g
Sat. Fat 2.3g
Carbohydrate 56g
Fibre 7.5g

You need beautifully sweet, ripe tomatoes for this soup, so, if using canned, try to buy the best you can afford. If they seem slightly on the acidic side, you can add a pinch of sugar. Don't worry about the fact that you are discarding the crusts from the bread – you can leave them to dry (putting them in a low oven will speed this up) and blitz them for breadcrumbs.

Serves 6

Heat the olive oil in a large, heavy-based saucepan and add the garlic. Cook gently for a couple of minutes, making sure the garlic doesn't brown, just softens slightly. Add the tomatoes, then simmer for 30 minutes, stirring occasionally, until the tomatoes become concentrated. Season well with salt and pepper, then add 300ml (10fl oz) water and bring to the boil.

Cut most of the crusts from the bread and discard. Tear or cut the remaining bread into large chunks. Put the bread into the tomatoes and stir until the bread absorbs the liquid, adding more boiling water if it's too thick. Remove from the heat and allow to cool slightly.

Tear any very large basil leaves. Stir into the soup and drizzle in a generous amount of extra virgin olive oil – between 3 and 5 tablespoons should be about right. Allow the soup to stand before serving so that the bread absorbs the flavours of the basil and the oil.

TIP

- Add more extra virgin olive oil to each bowl at the table to increase the energy content.

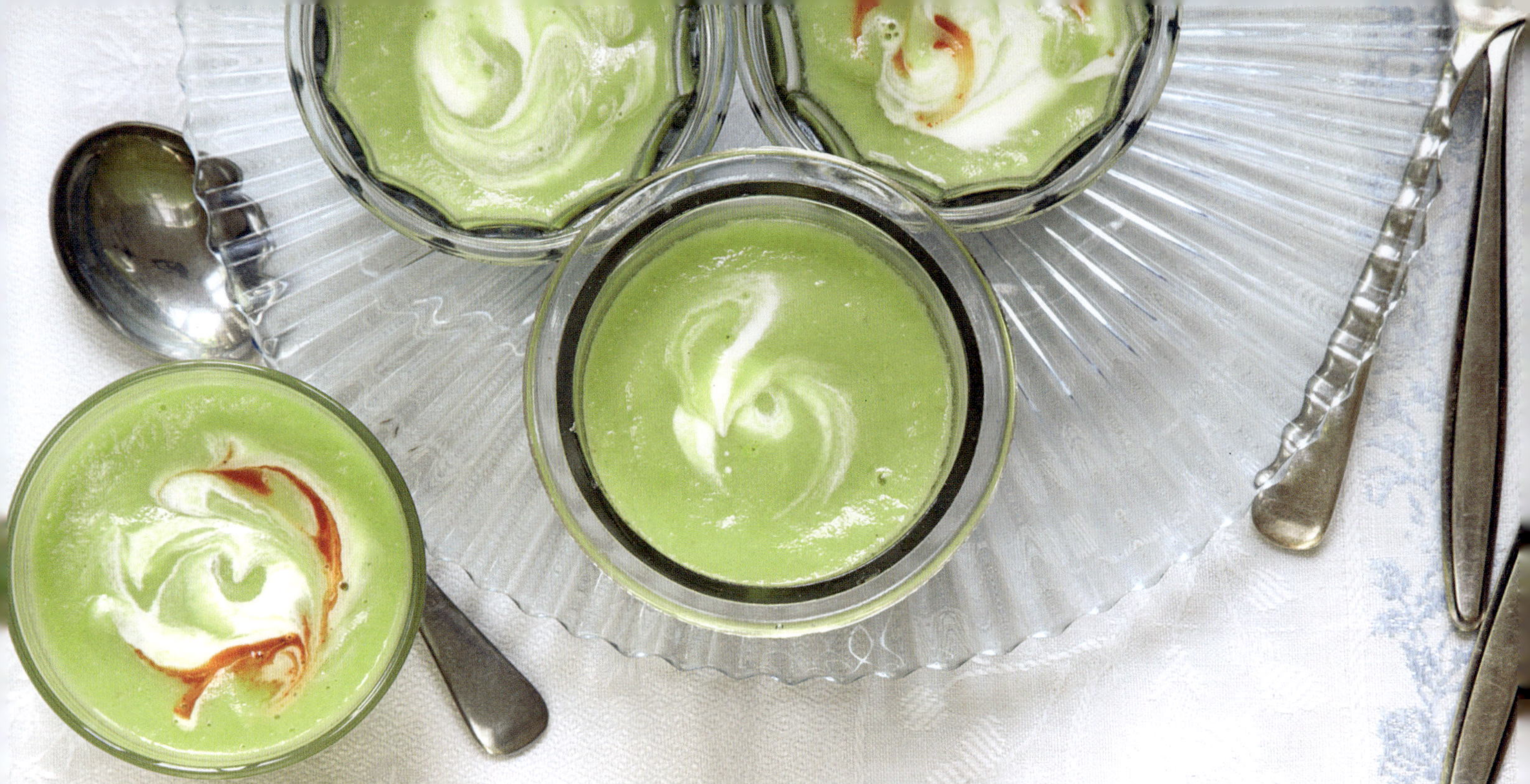

CHILLED AVOCADO SOUP

I know that some people do not like the idea of a chilled soup, but it is really very refreshing on a hot day when you need something easy to eat – and it can be packed full of good calories too. As you can see, this one is also ridiculously quick and easy to make. This recipe is very tasty eaten with garlic bread or soft flat breads. Miss out the Tabasco or hot sauce and lime if you have a sore mouth for a lovely soothing soup. I use white pepper here so as not to mar the colour with flecks of black, but black pepper could also be used. Avocados are an excellent source of vitamin E and monounsaturated fat.

Serves 4

2 very ripe avocados, *stoned and peeled*
500ml (17fl oz) chilled vegetable or chicken stock
2 tablespoons yogurt or crème fraîche
Juice of ½ lime
Dash of Tabasco or hot sauce *(optional)*
Salt and white pepper

Put the avocados and stock in a blender and blitz until smooth. Stir in the yogurt or crème fraîche. Decant into a bowl or saucepan. Season with salt and pepper, a squeeze of lime juice and a dash of Tabasco, if you like. Check the consistency – you might want to thin it down with a little more stock or water. Do not be heavy-handed, as it is important not to mask the flavour of the avocado.

Energy 230 kcal/956 kJ
Protein 4.8g
Fat 21.4g
Sat. Fat 4.8g
Carbohydrate 5.4g
Fibre 4.6g

Jo Pratt's
ROAST PEPPER SOUP
with Pumpkin Seed and Feta 'Croutons'

4 red peppers, *halved and deseeded*
3 carrots, *peeled and quartered lengthways*
1 long red chilli, *halved*
2 garlic cloves, skin on
500g (17³⁄₅oz) ripe tomatoes, *halved*
2 teaspoons paprika
3 tablespoons olive oil
800ml (27fl oz) hot vegetable stock
Sea salt and freshly ground black pepper

For the croutons:
100g (3½oz) feta cheese
50g (2oz) pumpkin seeds
1 tablespoon olive oil

Energy 356 kcal/1480 kJ
Protein 10.9g
Fat 23.6g
Sat. Fat 6.3g
Carbohydrate 26.2g
Fibre 9.6g

Nutritional content for ¼ recipe

'This hearty, flavoursome soup is packed with beta-carotene, vitamin E and super simple to prepare. Enjoy on its own, but if you're after something that takes this soup to another level, the salty/spicy/tangy/crunchy croutons add a real 'wow' to the finished dish, so they're well worth making.' *Jo Pratt*

Serves 4–6

Preheat the oven to 200°C/gas mark 6/400°F.

Put the peppers, carrots, chilli, garlic and tomatoes in a large roasting tray and toss them in the paprika and olive oil. Season with salt and pepper and roast in the oven for about 40 minutes until the vegetables are softened and beginning to char around the edges.

To prepare the croutons, break the feta into small chunks and gently mix in the pumpkin seeds, olive oil, chilli and sumac. Spread in a single layer on a non-stick baking tray and bake for 10–12 minutes, turning once. When cooked the feta should be starting to become golden in places and the pumpkin seeds will be crunchy and puffed up.

Put the roasted vegetables in a blender with the stock (squeezing the garlic out of its skin). This may need to be done in two batches, depending on the size of your machine. Blitz to a chunky or smooth consistency, whichever you prefer, and transfer to a clean saucepan.

Heat the soup gently, then ladle it into bowls and scatter over the croutons.

TIPS

- This soup will freeze very well, but the croutons are best made fresh.
- If you want a faster meal after defrosting, you could just crumble feta cheese into the soup or use bread croutons.

CHICKEN NOODLE SOUP WITH MATZO BALLS

1 free-range chicken
2 litres (68fl oz) hot chicken stock
1 large onion, *cut into eight wedges*
2 large carrots, *cut into chunks*
3 sticks of celery
1 head of garlic, *cut in half horizontally*
Large sprig of parsley
Large sprig of thyme
Handful of spaghetti or vermicelli noodles (lokshen)
Salt and white pepper

Energy 337 kcal/1404 kJ
Protein 27.5g
Fat 18.0g
Sat. Fat 4.8g
Carbohydrate 17.1g
Fibre 3.1g

Nutritional content for soup only

A proper chicken broth is what many people turn to when they are feeling unwell. This is the classic version, but it is infinitely adaptable – see the end of the recipe for some ideas. And please, do try to add some carbohydrates to the soup, whether they're noodles or one of the other suggestions. Although this is a large portion it really does pack a whole meal into an easy-to-eat soup. It is brimming with protein, energy and beta-carotene.

Makes 8 portions (but is one of the best for keeping in the fridge or freezer, without the matzo balls)

Put the chicken in a large saucepan. Pour over the chicken stock, making sure the chicken is well covered. Bring the stock to the boil and start skimming off any mushroom-coloured foam that collects on the surface – when it turns white, stop skimming. Turn down the heat and simmer for 30 minutes.

Add all the vegetables, garlic and herbs, and simmer for a further 30 minutes or until the vegetables are tender. Season well with salt and white pepper. Strain the soup. Pull the chicken meat from the carcass and return about half of it to the soup. Keep the rest for something else. Return the vegetables to the soup as well, then add the spaghetti or vermicelli. Simmer for a further 10 minutes until the pasta is cooked (if using the matzo balls add them 5 minutes before the end of cooking time).

There are so many things you can add to this soup, as, really, it's a fortified, better-flavoured chicken stock so can be used as a base for almost anything. Add handfuls of any of the following:

Pasta – any kind, including stuffed pasta, such as tortellini
Rice and other grains, such as pearled spelt or barley, or quinoa
Potatoes or other root vegetables – diced or, if they are young new potatoes, left whole or sliced
Greens – lots of fresh chard, kale and spring greens
Meatballs – see the recipes on pages 94–95 for some ideas
Spice – a pinch of saffron is really good, particularly if you add rice
Lemongrass, garlic and ginger can transform the flavour, especially if you add a little coconut milk and soy sauce
Dumplings – of any sort, but the ones opposite, made from matzo meal, are very light and fluffy.

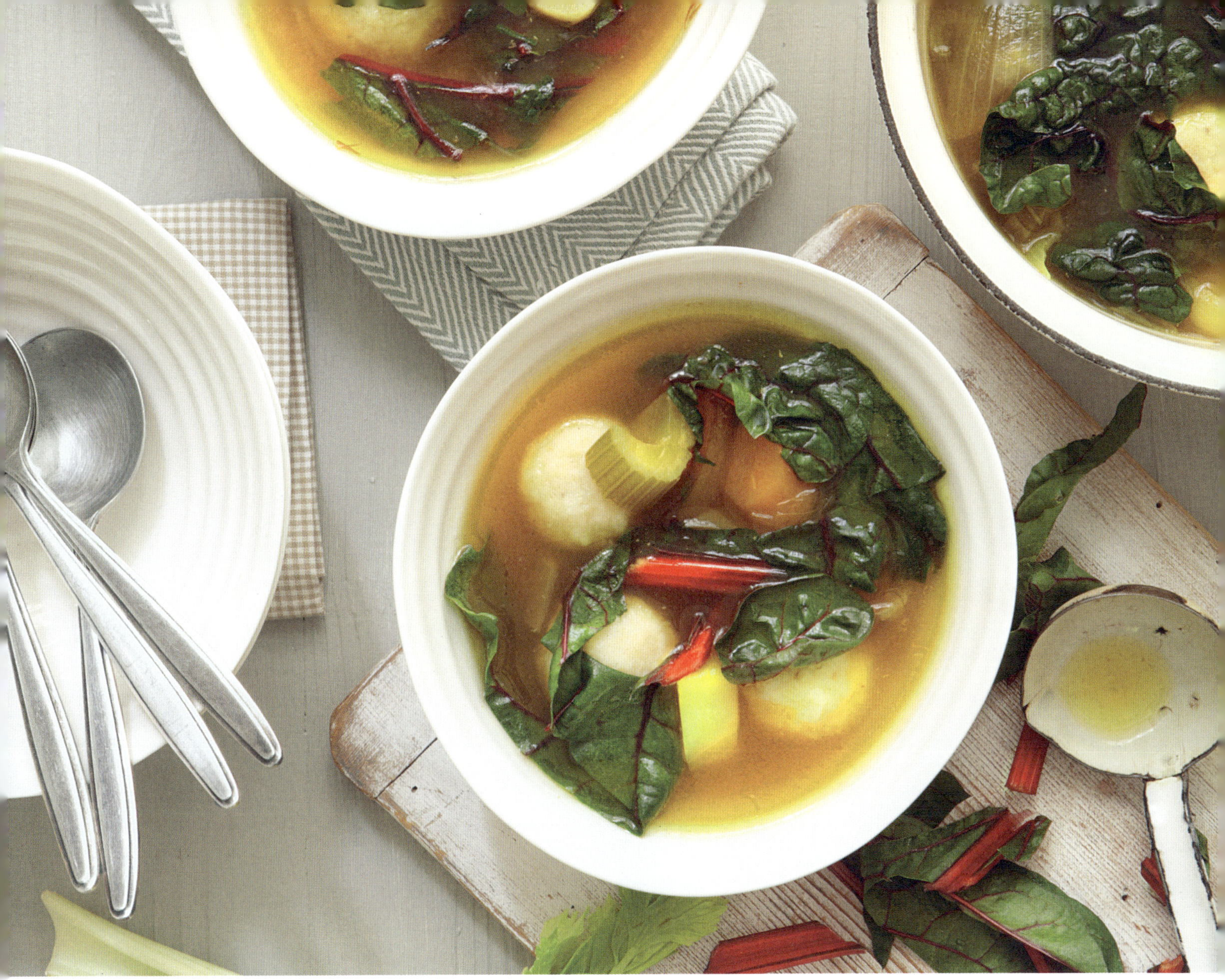

For the matzo balls:
110g (4oz) medium matzo meal
1 teaspoon baking powder
50g unsalted butter, *melted*
1 large free-range egg, *beaten*
Finely chopped parsley or dill
Salt and freshly ground
black pepper

Put the matzo meal and baking powder in a bowl and season with salt and pepper. Pour over 150ml (5fl oz) cold water. Mix thoroughly. In a separate bowl, mix the butter with the egg, then add this to the matzo meal along with the parsley. Leave to soak for about 20 minutes.

Form the mixture into balls the size of walnuts. They can be frozen at this point if you wish. Simmer in hot broth or water – when they float to the top they will be done.

Nutritional information for 1 portion of matzo balls only:
Energy 36 kcal/149 kJ **Protein** 0.8g **Fat** 2.0g
Sat. Fat 1.1g **Carbohydrate** 3.9g **Fibre** 0.2g

Thane Prince's SMOKED HADDOCK CHOWDER

750g (26½oz) smoked haddock fillet, *preferably undyed*
2 tablespoons olive oil
2 tablespoons unsalted butter
2 onions, *finely chopped*
2 leeks, *halved lengthways and thinly sliced*
3 sticks of celery, *thinly sliced*
4 potatoes, *peeled and diced*

To finish:
Double cream
Tabasco
Salt and freshly ground black pepper

Energy 425 kcal/1788 kJ
Protein 41.5g
Fat 13.7g
Sat. Fat 6.8g
Carbohydrate 36.2g
Fibre 6.9g

I can't think of many soups more traditional or comforting than this one. Thane rings the changes a bit with the entirely optional Tabasco – it's very subtly done, but add only if you aren't sensitive to chilli. The fish in this recipe is an excellent source of protein. Along with the potatoes and vegetables, it really is a meal in a bowl.

Serves 4

Place the fish in a single layer in a large pan, cover with cold water and bring to the boil. Simmer for 1 minute, then turn off the heat. Leave for 10 minutes.

Remove the fish from the pan and, when it is cool enough to handle, carefully remove all the skin and bones. Try to keep the flakes of fish as large as possible as they will break up as you reheat them. Reserve the cooking water.

Heat the oil and butter in a large saucepan. Add the onions, leeks, celery and potatoes and fry for a few minutes until starting to colour. Pour over the reserved cooking liquid. Reduce the heat to a simmer and cook for 10 minutes until the vegetables have softened.

Using a potato masher, lightly mash the soup to break up some of the cubes of potato and release some of the starch. Add cream to taste and check for seasoning (remember the haddock will be salty). Add a few drops of Tabasco for a chilli hit, or put this on the table for people to add themselves.

Stir in the parsley and finally add the large flakes of fish. Bring the soup up to a simmer, then cook for a further minute and serve in warm bowls.

TIP

- This isn't the best soup to freeze, as the fish can break up too much and the potatoes don't have the best texture when defrosted. To get round this, blitz instead, before or after reheating, for a smooth, creamy fish soup. You may need to add a little more liquid.

Stanley Tucci's
COD BAKED WITH TOMATOES

4 tablespoons extra virgin olive oil
1 medium onion, chopped
1 to 2 cloves garlic, chopped
sea salt
400g (14 oz) can whole San Marzano tomatoes, crushed by hand
1 bay leaf
85g (3 oz) good quality black olives
freshly ground black pepper
4 to 6 cod fillets (approx **150g (5oz)** each)
1 tablespoon chopped fresh flat-leaf parsley

Energy 293 kcal/1125 kJ
Protein 29g
Fat 17g
Sat. Fat 2.5g
Carbohydrate 7.8g
Fibre 2.0g

This *merluzzo al forno* is a version of a classic Livornese dish. You can make it with any firm, white fish, like red snapper or halibut, but I like it best with cod. Capers can be added for more acidity.

Serves 4 to 6

In a saucepan, heat 3 tablespoons of the olive oil over medium heat. Add the onion and the garlic and cook until soft but not coloured, 5 to 7 minutes. Add a little salt and stir through until the mixture is well coated with the oil and onions. Meanwhile, crush the tomatoes in a bowl with your hands. Add them to the saucepan, together with the bay leaf and salt. Stir everything together, bring to a boil, and then reduce the heat to a simmer and cook for 15 to 20 minutes. Stir in the olives, remove from the heat, and season with salt and pepper.

Preheat the oven to 175°C/ gas mark 4/350°F.

Spoon a thin layer of the sauce into a baking dish. The lay the fish on top and spoon the remaining sauce over the top. Make sure all the fish has at least a light covering of sauce. Drizzle with the remaining 1 tablespoon olive oil, cover with aluminium foil and bake for 15 to 20 minutes, until the fish is almost cooked through. Remove from the oven and allow to rest so that the fish keeps cooking in the sauce's residual heat and remains moist. Garnish with the parsley and serve.

Jane Baxter's ORECCHIETTE
with Purple Sprouting Broccoli

2 tablespoons olive oil
4 garlic cloves, *finely sliced*
2 dried chillies, *stalks removed and sliced*
8 anchovy fillets
400g (14oz) purple sprouting broccoli
350g (12⅖oz) orecchiette
Salt and freshly ground black pepper
Grated Parmesan cheese, *to serve*

Energy 300 kcal/1272 kJ
Protein 15.3g
Fat 5.3g
Sat. Fat 0.5g
Carbohydrate 51.2g
Fibre 4.7g

Orecchiette are one of the more unusual types of pasta, but you can use any short pasta you like. Small shells would also be good as they will hold the sauce well. The strong flavours make this a favourite for those with tired palates. It is excellent for folate and beta-carotene, with the anchovies providing some calcium.

Serves 4

Preheat the oven to 200°C/gas mark 6/400°F.

Heat the olive oil in a saucepan and add the garlic and chillies. Cook over a low heat until the garlic has softened a little but not browned. Add the anchovies, remove the pan from the heat and stir vigorously so the anchovies melt into the oil.

Bring a large saucepan of water to the boil and add salt. Add the sprouting broccoli and cook for about 4 minutes until just tender. Drain and roughly chop the stems. Add the broccoli to the garlic, chilli and anchovy mix, and cook over a low heat for about 5 minutes.

Meanwhile, cook the orecchiette for about 12 minutes (or according to packet instructions) until almost cooked but a little al dente. Drain well and place in the pan with the sprouting broccoli and sauce. Taste for seasoning – the anchovies will make it quite salty already – and add salt and black pepper as necessary. Serve with lots of grated Parmesan.

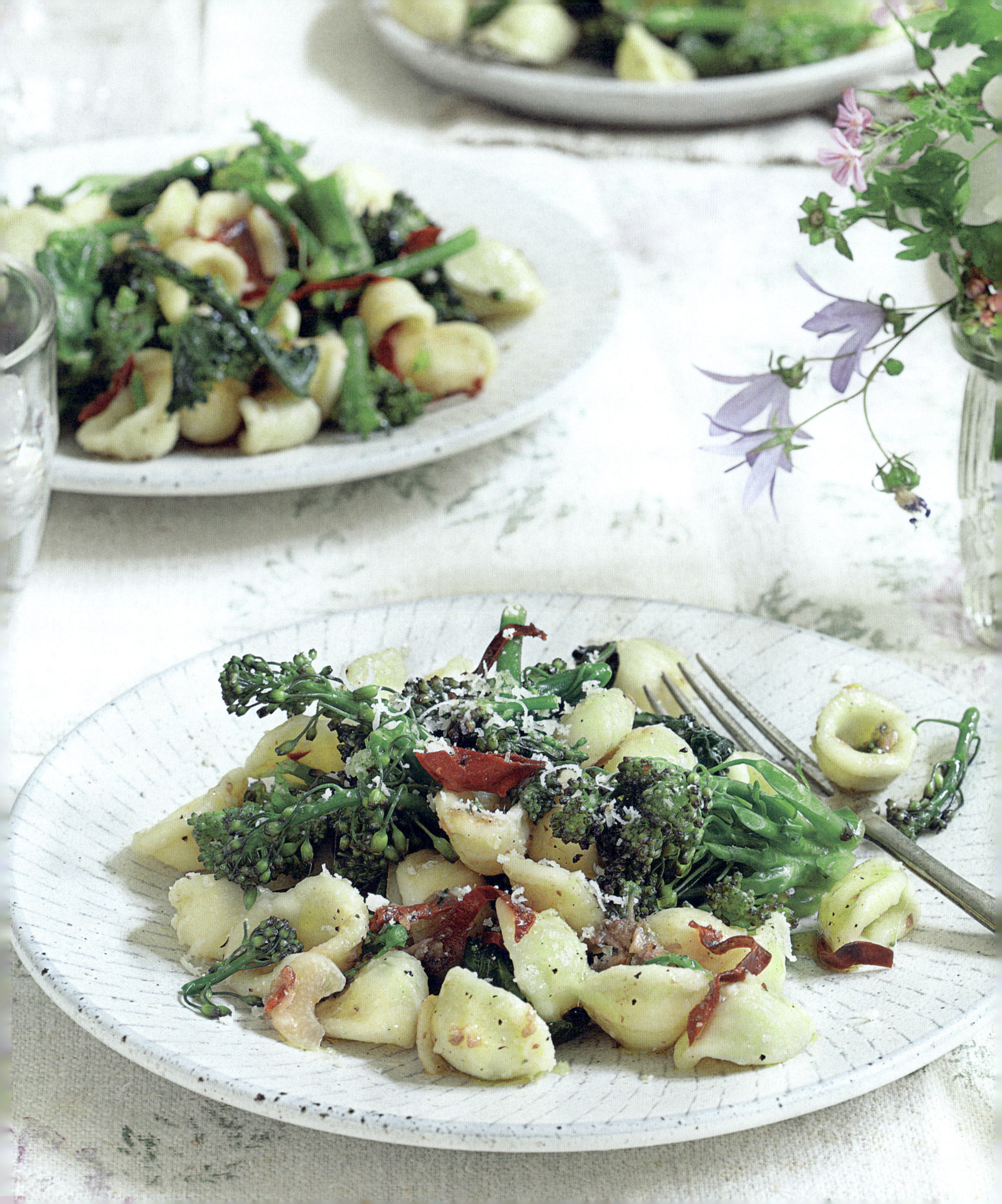

BAKED EGGS

For each egg:
Unsalted butter, for greasing
1 large free-range egg
1 tablespoon single cream
1 tablespoon grated hard cheese, *such as Cheddar or Gruyère*
Salt and freshly ground black pepper

Ideas for fillings:
Ham, good-quality bacon or chorizo, *cubed and fried*
Flaked hot smoked salmon or trout
Cooked smoked haddock
Wilted spinach, *with a grating of nutmeg*
Mushrooms, *fried in garlicky butter*
Diced tomatoes

To serve:
Toast soldiers
Steamed asparagus spears
Steamed tenderstem broccoli

These are endlessly versatile little pots; you really can put in anything you fancy. You can cook them in either individual ramekins or those slightly larger oval shaped ones. Try to use a cheese with a good melting quality – Gruyère is ideal. Eggs are an excellent source of nourishment, high in protein and a good source of iron and vitamin D. Don't worry about the cholesterol in eggs; more recent research has shown that cholesterol in foods is not a major influence on blood cholesterol and health. This is a great basic recipe that can be adapted to suit your changing tastes.

Preheat the oven to 160°C/gas mark 3/325°F.

Butter each ramekin generously. Add one or more of the filling suggestions and season with salt and pepper. You can combine these as much as you like. For example, spinach will work with any meat or fish; chorizo is lovely with tomato.

Break an egg into each ramekin, pour over the cream, then sprinkle with cheese. Put the ramekins on a baking tray. For a just-set white with a runny yolk, bake for 10 minutes. For a firmer yolk, bake for a couple of minutes longer.

Serve with toast soldiers, lightly steamed asparagus or tenderstem broccoli.

Nutritional Information for the basic egg recipe:
Energy 284 kcal/1179 kJ **Protein** 18g **Fat** 23.4g
Sat. Fat 12.3g **Carbohydrate** 0.6g **Fibre** 0g

Creamed Spinach with Eggs

Large knob of unsalted butter
1 onion, *finely chopped*
300g (10½oz) spinach, well washed or **420g (15oz)** frozen spinach, *defrosted and drained*
Pinch of turmeric
Pinch of cumin
Pinch of cinnamon

This is a kind of variation of the baked eggs, but much richer and substantial. It's a comfort food classic to which I've added very little spice, as that's what my mother-in-law does – it really works. You can, of course, leave it out. You could also omit the eggs and just serve the spinach as a side dish. This combination of ingredients gives a highly nutritious dish with plenty of protein, iron, calcium, beta-carotene and vitamin E.

150ml (5fl oz) single cream
100g (3½oz) Cheddar or Gruyère cheese, *grated*
4 free-range eggs

Energy 308 kcal/1278 kJ
Protein 17.4g
Fat 24.3g
Sat. Fat 12.5g
Carbohydrate 5.7g
Fibre 2.8g

Put the butter in a large frying pan and melt. Add the onion and sauté over a low heat until softened and translucent. Add the spinach. Stir and bash down with a wooden spoon until it has collapsed and is wilting, then sprinkle over the spices. Season with salt and black pepper. Cook until all the water has evaporated.

Add the cream and continue to stir over a low heat, reducing the amount of liquid until the spinach is quite firm, then stir in half the cheese. Stir until the cheese has melted. Make 4 wells in the spinach mixture, break an egg into each, then cover the eggs with the remaining cheese. Cook for a couple of minutes on the hob, then place under a hot grill (you may need to protect the handle of your frying pan). Cook until the cheese has melted and browned, and the egg whites are just cooked through.

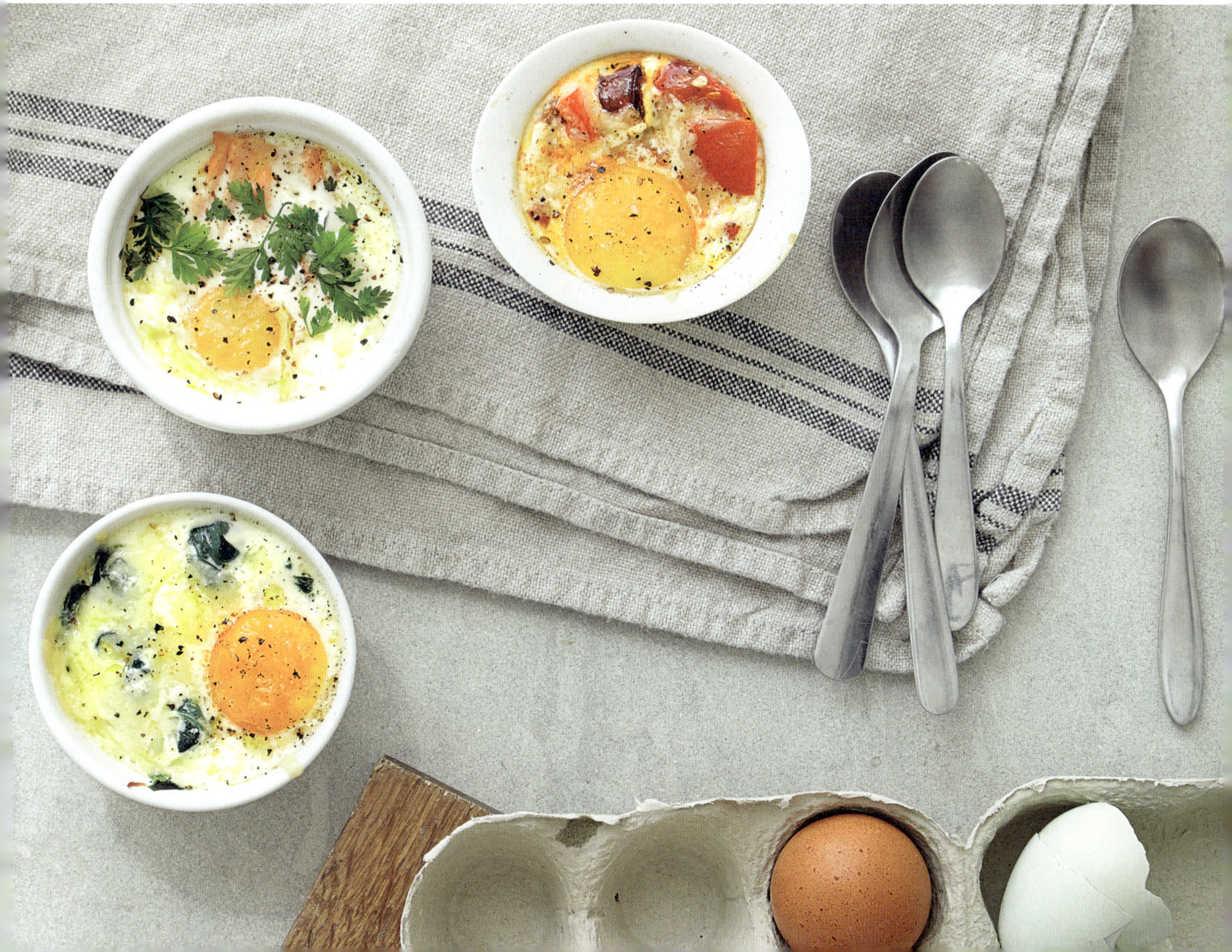

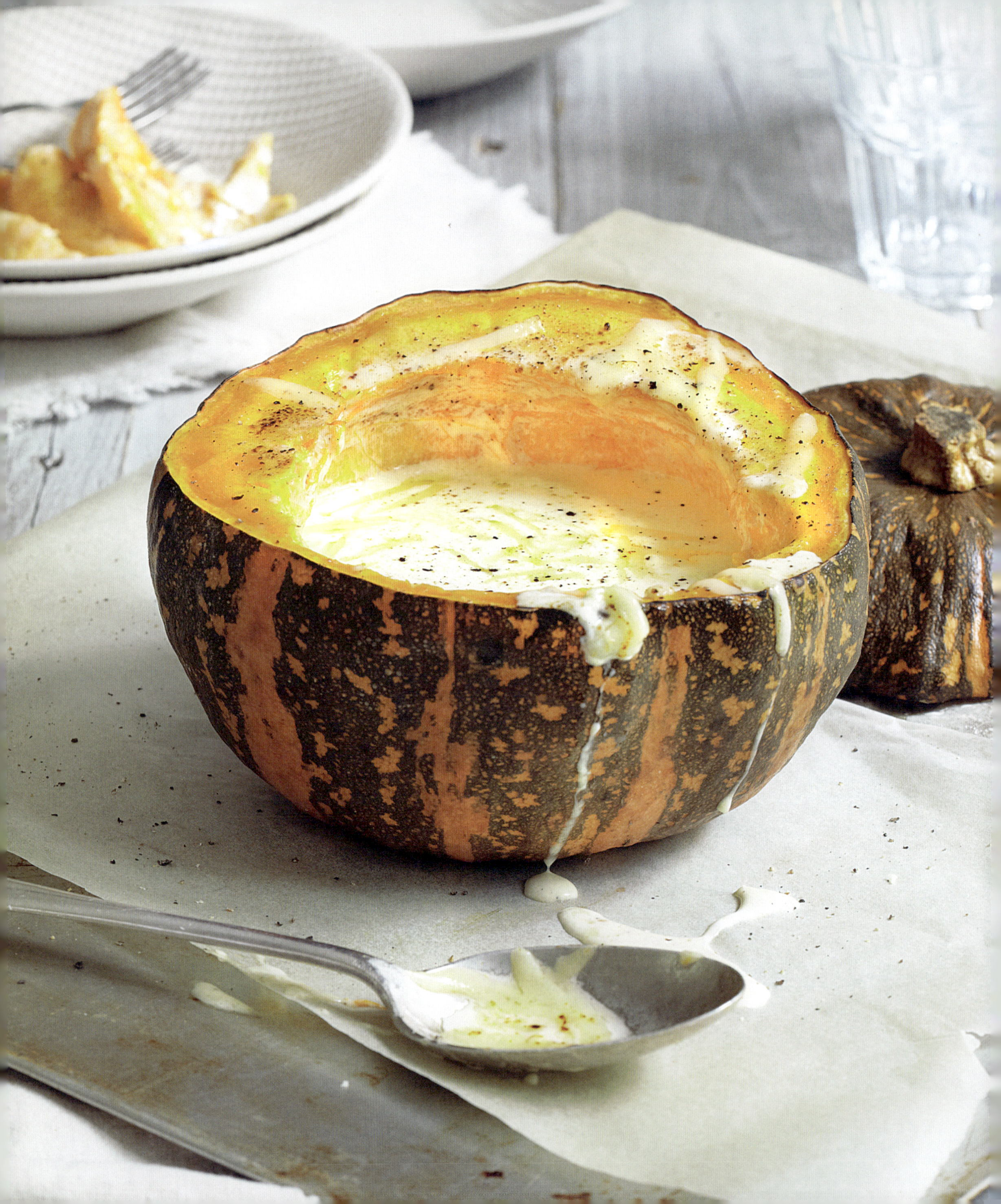

Hugh Fearnley-Whittingstall's
WHOLE PUMPKIN
Baked with Cream

1 medium (3–4kg) pumpkin, *or 4 small squashes*
Up to **250g (9oz)** Gruyère cheese, *grated (depending on the size of your pumpkin)*
Up to **1** litre single cream (ditto)
Freshly grated nutmeg
Knob of unsalted butter
Sea salt and freshly ground black pepper

Energy 757 kcal/3140 kJ
Protein 32.2g
Fat 62.6g
Sat. Fat 39.5g
Carbohydrate 16.5g
Fibre 7.8g

This recipe does say to fill to two-thirds full, but this makes it quite rich; you can just add as much cheese and cream as you think you can cope with. This soup really is the king of all soups. It has a generous amount of protein and is brimming with vitamins such as beta-carotene and vitamin E as well as providing plenty of energy.

Serves 4

Preheat the oven to 190°C/gas mark 5/375°F. Slice the top off the pumpkin or squashes three-quarters of the way up, and retain it – this is your lid. Scoop out all the seeds and surrounding fibres from the pumpkin. Place the scooped-out pumpkin on a baking tray or in an ovenproof dish (which must have sides, to catch any leaking cream – an accident that shouldn't, but can, happen).

Put enough grated Gruyère into the empty cavity of the pumpkin to fill about a third of it, then pour in the cream until the cavity is two-thirds full. Add a few gratings of nutmeg, a little salt and plenty of black pepper. Throw in a knob of butter and replace the lid, so the pumpkin is whole again.

Place in the oven and cook for 45 minutes and up to 1¼ hours, depending on the size of the pumpkin. Test for doneness by removing the lid and poking at the flesh from the inside. It should be nice and tender. At this point, the skin may be lightly burnt and the whole thing just beginning to sag a bit. Be wary – when the pumpkin is completely soft and cooked through, there is a real danger of collapse. The larger the pumpkin, the bigger the danger. Don't panic if it happens – it will look a bit deflated but will still taste delicious.

Serve small squashes individually in bowls, with spoons to scoop out the flesh. Serve the larger pumpkin by scooping plenty of flesh and the creamy, cheesy liquid (the Gruyère will have melted into lovely long, messy strings) into warmed soup bowls. Either way, serve piping hot.

STUFFED JACKET POTATOES

Serves 1

250g (9oz) baking potato(es)
20g butter or spread
a splash milk
6g cheese, grated (cheddar or other cheeses can be used)
pinch flat-leaf parsley, chopped
pinch nutmeg, finely grated
Salt and freshly ground black pepper

Energy 313 kcal/1309 kJ
Protein 8g
Fat 17g
Sat. Fat 2.5g
Carbohydrate 7.75g
Fibre 1.95g

Bake your chosen potatoes in their jackets at 210°C/gas mark 8/450°F for approximately 75–90 minutes. King Edwards and Desiree potatoes are the two best types for soft fluffy insides as they are less waxy than some varieties. Once cooked, remove from the oven and turn the oven up to 235°C/gas mark 8/455°F.

Slice the potatoes in half lengthways. Using a large spoon, scoop out the inner potato into a bowl or pan that you can use for mashing – leave only a little of the inner potato to protect the skins from breaking up. Place the potato skins on to a lightly greased baking tray. You can return them to the hot oven to crisp up a bit if you wish (whilst working on the filling) but this step is not essential.

Add in the butter or spread, parsley, nutmeg to the scooped-out potato in your bowl, and mash. Add milk to get to the correct consistency – it should be a smooth, soft, thick, creamy paste like consistency. Season with salt and pepper.

Spoon in the mashed potato and press down into the potato skins (use an oven cloth as they'll be hot) so that they are level. Once you have filled all the potato skins, top them with the grated cheese. Place the tray on the top shelf of your preheated oven and cook for about 15 minutes or until golden brown. You can also finish under the grill, if required.

Variations

There really are so many variations to the basic recipe above. Below are some ideas to try out - you can even combine some of these combinations!

- For a creamier and more nutritious mash, substitute the milk with a little cream and/or an egg yolk.
- Add any of the following topping with cheese – ham, diced corned beef, chopped spring onions, chives, smoked mackerel and cream cheese, feta cheese and chopped olives, grilled, chopped bacon, smoked salmon/trout and dill, tinned tuna, sundried tomatoes, smoked paprika (to inject a little warmth), garlic mushrooms, sliced tomatoes and extra cheese, finely diced onions or peppers cooked in a little butter. .
- Stir some good old baked beans in tomato sauce into your mash. NB: Will likely not need much milk (if any).
- Add Boursin cheese to your potato mix for a creamier garlic and herb experience. NB: May not need much milk.
- If you have any left-over cooked mince (Bolognese or Chilli, meat or veg!) mix it in with your mash.
- Top with different cheeses or combinations of cheeses, such as: Mozzarella, Saint Paulin, Gouda, Raclette, Goats cheese, Red Leicester, Brie, Stilton, Parmesan, Sage Derby, smoked cheese, Emmental, Gruyere, Wensleydale, etc.

TIP

- If you are short on time then you can prepare this in advance (or even the day before) and keep in the fridge. When required reheat in a microwave.

Maggie Beer's CAVOLO NERO

1 bunch (about 700g (25oz)) cavolo nero, *washed and chopped*
50g (2oz) unsalted butter
1 tablespoon extra virgin olive oil
2 small shallots, *finely sliced*
½ quince, peeled, *cored and coarsely grated*
½ teaspoon lemon juice

This is a lovely side dish to eat in the winter months. Cavolo nero is an excellent source of beta-carotene and phytonutrients that are abundant in the brassica family. The extra butter and oil give additional energy.

Serves 4 as an accompaniment

Bring a large saucepan of water to the boil. Add the cavolo nero and blanch for 3 minutes or until just tender – how long it takes will depend on the age of the cabbage. Drain well and squeeze out any excess moisture.

Heat the butter in a large frying pan over a medium heat until it has turned a nut-brown colour, then add the olive oil to inhibit burning. Add the shallots and the quince, and cook over a low heat until tender and golden. Add the lemon juice and the blanched cavolo nero, then toss to combine and serve.

Energy 164 kcal/676 kJ **Protein** 5.2g **Fat** 14.4g
Sat. Fat 7.1g **Carbohydrate** 3.3g **Fibre** 5.1g

SMOKED TROUT WITH POTATO SALAD

½ cucumber, *peeled*
10 small new potatoes, *steamed or boiled*
2 tablespoons yogurt
1 tablespoon soured cream or crème fraîche
1 teaspoon Dijon mustard *(optional)*
½ teaspoon white wine vinegar
Pinch of sugar
A few chives, finely cut
Small bunch of dill
A few tarragon leaves
Salt and freshly ground black pepper
2 cooked trout fillets (approx.120g (4oz) each)

Smoked trout is a quite delicately flavoured fish, so this salad is deliberately quite mellow without any strong, astringent ingredients. If you do want to pep it up a bit, add the mustard. And if you can handle them, a few cornichons or capers wouldn't go amiss. Although trout is an oily fish, the fat content is low and it is an excellent source of protein for a light meal.

Serves 2

Halve the cucumber lengthways, scoop out the seeds using a teaspoon and cut the flesh into crescents. Put in a bowl. Cut the potatoes into rounds and add to the cucumber. In a separate bowl, mix the yogurt and soured cream together. Add the mustard, if using, vinegar and sugar and season with salt and pepper. Pour this mixture over the cucumber and potatoes. Stir to combine. Add the herbs and stir again. Serve the potato salad with the trout fillets.

Energy 291 kcal/1217 kJ **Protein** 31g **Fat** 11g
Sat. Fat 3.1g **Carbohydrate** 17.3g **Fibre** 2.3g

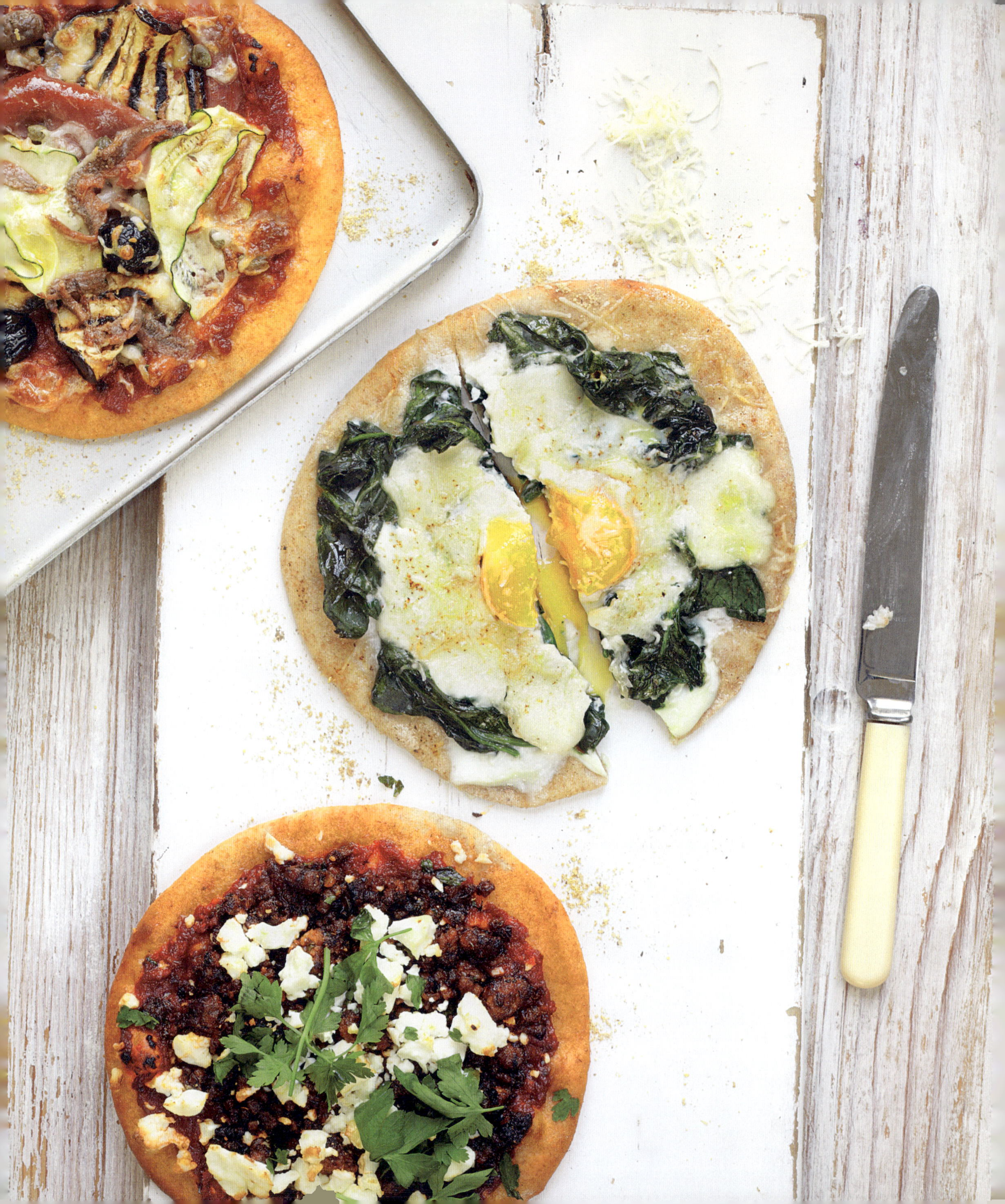

FLATBREAD PIZZAS

150g (5½oz) plain or wholemeal flour
1½ teaspoons baking powder
½ teaspoon salt
150ml (5fl oz) Greek yogurt
Semolina or cornmeal,

Energy 183 kcal/772 kJ
Protein 5.8g
Fat 4.3g
Sat. Fat 2.6g
Carbohydrate 32.1g
Fibre 1.6g

These yogurt-enriched flatbreads are slightly more calorific than using a yeasted dough, but are much lighter, so easier to eat if you are struggling to find an appetite. The dough is also easier to work with, as it's not so elastic. It will keep well in the fridge. You can use any traditional pizza toppings here, but I have included a very quick cheat's way of making an instant tomato sauce, as well as some options that don't require tomato sauce at all (overleaf). These pizzas are ideal as a plain and savoury meal or snack. The different toppings can be used to really boost your energy, protein, vitamins and minerals. Meat, eggs and spinach are all particularly good sources of iron.

Makes 4 flatbread pizzas, each about 18cm

Mix all the ingredients except the semolina into a dough. If it seems quite sticky, add a little more flour. Knead for a minute or two until the dough is smooth and then wrap well in clingfilm and chill for at least 1 hour – you can leave it in the fridge for a day or two without it coming to any harm.

When you are ready to cook your flatbreads, heat your oven to its highest setting and put in an upturned baking tray or baking stone, if you have one, to heat.

Cut the dough into four pieces and roll each out very thinly, to a diameter of about 18cm (7 in).

Pile your choice of topping on top. Remove the baking tray or stone from the oven and dust with semolina or cornmeal if you have some. If you don't, putting a piece of baking parchment on top of the tray when you heat it will stop the pizza from sticking.

Slide the flatbread onto the tray and put back into the oven. Turn the heat down to 200°C/gas mark 6/400°F and cook for 8–10 minutes, until they are well browned around the edges and on the underside.

TIP

- You can make a larger quantity of dough and freeze it. The best way to do this is to portion it out and wrap individually in clingfilm, so if you fancy making just one pizza for yourself you can do so without having to make a whole batch. Simply remove from the freezer and defrost before using.

QUICK TOMATO SAUCE

Enough for 4 flatbreads

Flatbread pizzas recipe (page 87)
4 tablespoons tomato purée
2 tablespoons olive oil
2 garlic cloves, *crushed*
Pinch of sugar
Pinch of dried oregano
Salt and freshly ground black pepper

Mix all the ingredients together and spread over the pizzas. Then top with traditional pizza toppings. Try: coarsely grated or very finely sliced courgettes; grilled aubergines; mozzarella; ham or prosciutto; or olives, capers and anchovies.

Energy 67 kcal/276 kJ **Protein** 1.1g **Fat** 5.6g
Sat. Fat 0.8g **Carbohydrate** 3.3g **Fibre** 0.8g

SPINACH AND EGG TOPPING

Enough for 4 flatbreads

Flatbread pizzas recipe (page 87)
300g (10½oz) spinach *(seems a lot, but it will collapse down)*
1 ball of mozzarella cheese
4 free-range eggs
Grating of nutmeg
Grated Parmesan cheese *(optional)*

Blanch the spinach in a pan of boiling water for 1 minute, then drain and immediately refresh under cold running water. Squeeze out as much of the water as possible and chop roughly.

Pile the spinach onto the flatbreads, and sprinkle over the mozzarella. Turn the edges of the flatbreads up a little just in case the egg makes a dash for it, and make a well in the centre for the egg. Grate over a little nutmeg and some Parmesan, if you like.

Energy 123 kcal/511 kJ **Protein** 13.5g **Fat** 7.3g
Sat. Fat 4.6g **Carbohydrate** 1.2g **Fibre** 2.1g

'WHITE' PIZZA

Enough for 4 flatbreads

This recipe uses potatoes, but you could also use other white root vegetables, such as celeriac or Jerusalem artichoke.

Flatbread pizzas recipe (page 87)
6 small new potatoes, *sliced as thinly as possible, skin on*
1 block of firm mozzarella cheese **(100g / 3½oz)**, *grated*
Leaves from a sprig of rosemary or sage, *very finely chopped*
Olive oil
Salt and freshly ground black pepper

Bring a saucepan of water to a boil. Blanch the potatoes for a minute. Drain immediately and cool under cold running water. Spread the potatoes over the flatbreads, then sprinkle over the cheese and chopped herbs. Drizzle over a little olive oil and season.

Energy 114 kcal/476 kJ **Protein** 5.7g **Fat** 6.0g
Sat. Fat 3.6g **Carbohydrate** 9.7g **Fibre** 0.8g

SPICY LAMB FLATBREADS

Enough for 4 flatbreads

For a traditional Middle Eastern take on pizza, try this.

Flatbread pizzas recipe (page 87)
200g (7oz) minced lamb
2 tablespoons tomato purée
1 tablespoon olive oil
½ small onion, *finely chopped*
1 teaspoon ground cumin
1 teaspoon ground coriander
1 teaspoon sumac *(optional)*
1 garlic clove, *minced*
1 teaspoon dried mint
Chopped parsley
50g (2oz) feta, *crumbled (optional)*

Mix all the ingredients together except the chopped parsley and feta, trying to keep the mixture quite loose. Divide between the flatbreads and sprinkle over the parsley and feta, if using.

Energy 168 kcal/701 kJ **Protein** 12.6g **Fat** 12.2g
Sat. Fat 5.2g **Carbohydrate** 2.7g **Fibre** 0.5g

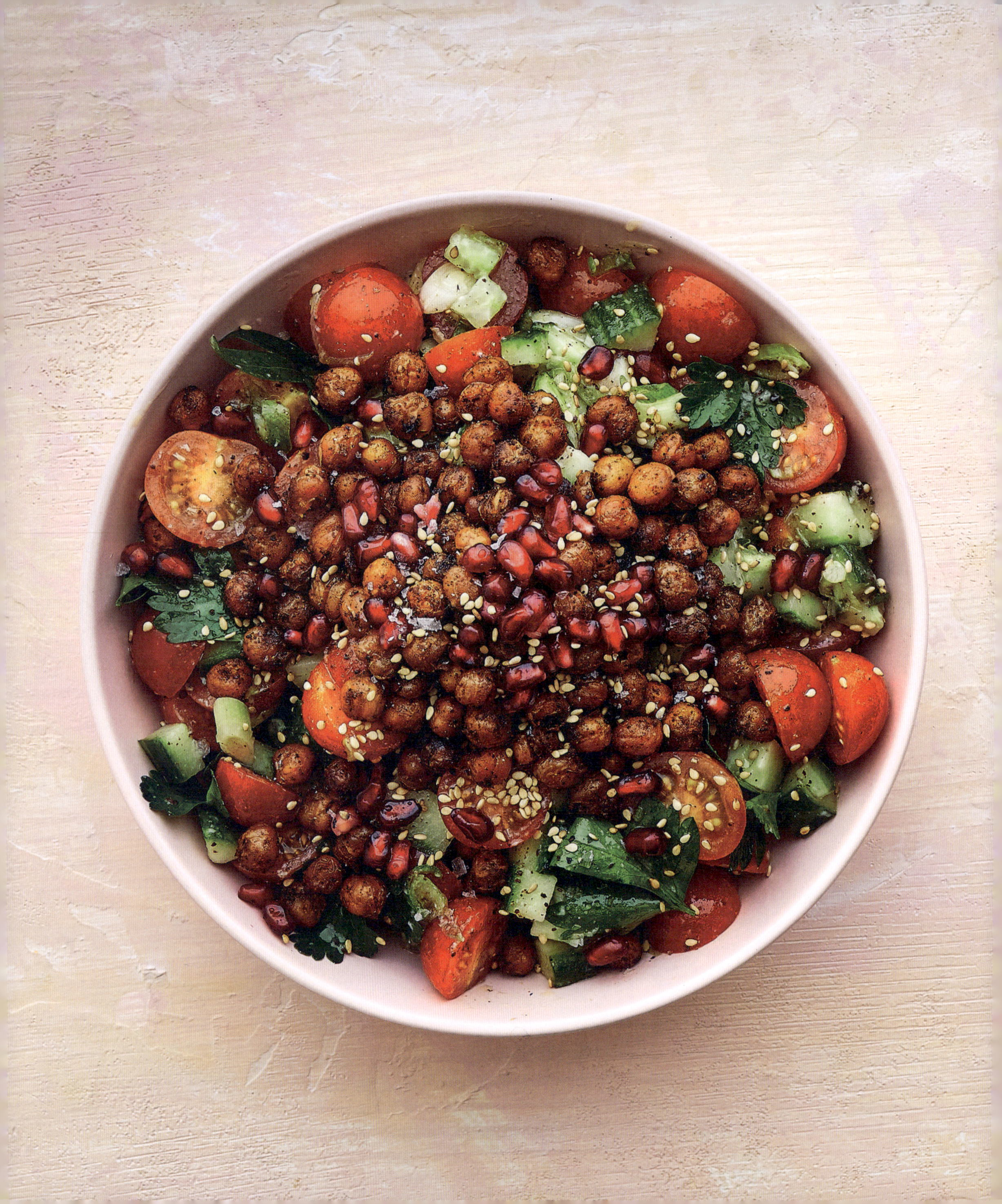

Divya Sharma's ROASTED CHICKPEA SALAD

This colourful vegan salad is big on flavour and texture. Great on its own or serve with grilled chicken, fish, halloumi cheese or roasted nuts to boost the protein.

Serves 4

2 x 400g (14oz) cans of chickpeas, rinsed and drained
2 tablespoons olive oil
3 teaspoons sumac
2 teaspoons smoked paprika
1 teaspoon salt
6 large garlic cloves, unpeeled
4 tablespoons extra-virgin olive oil
4 tablespoons lemon juice
300g (10oz) cherry tomatoes, halved
1 cucumber, coarsely chopped
5 spring onions, finely chopped

Energy 377 kcal/1577 kJ
Protein 9.9g
Fat 23.8g
Sat. Fat 4.1g
Carbohydrate 34.3g
Fibre 9.5g

Position a rack in the centre of the oven and preheat the oven to 200°C/gas mark 6/400°F. Line a large baking sheet with parchment paper.

Toss the chickpeas with the olive oil, 1 teaspoon of the sumac, the paprika and a pinch of the salt. Season with pepper.

Wrap the garlic cloves in a small sheet of foil and place on the same baking sheet. Roast, stirring the chickpeas halfway through the cooking time, for 25–30 minutes or until crisp and golden brown. Allow to cool.

Unwrap the roasted garlic and squeeze the flesh into a serving bowl, discarding the skins. Mash the garlic using a fork. Stir in the extra-virgin olive oil, lemon juice, remaining 2 tsp of sumac and the remaining salt.

Add the tomatoes, cucumber, spring onion and parsley and toss to coat. Sprinkle with the chickpeas and pomegranate.

SALMON (OR TOFU) WITH SOBA NOODLES

and Oriental Greens

Small piece of fresh ginger, *grated*
2 garlic cloves, *crushed*
1 tablespoon honey
2 tablespoons soy sauce
1 tablespoon mirin or sweet sherry
2 salmon fillets or **1** packet of firm tofu
100g (3½oz) dry soba noodles or **200g (7oz)** ready cooked
1 teaspoon sesame oil
2 teaspoons vegetable oil
2 spring onions, *sliced into rounds*
Bag of pak choi (about 6 heads) or other Chinese greens
1 teaspoon sesame seeds *(optional)*
Salt and freshly ground black pepper

Energy 729 kcal/3041 kJ
Protein 27.3g
Fat 24.7g
Sat. Fat 3.6g
Carbohydrate 94.7g
Fibre 1.3g

Nutritional value for recipe made with salmon

This is a very useful cold noodle salad. Tofu is a good alternative to salmon. You can use any greens here – asparagus, green beans or sprouting broccoli would all work well. Incidentally, packets of ready-cooked noodles are very useful to have in stock for instant meals. Add sesame oil, soy sauce and perhaps a pinch of Chinese five spice and you have an instant snack. Noodles are a great source of starchy carbohydrate and the salmon provides good protein. The vitamins – beta-carotene and folate – will depend on your choice of vegetables.

Serves 2

Put the ginger, garlic, honey, soy sauce and mirin in a bowl and mix together. Season with salt and pepper. Add the salmon fillets or tofu and turn over so all the sides are completely coated in the marinade. Leave for at least 30 minutes to marinate, but longer if you have it.

If you are using uncooked noodles, cook them according to the packet instructions. Drain and toss them in the sesame oil and leave to cool.

Heat the vegetable oil in a frying pan. Drain the salmon, reserving the marinade. Place the salmon, skin-side down, in the oil and fry for 3 minutes, then flip over and cook for a further couple of minutes. Remove from the pan.

Add the spring onions and pak choi to the pan, and sauté for a couple of minutes, then pour in the reserved marinade. Allow to sizzle for a minute or two, then add a splash of water. The greens should wilt down very quickly.

To serve, remove and discard the skin from the salmon and break the flesh into pieces. Pile on top of the noodles, then add the greens and pour over any liquid left in the frying pan. Serve sprinkled with the sesame seeds, if using.

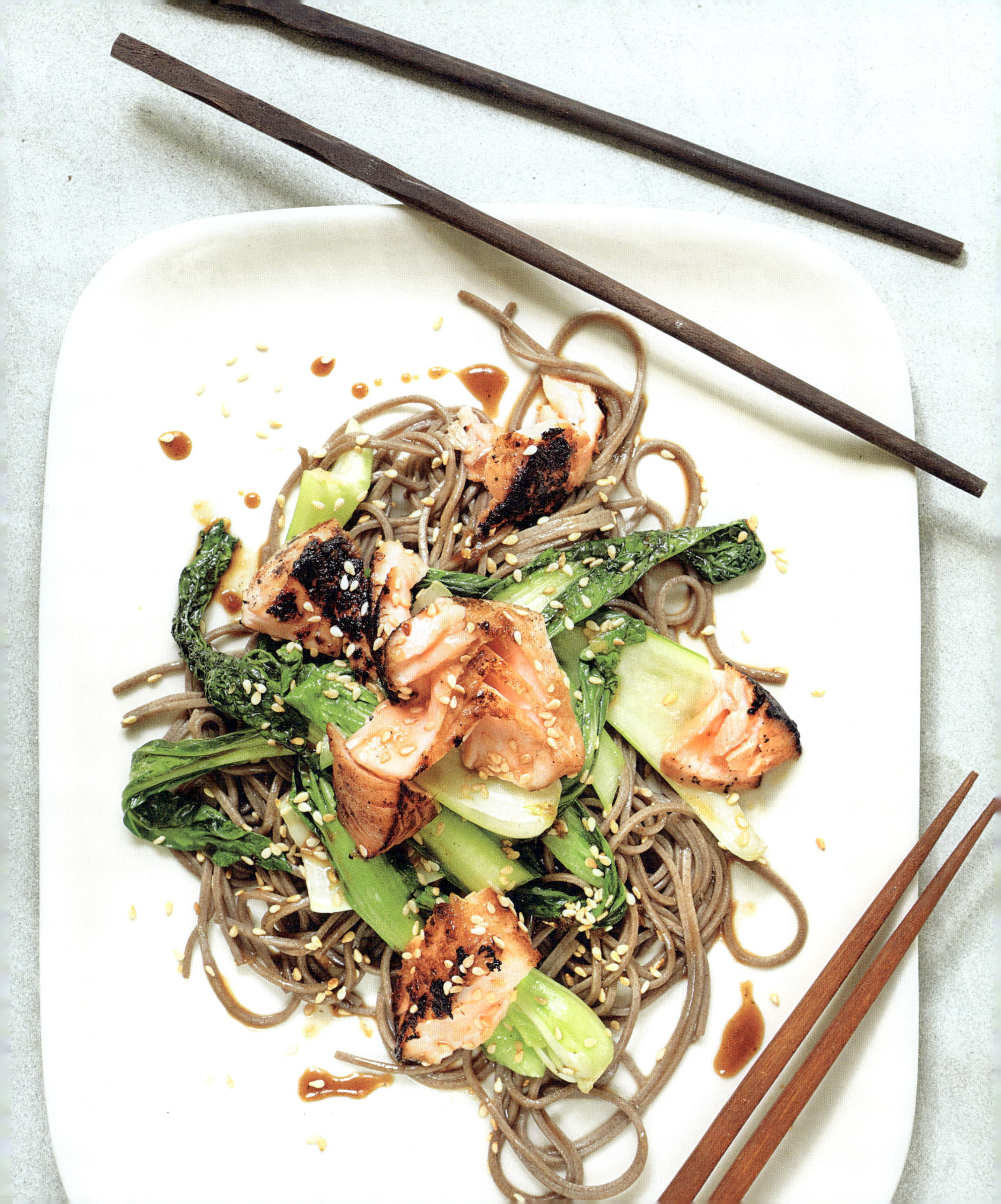

WAYS WITH MEATBALLS

1 tablespoon olive oil
1 onion, *finely chopped*
2 garlic cloves, *finely chopped*
300g (10½oz) minced beef
300g (10½oz) minced pork
100g (3½oz) breadcrumbs
75ml (2½fl oz) single cream, milk or yogurt
1 large free-range egg
1 teaspoon dried oregano
2 handfuls of fresh parsley leaves, *finely chopped*
Salt and freshly ground

Per meatball
Energy 96 kcal/402 kJ
Protein 7.0g
Fat 5.6g
Sat. Fat 2.2g
Carbohydrate 4.8g
Fibre 0.3g

Meatballs are probably the most useful thing to make as a batch, as they are so incredibly versatile. This basic recipe opens itself up to endless variations, so at the end of the recipe you will see a few of those along with some suggestions as to what to do with them. These particular meatballs are especially good as they are fortified with breadcrumbs and cream. This makes them very soft and more calorific if you need building up a bit. A great source of protein and iron, and very easy to control portions for those with a small appetite.

Makes 20

Preheat the oven to 220°C/gas mark 7/425°F. Line a baking tray with baking parchment or greaseproof paper.

Heat the oil in a frying pan and add the onion and garlic. Sauté for a few minutes over a low heat until the onion has softened. Remove from the heat and cool.

Put the meat, breadcrumbs, cream, egg and herbs in a large bowl. Season liberally with salt and pepper. Mix everything together thoroughly – the easiest way to do this is with your hands. Form the mixture into balls the size of golf balls – each weighing about 40g. Space these out on a baking tray. Bake in the oven for around 15 minutes until well browned and cooked through.

Variations:

The Slider
Instead of making balls, flatten the meatballs into little patties and turn into sliders (mini burgers). Children in particular will like assembling these if you get some mini burger buns. You can add slices of cheese to the burgers for the last 5 minutes of cooking for a cheese burger and serve with any of the usual condiments, just as you like.

Lamb Balls
You can use lamb mince instead of pork or beef: add dried mint or rosemary and lemon zest to the burger, then crumble in some feta cheese. Serve sliced into pitta breads with a yogurt and mint dressing.

Scandinavian Balls
The Scandinavian classic has to be one of the most comforting ways to serve meatballs. Make a beef gravy with stock and granules, add a drop of

cream and, if you have some, stir in some lingonberry jam (you can get it online or from IKEA) – otherwise use redcurrant jelly. Serve with lots of mashed potato.

Steamed Balls for Soup

Use the Lamb Balls mixture opposite and drop into a broth such as the Chicken Noodle Soup (page 74), or you could even add to a bowl of consommé. Simmer until cooked. An instant meal when you have ready-cooked meatballs in the fridge or freezer is to cook some instant noodles, drop into chicken consommé or stock, and add a bit of soy sauce or any other condiments you fancy. Add lots of fresh herbs – and serve your instant meatball and noodle soup.

Change the meat to a mixture of pork and chicken – you could even add some finely chopped prawns. Add lime zest, a little grated ginger, and perhaps some coriander stem. Mix the chicken consommé or stock with coconut milk, add soy or fish sauce, lime juice, fresh herbs and noodles.

Meatballs and Spaghetti

This is brilliant if you can cope with tomato sauce. All is not lost if you can't, however. You can simply slice into your favourite pasta bake with lots of vegetables. Make much smaller meatballs (you could even just use sausage meat) and slice into rounds.

The Vegetarian Option

You can make a vegetarian version of the meatball just by adapting the recipe opposite, swapping the meat for any type of bean or a firm lentil such as Puy. You can also introduce more protein by swapping the breadcrumbs for something like quinoa. Here is one idea:

1 tablespoon olive oil
1 onion, *finely chopped*
2 garlic cloves, *finely chopped*
600g (21oz) beans, cooked *– cannellini, black, kidney and pinto beans are all good*
100g (3½oz) quinoa, cooked
50g (2oz) crumbled feta or grated Parmesan cheese
2 free-range eggs, *beaten*
1 teaspoon dried mixed herbs
4 tablespoons fresh soft herbs, *finely chopped – parsley, mint, coriander or dill*
Zest of **1** unwaxed lime or lemon
Salt and freshly ground black pepper

Heat the olive oil in a frying pan and sauté the onion until soft. Add the garlic and cook for a couple of minutes. Take 200g of the beans and purée with the onion and garlic, until almost smooth. Put the rest of the beans in a large bowl and mash coarsely so they keep some texture. Add the puréed beans to this, along with all the other ingredients. Mix thoroughly. If you find the mixture is a little dry add a little water, milk or lemon juice, a tablespoon at a time. Proceed as opposite regarding shaping.

Nutritional Information per vegetarian meatball:
Energy 126 kcal/403 kJ **Protein** 8.5g **Fat** 2.5g
Sat. Fat 0.7g **Carbohydrate** 18.6g **Fibre** 7.2g

Maria Elia's WATERMELON, AVOCADO AND BLACK BEAN TACOS

with Greek Yogurt Crema

Juice of 1 orange
Juice of 1 lemon
Juice of 1 lime
Zest of ½ unwaxed orange
Zest of ½ unwaxed lemon
Zest of ½ unwaxed lime
½ red chilli, *finely chopped*
250g (9oz) watermelon, *deseeded and thinly sliced*
Sea salt

For the crema:
125ml (4¼fl oz) Greek yogurt
½ teaspoon ground cumin
2 teaspoons coriander seeds, *roasted and ground*
1 garlic clove, *finely chopped*
2 teaspoons finely grated orange zest
1 tablespoon freshly squeezed orange juice

For the tacos:
8 × 15cm (6in) corn or flour tortillas
½ can cooked black beans, *drained and rinsed*
8 cherry vine tomatoes, *quartered*
1 avocado, *diced into 1cm cubes*
15g (½oz) picked coriander leaves
1 small orange or blood orange,

This has a lot of ingredients in it, but don't let this put you off – it really is just a case of assembling and mixing, and most of it can be made in advance. It's well worth the effort! Packed with fresh ingredients, this is a great source of vitamins, especially vitamin C. This is ideal for poor appetites, as you can start with a small portion, with fillings of your choice, taking whatever you feel able to eat.

Serves 4

Combine the citrus juices and zests in a large non-reactive bowl or container. Add the chilli, ½ teaspoon sea salt and the watermelon. Mix thoroughly, then transfer to the fridge and marinate for at least 30 minutes or overnight.

To make the crema, mix all the ingredients together and refrigerate until required.

Pour the marinating watermelon into a sieve and drain off any excess juice.

To assemble, heat a griddle pan or grill and heat the tortillas on both sides.

Spoon a little crema down the centre of each tortilla, then top with drained watermelon, black beans, tomatoes, avocado, coriander leaves, orange, spring onions and chilli. Serve two per person, or one for a small appetite, with a wedge of lime.

Variation

Use 250g (90z) boneless, finely sliced skinless sea bream or sea bass fillets to replace the watermelon and marinate in the citrus zest and juices for 15 minutes. Alternatively, use a mix of half melon, half fish.

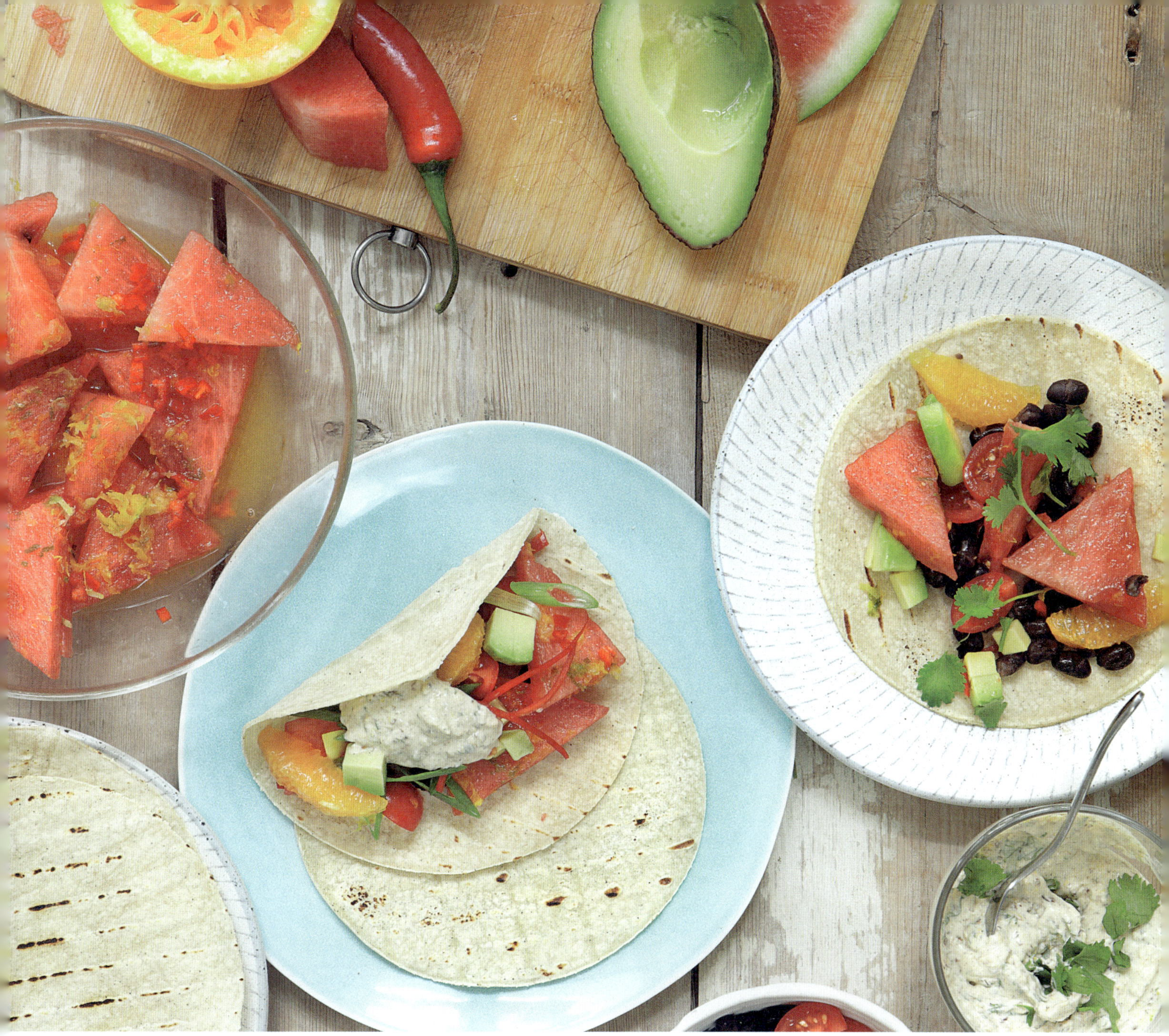

peel cut off and segmented
2 spring onions, *finely sliced*
1 red chilli, *deseeded and finely sliced*

To serve:

Nutritional information for each portion (2 tacos):
Energy 556 kcal/2353 kJ **Protein** 23.2g **Fat** 10.7g
Sat. Fat 3.7g **Carbohydrate** 99.2g **Fibre** 11.2g

Nutritional information for each portion (2 tacos) with sea bream:
Energy 586 kcal/2480 kJ **Protein** 28.7g **Fat** 11.6g
Sat. Fat 3.7g **Carbohydrate** 99.2g **Fibre** 11.2g

MAIN MEALS

With busy lives, many people wait until the evening to eat a main meal. Having cancer treatment can be tiring and waiting until the evening may mean you are too tired to eat or prepare food. Try eating at a time that suits you best – you can have a main meal in the middle of the day or an evening meal a little earlier than usual. Many of the recipes in this section can be frozen in individual portions to make it easy when you want something without the preparation. Family and friends may be able to help by preparing some food for you ahead of your treatment. If you struggle to eat drier foods try to choose meals that have a sauce or gravy. You can freeze extra gravy or sauce in individual portions to use at another time.

Fish and seafood

- Poached or baked fillet of fish, such as salmon, cod or haddock – make a sauce by warming crème fraîche with pesto or lemon, serve with mashed potato as a fish pie
- Smoked haddock chowder with sweetcorn, potato and cream
- Marinated cooked salmon served with stir-fried vegetables and noodles or rice
- Bake salmon wrapped in a foil parcel with lemon juice, serve with couscous and roasted vegetables
- Grilled white fish such as sea bass or plaice served with a salsa of tomatoes, coriander and olive oil
- Cooked prawns in a tomato and garlic sauce; serve with rice or noodles

Chicken

- Chicken fillet with cream cheese wrapped in prosciutto, serve baked with jacket potato and vegetables or salad
- Chicken fillet topped with cream cheese and mustard, grilled until golden brown

Meat

- Sausages with mashed potatoes and baked beans
- Cottage pie or shepherd's pie – try using frozen mashed potato on either of these to make cooking quick and easy; alternatively, freeze any extra mashed potato for use at a later date, then defrost in the fridge and add extra butter, crème fraîche or cream for the best texture
- One-pot meals such as corned beef hash or beef casserole
- Skewer lamb loin marinated in soy sauce, cumin, paprika and olive oil – grill and serve with a salad and rice

Vegetarian

- Stuffed peppers – use cooked rice mixed with pesto and cheese
- Cheese soufflé: although a soufflé may seem complicated, there are recipes for twice baked soufflés that can be frozen after the first baking and then just reheated before serving
- Risotto: use butternut squash, mushrooms, tomatoes or mixed vegetables with short grain rice and keep the risotto moist – add extra cheese before serving, such as Parmesan or goat's cheese
- Ratatouille – add a sprinkle of cheese and serve with baked potato or rice
- Vegetarian sausages – serve with mashed potatoes and cooked red onions or baked beans
- Vegetable casserole or stew
- Savoury flan – cheese and onion or cheese and tomato; buy ready-made pastry if you are too tired to cook
- Vegetable curry – use fragrant spices and avoid chilli if your mouth is sore, serve with cooked rice or Indian bread such as naan or roti

The Royal Marsden's CHICKPEA AND SWEET POTATO MONGOLIAN STEW

350g (12⅓oz) or **2** large sweet potatoes, *peeled and cut into 2cm cubes*
1 tablespoon vegetable oil
1 large onion, *diced*
2 bay leaves
1 teaspoon ground cinnamon
2 garlic cloves, *minced*
1 teaspoon cumin seeds
2½ teaspoons ground turmeric
2½ teaspoons garam masala
4 fresh tomatoes
Bunch of fresh coriander
100g (3½oz) Greek yogurt
400g (14oz) can chickpeas, *drained and rinsed*
150g (5½oz) soya beans
1 vegetable stock cube
275ml (9fl oz) single cream
Salt and freshly ground black pepper

Energy 374 kcal/1569 kJ
Protein 19.0g
Fat 18.1g
Sat. Fat 6.5g
Carbohydrate 37g
Fibre 12.7g

This delicious vegetarian stew contains lots of fragrant spices without any heat. This is a popular dish from the hospital menu providing plenty of protein and energy from the chickpeas and vegetables in a smooth, creamy sauce. It is packed with vitamins, being high in beta-carotene, vitamin E, folate and iron. Serve with rice.

Cool and freeze individual portions for a quick and easy meal when you are too tired to cook.

Serves 6

Boil the sweet potatoes in a large saucepan until three-quarters cooked, about 15 minutes, then strain and set aside (the potatoes should still be firm).

Heat the oil in a saucepan on a medium heat and fry the onion, bay leaves and cinnamon until the onion is transparent. Add the garlic, cumin, turmeric and garam masala, and sweat for about 4 minutes.

Meanwhile, in a blender, whizz the tomatoes and coriander (reserving a few leaves for the garnish).

Add half the yogurt to the onion and cook for a further 5 minutes. Add the blended tomatoes and coriander. Add the chickpeas, sweet potato, soya beans and vegetable stock, and up to 500ml (17fl oz) hot water, if required. Bring to the boil and then simmer for 5 minutes.

Stir in the rest of the yogurt and the cream, and heat through. Season and garnish with chopped fresh coriander.

Mary Contini's
SPINACH AND RICOTTA CRESPELLE

'A delicious recipe that can be prepared ahead of time. You need savoury pancakes, a filling of spinach and ricotta, and a fresh tomato sugo and a béchamel sauce to bake them with. It is simple to assemble and a dish that will be fresh and easy to enjoy.' *Mary Contini*

Elements to this dish will freeze very well – so it might be worth making a couple of batches of both the pancakes and tomato sauce. That way if you want to use them for this, you just have the spinach and ricotta to mix together and a very simple béchamel to make – or you could of course use them for other things. This dish is a lovely blend of flavours and good, soft textures that are easy to eat. It is good for protein and packed with beta-carotene, calcium, vitamin E and folate.

Serves 6

For the crespelle/crêpes:
100g (3½oz) plain flour, *sieved*
300ml (10fl oz) semi-skimmed milk
2 large free-range eggs
Salt and freshly ground black pepper
Unsalted butter or olive oil, *for frying*

For the spinach and ricotta filling:
350g (12⅓oz) fresh ricotta cheese
3 tablespoons grated Parmigiano Reggiano, *plus extra for sprinkling*
1 free-range egg yolk, *beaten*
1 teaspoon caster sugar
250g (9oz) fresh spinach, *boiled in salted water, squeezed dry and shredded (or 125g frozen spinach)*
2 tablespoons chopped fresh organic herbs – *parsley and basil with a few mint leaves*
Generous grating of fresh nutmeg
Squeeze of lemon juice
Salt and plenty of freshly ground black pepper

For the fresh tomato sauce:
750g (26⅓oz) ripe sweet tomatoes
3–4 tablespoons extra virgin olive oil
2 garlic cloves, *sliced*
Bunch of fresh basil

To make the crêpes, whizz all the ingredients together in a liquidiser. Heat a good non-stick frying pan and smear with a small amount of butter or olive oil. Add a ladle of pancake batter, just enough to coat the bottom of the frying pan. Cook the pancake slowly until it starts to brown underneath and you start to see little bubbles forming on the surface. Flip it over and cook on the other side. Remove and leave on a plate to cool. Make all the batter into pancakes and stack on the plate, piled high. Once they are cool they can be covered with clingfilm and refrigerated for up to 5 days.

To make the spinach and ricotta filling, use a fork to loosen the ricotta. Add the rest of the ingredients together and mix with a fork. Check the flavour and add salt and pepper to taste. If the filling seems too dry, add a tablespoon of milk to loosen.

To make the tomato sauce, make a cross on the base of each tomato, then drop into just-boiled water for 10 seconds. Drain – the skins should now easily peel off. Roughly chop the tomatoes and put them in a shallow pan. Add the oil and garlic, and allow to simmer for 20 minutes until the tomatoes collapse and the sauce thickens. Season to taste and add lots of fresh basil to lift the flavour.

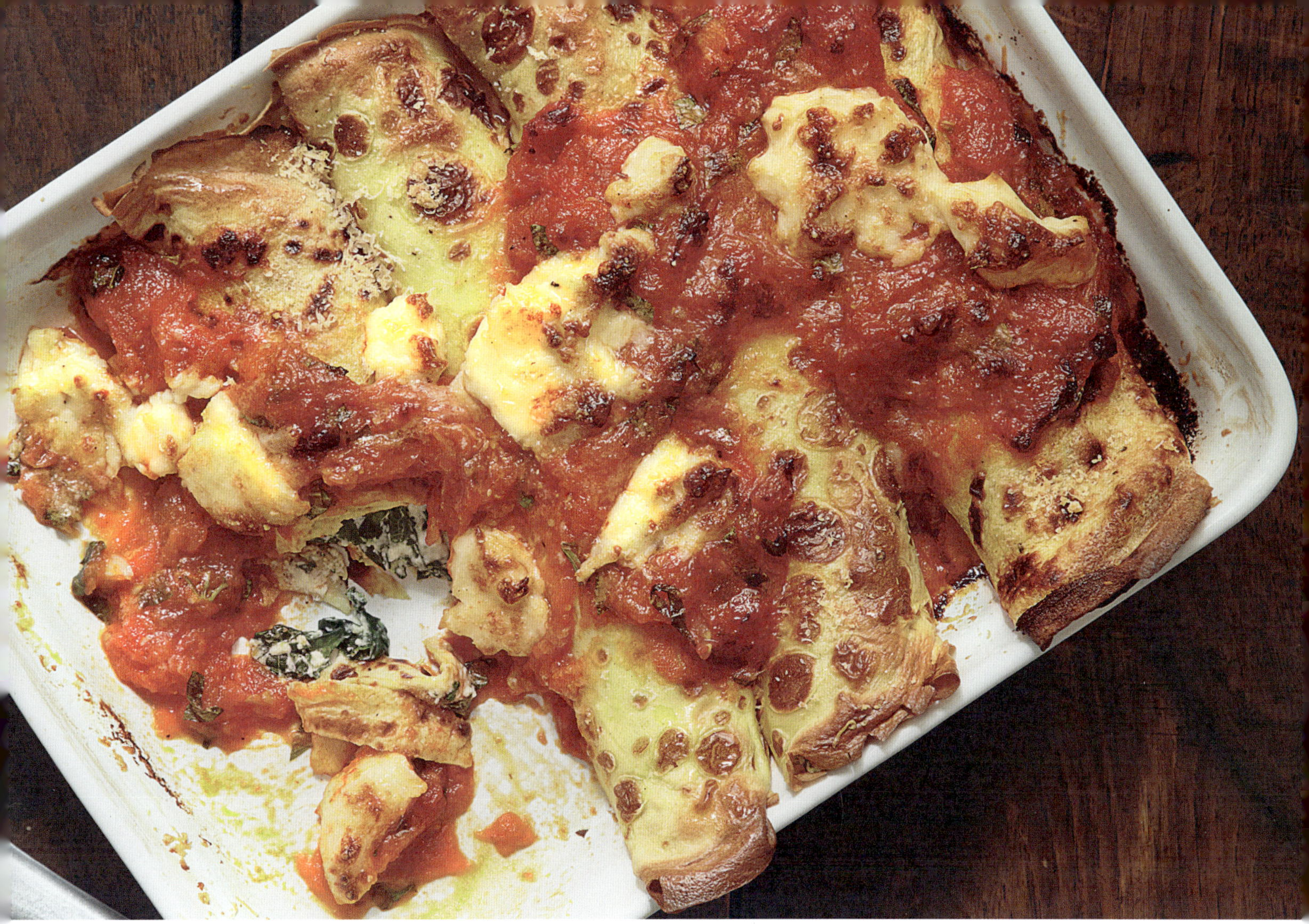

Salt
For the easy béchamel sauce:
500ml (17fl oz) milk
50g (2oz) unsalted butter
50g (2oz) plain flour
Freshly grated nutmeg
Salt and freshly ground black pepper

Energy 477 kcal/1991 kJ
Protein 20.8g
Fat 30.8g
Sat. Fat 15.2g
Carbohydrate 32.2g
Fibre 4.2g

To make the easy béchamel, whizz all the ingredients in a blender or food-processor. Pour into a saucepan and bring up to a gentle simmer, stirring until it thickens. Season to taste and set aside.

Preheat the oven to 200°C/gas mark 6/400°F. To assemble the crêpes, grease a large gratin dish with butter or olive oil. Take a crêpe, spread it with some of the spinach and ricotta filling, then spoon over some of béchamel. Don't worry if there are any lumps in the béchamel – these will magically disappear once it bakes. Sprinkle with grated Parmigiano. Turn the edges in top and bottom to fit your gratin dish, roll it up like a wrap, then place in the dish.

Repeat with the remaining pancakes. Pour over the tomato sauce and any last scrapings of béchamel and sprinkle with parmesan and some fresh basil leaves. Bake in the preheated oven for around 40 minutes, until piping hot.

Jack Monroe's
BARLEY RISOTTO WITH BEETROOT AND PEAS

with Lemon-Chilli Oil

500g (18oz) fresh beetroot, *peeled and diced (or use vacuum-packed and skip the first step)*
1 litre hot chicken or vegetable stock
25g (1oz) unsalted butter
1 onion, *finely sliced*
2 garlic cloves, *crushed*
250g (9oz) pearl barley
100ml (3½fl oz) red or white wine or water
200g (7oz) frozen petits pois or other small green vegetable *(green beans, broad beans, tenderstem broccoli, sugar snaps...)*

For the oil (optional):
Zest and juice of **1** unwaxed lemon
2 tablespoons groundnut oil
Pinch of dried chilli flakes

Small bunch of parsley, *chopped, to serve*

Energy 437 kcal/1839 kJ
Protein 11.0g
Fat 13.1g
Sat. Fat 4.8g
Carbohydrate 68.9g
Fibre 7.1g

'I love this risotto – a feast for both the eyes and the tastebuds – with wholesome, nutty flavours from the pearl barley and groundnut oil, deep earthy goodness from the beetroot and a pop of spring freshness with each tiny petit pois… If you're stuck for time or pans, you can fling the beetroot in with the onion at the start, and the vacuum-packed varieties work just as well as big knobbly fresh ones.' *Jack Monroe*

The lemon and chilli oil is purely optional, but is definitely worth adding if you aren't suffering with a sore mouth. This dish provides a bountiful selection of vitamins, including folate, beta-carotene and vitamin E.

Serves 4

Put the beetroot in a saucepan and cover with some of the stock. Bring to the boil, then reduce to a simmer and cook until tender – about 15 minutes.

Melt the butter in a large, shallow saucepan or frying pan. Add the onion and garlic, and cook over a low heat until the onion is soft and translucent. Add the pearl barley and stir for a minute until well coated with the butter, then add the wine or water. Turn the heat up to medium for a minute and allow the wine to bubble and reduce. When the beetroot is tender, blitz in a blender with the remaining stock. Add this, a ladleful at a time, allowing the barley to absorb most of the liquid before adding the next ladleful. Repeat until the pearl barley is soft, swollen and slightly sticky – this will take about 30 minutes.

Toss in the frozen peas and stir through. Cook for a couple of minutes.

To make the lemon-chilli oil (if using) mix the lemon juice and zest with the oil and chilli, then drizzle this over the top of the risotto. Serve with lots of freshly ground black pepper and some chopped parsley.

TIP

- This risotto will freeze well – just make sure you do so as soon as it has cooled to room temperature.

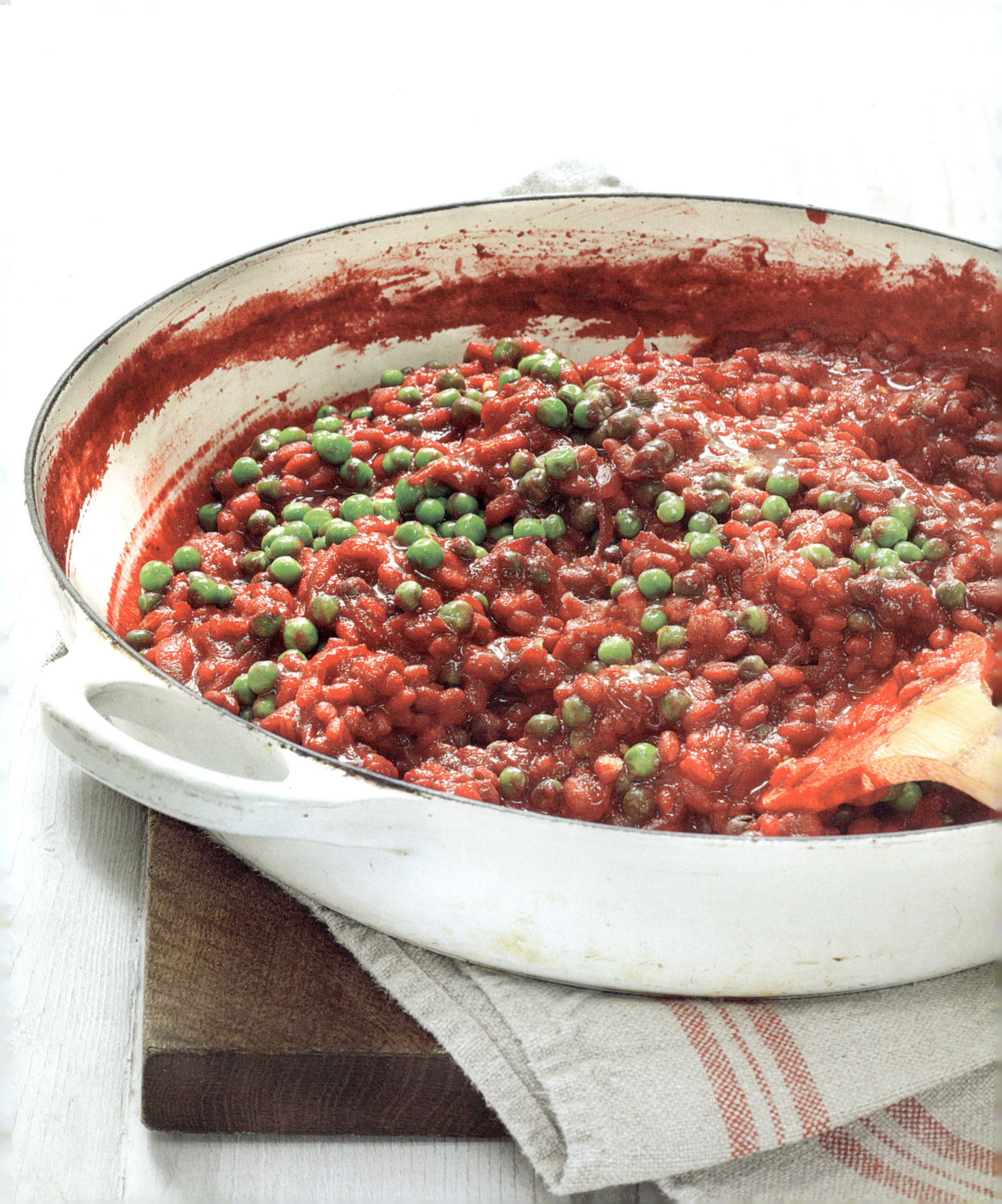

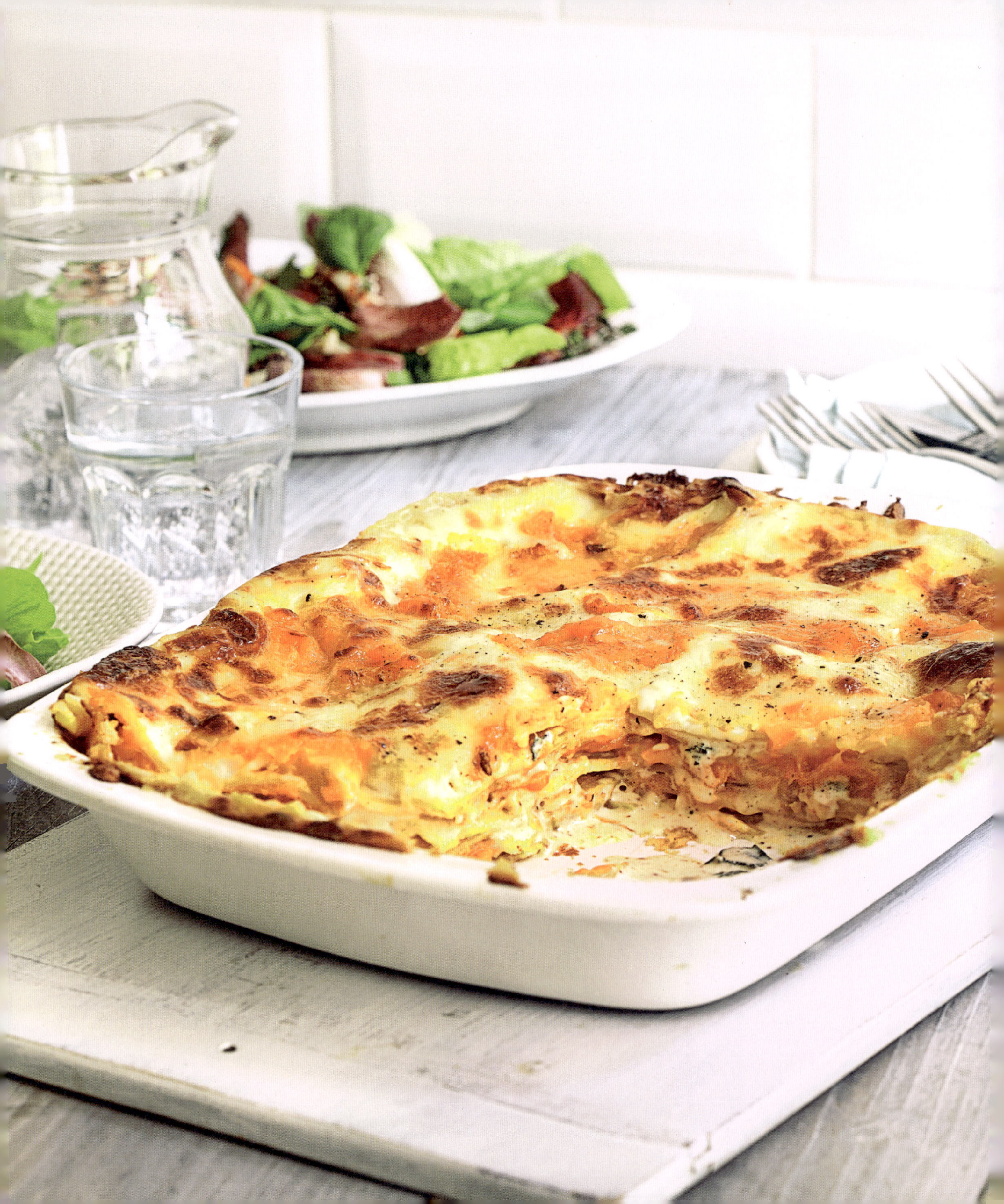

Jamie Deen's AUTUMNAL BUTTERNUT SQUASH LASAGNE

1 butternut squash, about **1.3kg (46oz)**, *peeled, deseeded and cut into 2.5cm cubes*
2 tablespoons olive oil
350ml (12fl oz) hot chicken or vegetable stock, *either bought or homemade*
100g (3½oz) unsalted butter, *plus extra for greasing*
8 fresh sage leaves, *plus extra to garnish*
100g (3½oz) plain flour
1.1 litres (37fl oz) full-fat milk
Freshly grated nutmeg
250g (9oz) no-precook lasagne sheets
170g (6oz) firm mozzarella cheese, *grated*
50g (2oz) Parmesan cheese, *finely grated*
Salt and freshly ground black pepper

Energy 506 kcal/2115 kJ
Protein 17.1g
Fat 30.4g

This makes a very generous quantity of lasagne and should serve eight. However, you can easily make up smaller lasagne and freeze until you want them. The balance of butternut squash and cheese ensures this is high in protein, calcium, beta-carotene and vitamin E. Serve with a crisp salad for extra vitamin C.

Serves 8

Preheat the oven to 200°C/gas mark 6/400°F. Line a baking tray with foil. Put the squash on the tray and drizzle with the oil. Toss well and season with salt and pepper. Roast for about 30 minutes until soft. Transfer to a food-processor with the stock and blend until smooth.

Grease a 23 x 33cm baking dish with butter. Reduce the oven temperature to 190°C/gas mark 5/375°F.

Melt 70g (2½oz) of the butter in a large saucepan over a medium heat. Twist and bruise the sage leaves to release their flavour and drop into the butter, stirring, flipping and bruising the leaves with a wooden spoon, until they are crisp but the butter is not yet brown. Using a slotted spoon, transfer the sage leaves to a plate and set aside.

Sprinkle the flour over the butter and stir over a medium heat for about 2 minutes until they are well combined and the flour has cooked a little. Slowly pour in the milk, whisking constantly. Return the sage to the sauce. Bring to the boil, whisking constantly, then reduce to a simmer and cook for 15 minutes. Stir every few minutes to make sure the sauce isn't catching on the bottom. Check for seasoning and add a little grated nutmeg.

Ladle a thin layer of the sage cream sauce into the base of the buttered dish. Lay four lasagne sheets in the pan, overlapping slightly. Add another ladleful of the sauce to cover the pasta, top with a quarter of the squash purée, then sprinkle with a quarter each of the mozzarella and Parmesan. Repeat the layering twice more, then ladle on the remaining white sauce and dollop the lasagne with the squash purée. Sprinkle with the remaining mozzarella and Parmesan and garnish with a few sage leaves. Dot the remaining 30g butter on top. Cover the lasagne tightly with foil and bake for 40 minutes. Remove the foil and bake for a further 20 minutes until golden and bubbling.

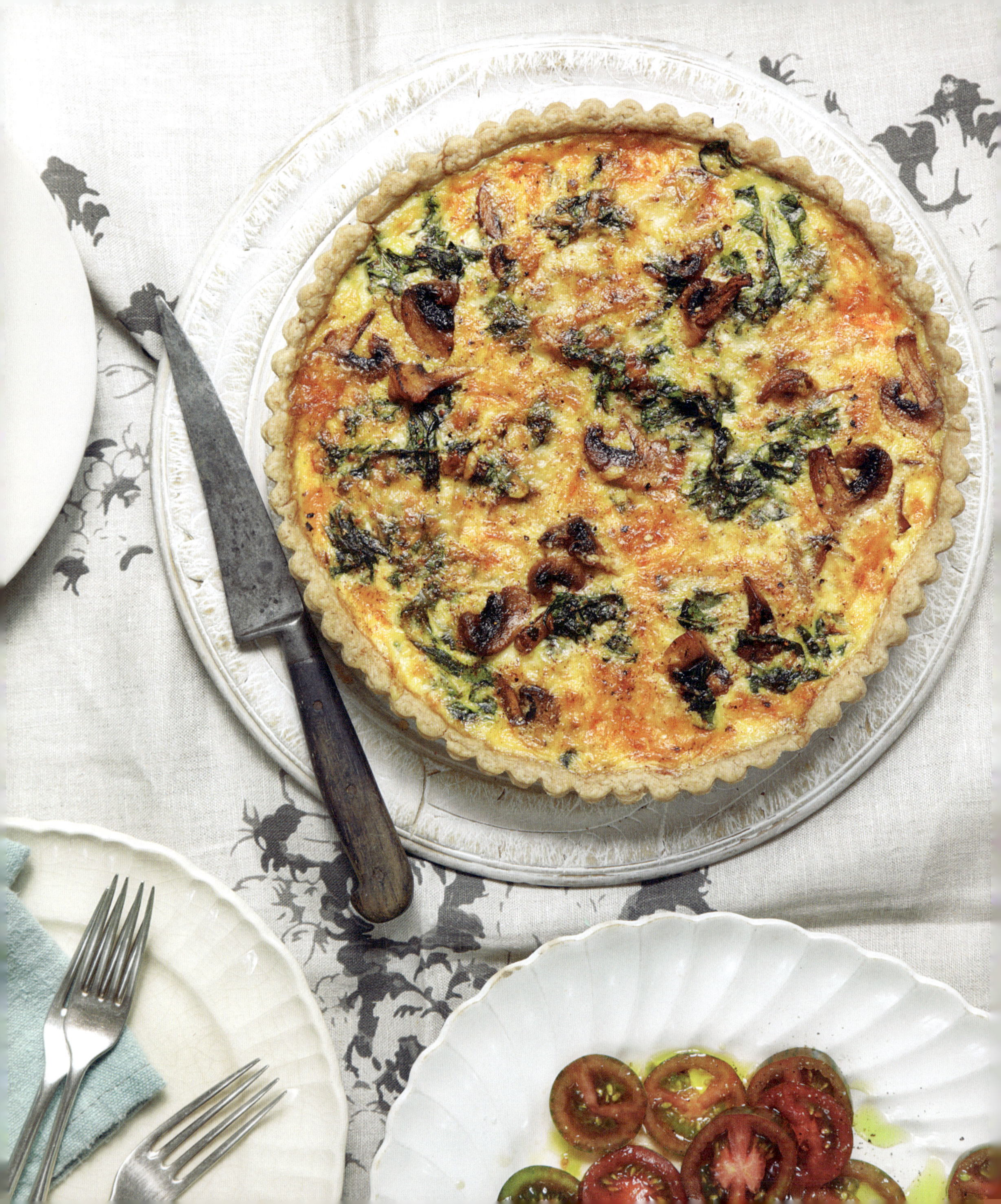

MUSHROOM AND SWISS CHARD TART

For the pastry:
225g (8oz) spelt flour
65g (2⅓oz) unsalted butter, *chilled and diced*
65g (2⅓oz) Trex or other solid vegetable fat

For the filling:
1 tablespoon olive oil
200g (7oz) mushrooms, *sliced*
200g (7oz) Swiss chard, *stems and leaves separated and shredded*
1 garlic clove, *crushed*
75g (2⅗oz) melting cheese, *such as Gruyère*
Grated nutmeg
4 free-range eggs, *beaten*
150ml (5fl oz) whole milk
150ml (5fl oz) double cream or crème fraîche
Salt and freshly ground black pepper

Energy 585 cal/2431 kJ
Protein 14.6g
Fat 45.4g
Sat. Fat 23.3g
Carbohydrate 32.0g
Fibre 2.1g

I've chosen a spelt flour pastry here, but you can use plain flour if you prefer. This makes one large tart, but it's a good one to make individually and freezing. This way you can vary the filling as much as you like. Any Mediterranean-type vegetables will be good in this, as would smoked fish, bacon or chicken. I particularly like the combination of butternut squash, asparagus and chicken. It provides a great range of nutrients such as protein, calcium, iron, beta-carotene and vitamin E.

Makes a 25cm tart or 6 individual tartlets

Preheat the oven to 200°C/gas mark 6/400°F.

To make the pastry, sift the flour into a bowl and rub in the fats. Season with salt. Add just enough cold water to bind, and stir with a knife until the pastry starts to come together. Using minimal contact, bring the dough together into a ball and knead very slightly until smooth. Wrap in clingfilm and chill for 30 minutes.

Roll out the pastry and use it to line a deep 25cm (9¾in) flan tin or six individual tartlet tins. Line the pastry with greaseproof paper and cover with baking beans. Blind bake in the oven for 15 minutes, then remove the paper and beans, and return to the oven for about 3 minutes or until the base is lightly golden. Set aside.

To make the filling, heat the olive oil in a large frying pan over a medium heat and add the mushrooms and the Swiss chard stems. Fry until softened and until any liquid from the mushrooms has evaporated. Add the garlic and chard leaves with a splash of water and cook until they have wilted down a bit and are soft enough to eat. Season with salt and pepper.

Spread the mushrooms and chard over the pastry case. Sprinkle over the cheese, then grate over a little nutmeg. In a small bowl, mix the eggs with the milk and cream. Pour this over the filling. Bake for about 30–35 minutes until just set. You want a very slight wobble to the centre.

Serve with a tomato salad if you can take tomatoes, or a green salad if you can't.

POACHED FISH IN PARSLEY SAUCE

300ml (10fl oz) milk
½ onion, *sliced*
2 cloves
1 bay leaf
½ teaspoon white peppercorns
1 blade of mace *(optional)*
1 heaped **teaspoon** cornflour
1 tablespoon crème fraîche
Large knob of unsalted butter *(optional)*
2 thick fish fillets – about **150g (5½oz)** each *(cod, haddock and pollack are all good)*
Small bunch of curly parsley, leaves only, *finely chopped*

Energy 335 kcal/1401 kJ
Protein 33.4g
Fat 12.8g
Sat. Fat 7.4g
Carbohydrate 24.0g
Fibre 0.8g

This is a classic nursery dish and might be considered quite old fashioned, but there is a reason it has endured – made properly it is sublime – delicate fish, falling softly into flakes, enveloped in the gentle aromas of the sauce. This is a very quick method: the fish cooks while the sauce is being made, rather than before, to ensure it stays tender and moist. This is an excellent dish for protein and calcium. Increase the energy by serving with a portion of soft, mashed potato.

Serves 2

Put the milk in a small saucepan, then add the onion, cloves, bay leaf, peppercorns and, if using, the mace. Bring almost to the boil, then remove from the heat and leave to infuse for a few minutes. Strain into a clean saucepan. Mix the cornflour with a little cold water and whisk it into the milk. Simmer until the sauce has thickened, then whisk in the crème fraîche and the butter, if using.

Meanwhile, bring a saucepan of water to the boil and season with salt. Lower in the fish fillets, turn the heat right down and simmer for about 5 minutes until cooked through. Remove from the saucepan and drain thoroughly. Serve with the sauce and garnish with the chopped parsley.

Optional extras: the beauty of this sauce is its mellowness, but you can add pep to it with mustard or capers, or make it sweeter with tarragon. A splash of wine, vermouth or pastis when you cook the fish wouldn't go amiss either.

Joe Woodhouse's
SAVOY CABBAGE GRATIN

The beautiful golden crust on top with crispy cabbage edges hides a creamy, cheesy, mustard-spiked sauce below. The cabbage goes wonderfully with the chestnuts and makes this a great wintertime dish. The richness is kept in check by the acidity from the mustard and this, combined with the wine, makes for a rather alpine-style eating experience. It is important with this recipe to use good-quality wine as it shines through in the finished dish; a dry or oxidative white wine is best.

Serves 4

1 Savoy cabbage (about **800g/1lb 12oz**), trimmed of any tough leaves and the dry base, cut through the stem into eight wedges
2 tablespoons olive oil
50g (1¾oz) unsalted butter
4 onions (about **600g/1lb 5oz**), roughly diced
4 garlic cloves, roughly chopped
100ml (3½fl oz) good-quality white wine or sherry
200g (7oz) crème fraîche
1 tablespoon Dijon mustard
100g (3½oz) cheese, grated (such as Gruyère or Comté)
200g (7oz) cooked chestnuts, roughly broken up
sea salt flakes and black pepper

Preheat the oven to 180°C/gas mark 4/350°F.

Place the cabbage wedges on a roasting tray, drizzle with the oil and season with salt. Roast in the oven for about 45 minutes until tender and the edges are beginning to colour.

Meanwhile, melt the butter in a medium saucepan with a lid over a medium heat. Add the onion, garlic and salt. Cook, covered, for 15–20 minutes until soft but without colour, checking occasionally and giving everything a good stir.

Add the wine or sherry and allow to bubble off, stirring, for 2 minutes.

Put the mixture in a blender and add the crème fraîche, mustard and half the cheese. Blend until smooth, check the seasoning and adjust accordingly.

Spoon some of this sauce onto a suitable dish for the gratin. Add the cabbage wedges, cut-side down, in one layer. Scatter over the chestnut pieces. Coat everything well with the rest of the sauce. Finish with the remaining cheese. Bake in the oven for 30–40 minutes until the sauce is bubbling and slightly thickened.

Heat the grill to a high heat. Grill for a final 5–10 minutes to get the top lovely and golden. Crack over black pepper and serve with a salad, to drag around in the gratin juices.

Energy 690 kcal/2886 kJ
Protein 16g
Fat 46g
Sat. Fat 26g
Carbohydrate 51.5g
Fibre 10.7g

ONE-POT ROASTED FISH WITH FENNEL AND NEW POTATOES

500g (18oz) new or salad potatoes, *halved*
1 large fennel bulb, *cut into 8 wedges*
150ml (5fl oz) white wine or water
Small bunch of parsley, *finely chopped*
Zest of **1** unwaxed lemon *(optional)*
25g (1oz) unsalted butter
4 thick fish fillets – *salmon is good*
1 tablespoon olive oil
Salt and freshly ground black pepper

Wedges of lemon, *to serve (optional)*

Energy 364 kcal/1520 kJ
Protein 22.5g
Fat 19.3g
Sat. Fat 5.7g
Carbohydrate 20.4g
Fibre 1.7g

Nutritional value for salmon. A white fish would provide a lower fat and energy content.

This dish will serve four – if you want to halve the quantities, I suggest you cook the same quantity of potatoes and fennel, then remove half before adding just two fish fillets so you have a good side dish for another day. Oily fish such as salmon is a good source of omega-3 fatty acids, and this recipe also provides a good source of vitamins D and E.

Serves 4

Preheat the oven to 200°C/gas mark 6/400°F.

Bring a large saucepan of water to the boil and add the potatoes, fennel and a pinch of salt. Return to the boil and simmer for about 5–6 minutes until starting to soften. Drain thoroughly.

Put the potatoes and fennel in a roasting dish and spread out evenly. Pour over the white wine, half the parsley and the lemon zest, if using, and give a quick stir to combine everything. Dot over the butter and season with salt and pepper. Put in the oven and bake for about 30 minutes, checking regularly to make sure nothing is catching. When the vegetables have taken on a light golden-brown colour, test with a sharp knife – they should at this point be tender. Add a splash of water if everything seems too dry.

Rub the skin side of the fish fillets with the olive oil and season. Place, skin-side up, on top of the potatoes and fennel. Bake for 10–15 minutes, depending on the thickness of your fish fillets.

Serve immediately with any buttery juices spooned over and the rest of the herbs sprinkled on top.

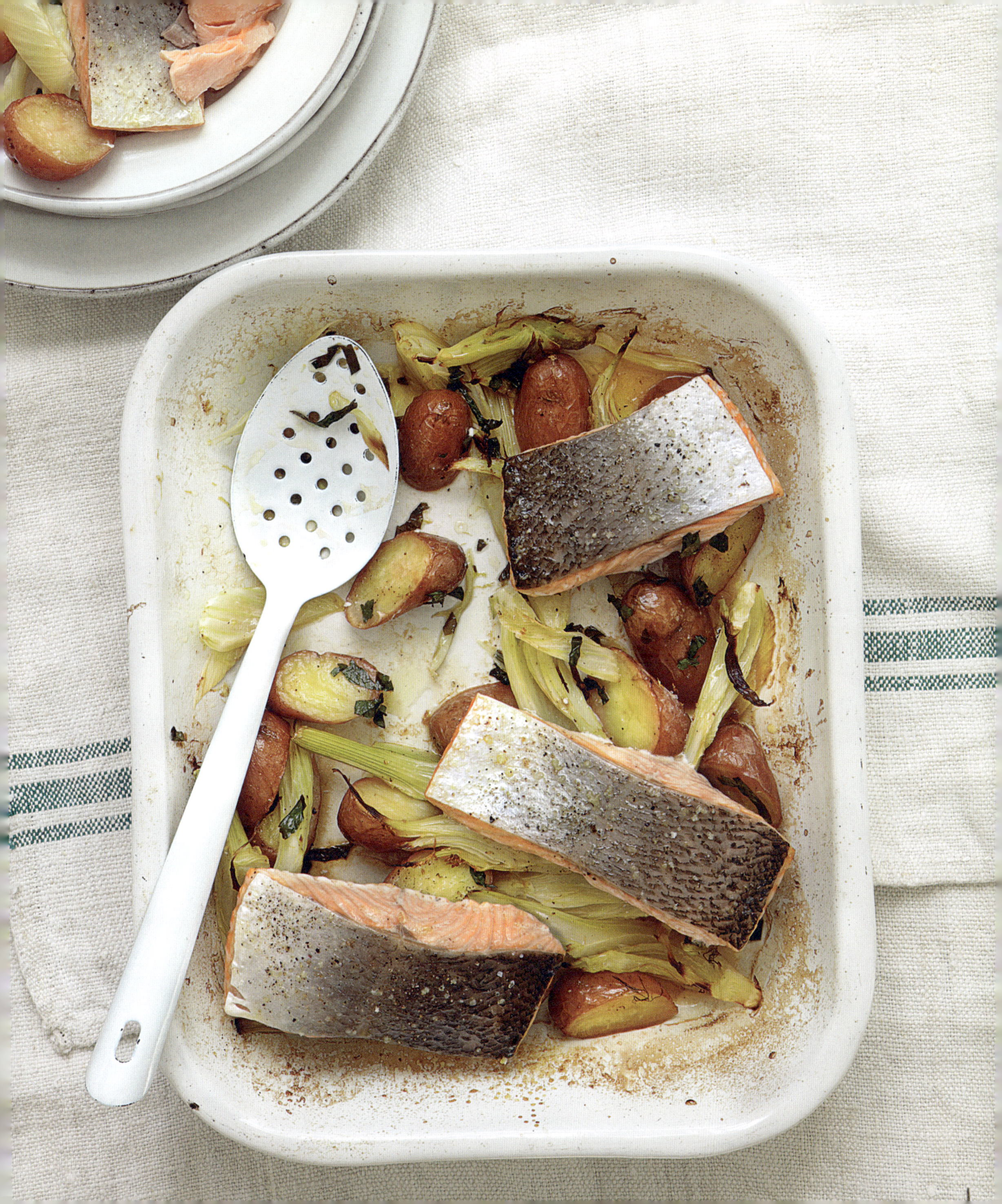

Paul Merrett's MACKEREL CHERMOULA ON A ROASTED BUTTERNUT SALAD

4 very fresh, decent-sized mackerel fillets
Olive oil, for frying

'Please don't feel you have to use mackerel if it's not your kind of fish – any would work well, but I think oily mackerel goes particularly well with the preserved lemon and paprika.' *Paul Merrett*

The oily fish and vegetables provide an excellent range of nutrients. It is particularly high in vitamin D and a good source of beta-carotene, vitamin E and niacin.

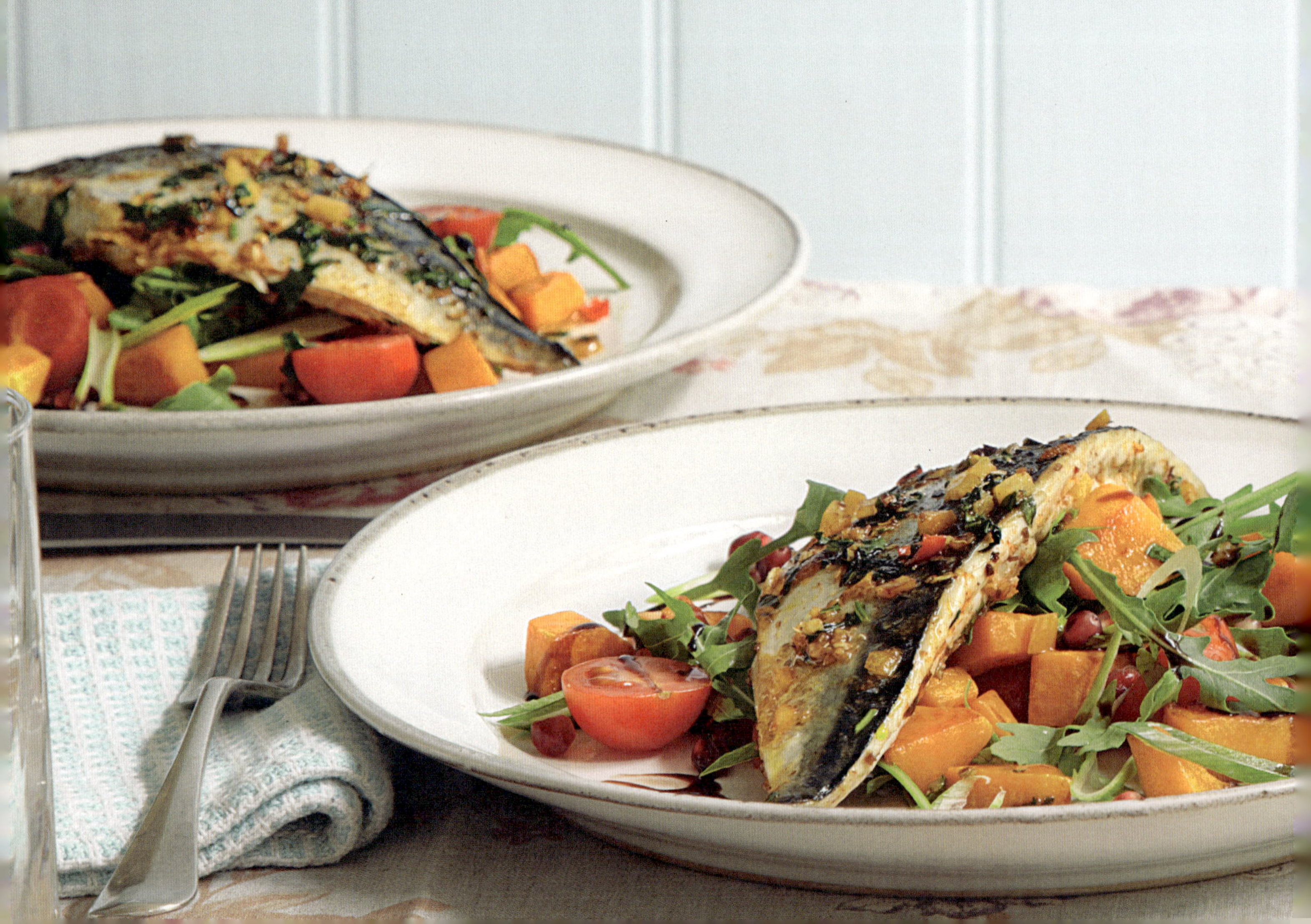

For the chermoula paste:
1 teaspoon coriander seeds
1 teaspoon cumin seeds
2 garlic cloves, *crushed to a paste*
Good pinch of saffron
2 tablespoons finely chopped flat-leaf parsley
2 tablespoons finely chopped fresh coriander
½ teaspoon salt
½ teaspoon paprika
1 small red bird's eye chilli, *very finely chopped*
2 preserved lemons, *skin only, very finely chopped*
2 tablespoons olive oil

For the salad:
2 tablespoons olive oil
½ butternut squash, *peeled and diced*
Handful of rocket leaves
8 cherry tomatoes, *cut into wedges*
4 spring onions, *finely sliced on an angle*
Seeds from **½** pomegranate
Splash of balsamic vinegar

Serves 4

To make the chermoula paste, heat a frying pan and toast the coriander seeds and cumin seeds. Leave to cool, then grind to a powder using a pestle and mortar. Tip into a bowl.

Add the garlic, saffron, chopped herbs, salt, paprika, chilli and preserved lemon. Stir well, then mix in the olive oil.

Spoon half the chermoula paste into a dish and lay the mackerel fillets on top. Spoon the remaining paste over the top to cover the fish. Leave to marinate for 15 minutes.

To make the salad, heat the oil in a frying pan over a medium-high heat, tip in the butternut and cook for 5–6 minutes until golden brown and cooked through. Transfer to a bowl and add the rocket, tomatoes and spring onions. Using a spoon, dig out the pomegranate seeds from the skin and tip into the salad. Add a splash of balsamic vinegar and arrange onto four serving plates.

When you're ready to cook the fish, heat the oil in a non-stick frying pan over a high heat. Place the mackerel fillets, skin-side down, into the pan and cook for 3–4 minutes or until the skin has coloured. Flip the mackerel over and cook for a further 3–4 minutes or until the fish is cooked through.

Towards the end of the cooking time, tip any remaining chermoula into the frying pan with the mackerel.

Place the mackerel fillets on top of the salad and serve, spooning over the chermoula from the pan.

Energy 619 kcal/2571 kJ **Protein** 43.3g **Fat** 47.2g
Sat. Fat 8.9g **Carbohydrate** 6.7g **Fibre** 2.4g

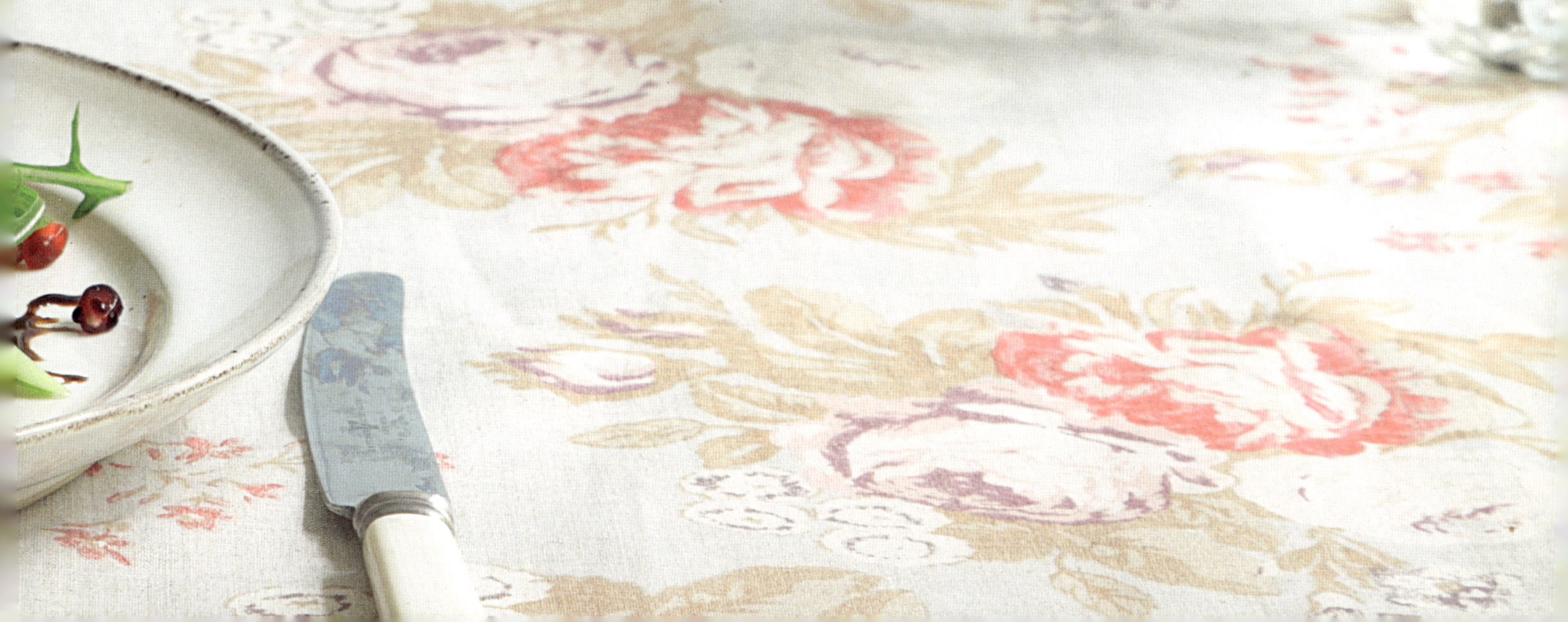

A SIMPLE FISH PIE

For the mashed potato:
1 kg (35oz) potatoes, *peeled and cut into chunks*
Large knob of unsalted butter

For the filling:
400ml (13½fl oz) milk
¼ onion, *chopped*
1 clove
1 bay leaf
1 teaspoon mustard
1 tablespoon cornflour
2 tablespoons crème fraîche
Small bunch of dill, parsley, tarragon or chives
2 teaspoons ouzo *(optional)*
400g (14oz) pack of diced fish (or equivalent firm fish)
100g (3½oz) raw prawns
2 hard-boiled eggs, *peeled and finely chopped (optional)*
2 tablespoons capers, *drained and chopped (optional)*
25g (1oz) Cheddar cheese, *grated*
Salt and freshly ground black pepper

Energy 251 kcal/1054 kJ
Protein 18.7g
Fat 7.7g
Sat. Fat 4.0g
Carbohydrate 27.9g
Fibre 2.2g

You can buy fish packs, containing a mixture of white and smoked fish. I like to add prawns as well, but, really, use any combination you like. This pie is ideal for a sore mouth or when you are too tired to tackle foods that need more chewing. Fish is a great alternative to meat and, along with the sauce, the eggs and cheese provide plenty of protein and calcium.

Serves 8

Preheat the oven to 200°C/gas mark 6/400°F.

Put the potatoes in a large saucepan, cover with water and add salt. Bring to the boil and simmer until tender, about 10 minutes. Drain thoroughly, then return to the saucepan with the butter and mash.

To make the filling, put the milk in a non-stick saucepan with the onion, clove and bay leaf, and bring to the boil. Whisk in the mustard and cornflour, and stir over a low heat until thickened. Stir in the crème fraîche and your choice of herb. Season with salt and pepper and add the ouzo, if using. Remove the onion, clove and bay leaf.

Put the fish and prawns in a pie dish and pour over the sauce. Gently turn it all over so the seafood is completely covered. Sprinkle over the eggs and capers, if using, and lightly combine with the top layer of the sauce.

Using a palette knife or similar, spread the mashed potato over the filling, making sure there are no gaps anywhere. Rough up the surface with a fork and sprinkle over the cheese. Bake the pie for about 25 minutes until the cheese has browned and everything is piping hot. Alternatively, if you want to freeze it's best to do this uncooked, so you aren't cooking the fish twice.

TIP

- This is a great recipe to portion out and freeze. You can make individual portions in ramekins, or two or more portions in foil trays.

ONE-POT CHICKEN WITH LEEKS, NEW POTATOES AND GRAPES

1 tablespoon olive oil
6 chicken thighs
500g (18oz) new potatoes, *sliced*
2 leeks, *sliced into rounds*
150ml (5fl oz) white wine (or omit and use 300ml (10fl oz) chicken stock altogether)
150ml (5fl oz) hot chicken stock
Small bunch of tarragon, *left whole*
100g (3½oz) seedless grapes
Salt and freshly ground black pepper

Energy 391 kcal/1637 kJ
Protein 23.9g
Fat 19.0g
Sat. Fat 4.8g
Carbohydrate 26.7g
Fibre 4.2g

This is a very mellow dish, especially with the addition of grapes, which is wonderful. If you want a thinner gravy, you can decant everything from the casserole and reduce the remaining liquor by boiling fiercely – you could also add a knob of butter and a tablespoon of crème fraîche or cream if you wish. This is a good protein-rich 'all-in-one' meal with plenty of vitamins and minerals, including iron, zinc and B vitamins.

Serves 4

Preheat the oven to 200°C/gas mark 6/400°F.

Heat the oil in a large casserole. Fry the chicken thighs, skin-side down, until crisp and brown. Remove from the casserole and set aside. Add the potatoes and leeks. Fry for a few minutes just to start the softening process, then pour over the white wine and stock. Season with salt and black pepper, then lay the tarragon sprigs on top.

Top with the chicken, skin-side up. Put in the oven, uncovered, and bake for about 30 minutes. Add the grapes for the last 5 minutes. Check that the vegetables are tender and the chicken is cooked through. Remove from the oven. Serve with the cooking liquor spooned over.

TIP

- This will freeze well, in individual portions.

Mindy Fox's
WARM CHICKEN AND BARLEY SALAD

1 teaspoon coarse sea salt
150g (5⅕oz) pearl barley
60ml (2fl oz) plus **3½ tablespoons** extra virgin olive oil
150g (5½oz) shiitake mushrooms, *stems discarded and caps halved, if large*
225g (8oz) button mushrooms, *stems trimmed and mushrooms halved or quartered, if large*
1 large garlic clove, *finely chopped*
225g (8oz) large shreds roast chicken
4 tablespoons finely chopped flat-leaf parsley
2 tablespoons finely chopped chives
2 tablespoons finely chopped mint
115g (4oz) rocket
1 tablespoon red wine vinegar
Salt and freshly ground black pepper

Energy 519 kcal/2168 kJ
Protein 23.6g
Fat 31.5g
Sat. Fat 4.9g
Carbohydrate 37.6g
Fibre 2.7g

'Toothsome pearl barley with fresh herbs and earthy mushrooms makes a very satisfying, healthy salad. Resist fussing with the mushrooms once they are added to the frying pan so that they brown up well, with nice crisped-up edges.' *Mindy Fox*

This is a high-energy salad with protein, iron, zinc and beta-carotene.

Serves 4

Bring 2 litres water to the boil in a large saucepan with the coarse sea salt. Remove from the heat and add the barley, then return, reduce to a low boil and cook the barley for 40–45 minutes until tender yet still firm to the bite.

About 20 minutes before the barley is ready, cook the mushrooms. Heat the 60ml (2fl oz) of oil in a large, heavy frying pan over a medium-high heat. Add about one-third of the mushrooms and stir once or twice, then cook without stirring for about 3 minutes until the mushrooms begin to brown. Push the mushrooms to the side of the pan, add another third and continue in the same manner until all the mushrooms are in the pan and nicely browned, about 10 minutes in total (if, towards the end, the first handful is browning too much, push them on top of the more newly added). Remove the pan from the heat. Add the garlic, then the chicken and toss to combine. Season with salt and pepper.

Drain the cooked barley and transfer to a large bowl; add 2 tablespoons of the remaining oil, the parsley, chives and mint. Then add the mushroom mixture and stir to combine. Season with salt and pepper.

In a second bowl, toss the rocket with the remaining oil and the vinegar. Season to taste with salt and pepper. Serve the rocket with the warm barley and mushrooms.

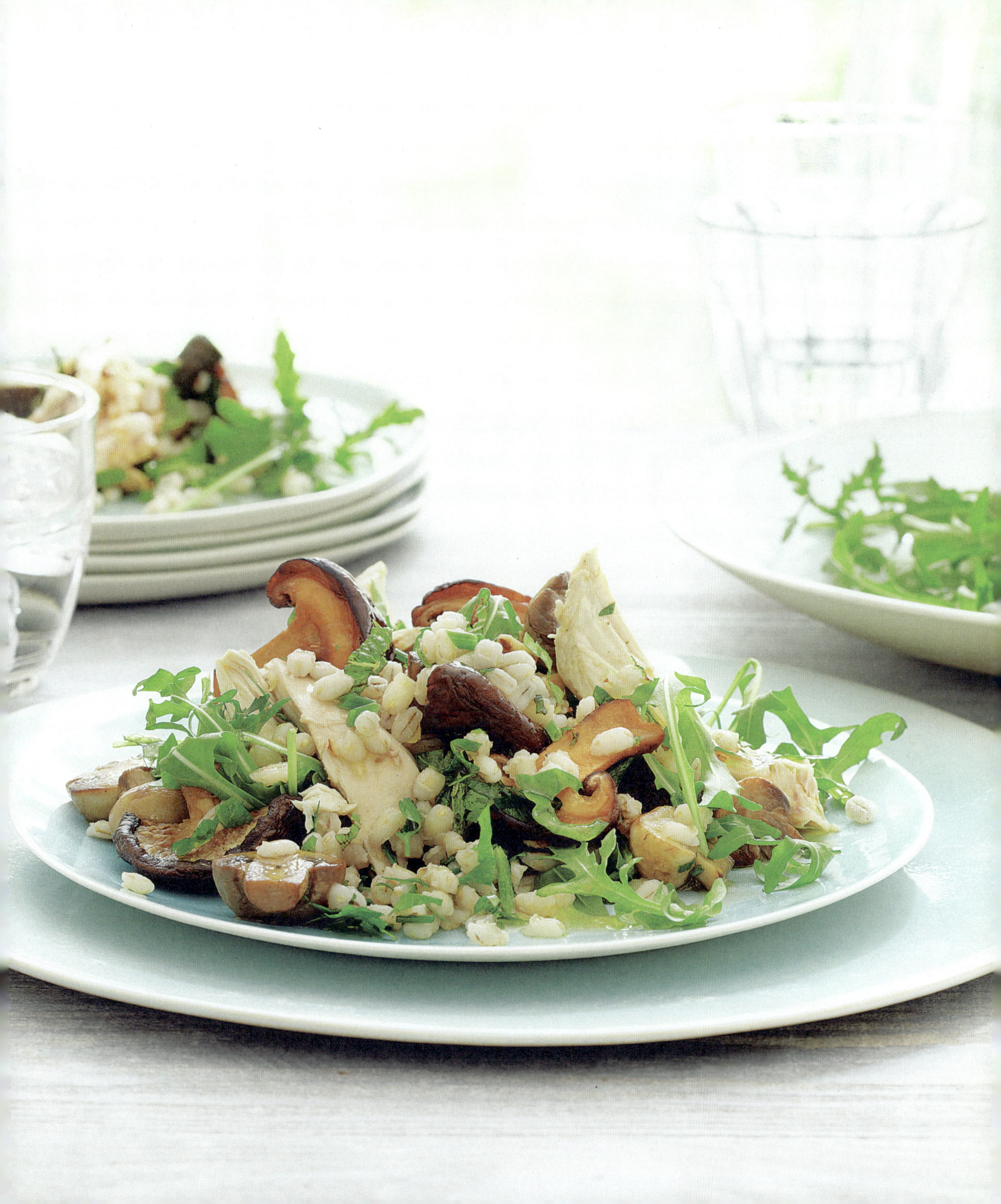

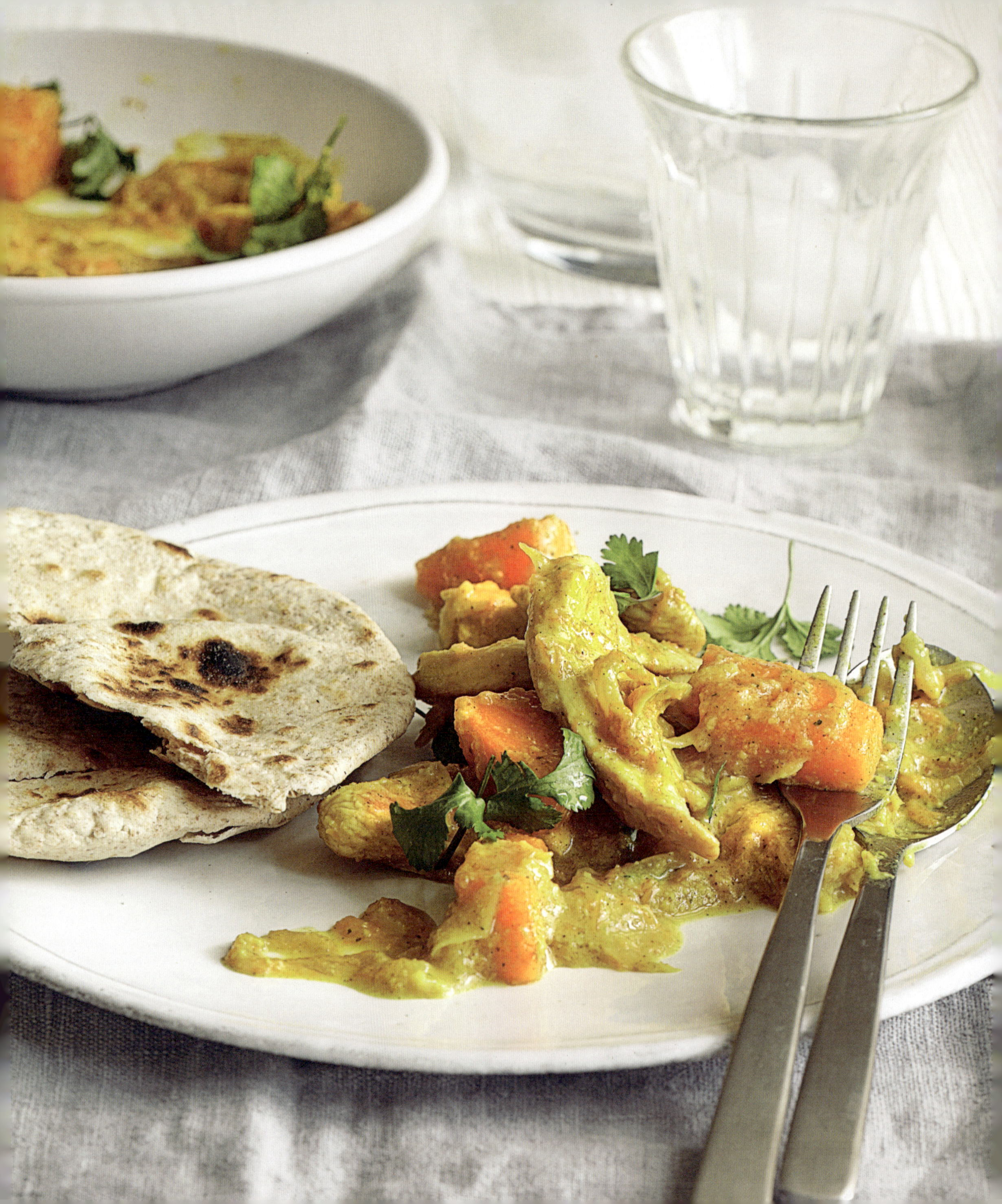

CHICKEN AND PUMPKIN CURRY

50g (2oz) unsalted butter
2 onions, *thinly sliced*
½ teaspoon ground cardamom
½ teaspoon ground fenugreek
½ teaspoon turmeric
¼ teaspoon cinnamon
2 garlic cloves, *finely chopped*
½ teaspoon finely chopped fresh ginger
50g (2oz) almonds or cashews, *ground*
200g (7oz) peeled pumpkin flesh, *cut into 3cm cubes*
4 chicken thigh fillets or **2** chicken breasts, *cut into bite-sized pieces*
225ml (7⅗fl oz) hot chicken stock or water
1 bay leaf
75g (2½oz) Greek yogurt
A few coriander leaves
Salt

Energy 318 kcal/1319 kJ
Protein 9.7g
Fat 23.8g
Sat. Fat 9.5g
Carbohydrate 9.7g
Fibre 2.3g

This is a creamy curry, with very mild, sweet spices and no chilli, so will hopefully be comfortable to eat if you have a sore mouth. If you don't, or if this is going to be eaten by more than one person, you can add a little chilli powder along with the other spices, or simply serve it with some sliced mild green chillies, which can be added at the table. You could also use a very mild curry powder or paste instead of the spices, if you wanted.

This combination of chicken, pumpkin and nuts combine to provide good sources of protein, beta-carotene and vitamin E.

Serves 4

Melt the butter in a large, heavy-based saucepan and add the onions. Cook slowly until they are soft and translucent but have not taken on any colour. Add all the spices, the garlic, ginger and ground almonds. Stir over a low heat for a couple of minutes, then add the pumpkin and chicken. Stir to coat, then pour over the stock or water. Season with salt and add the bay leaf. Cover, and simmer for about 15 minutes until the pumpkin and chicken are tender.

Add the Greek yogurt and simmer over the lowest of heat for a further 3–4 minutes. Taste for seasoning and adjust as necessary. Sprinkle over some roughly torn coriander leaves. Serve with flatbreads or some steamed rice.

TIP

- This curry will freeze, but bear in mind that both the ginger and chilli will intensify when frozen, so if you are particularly sensitive to either, be cautious when adding.

Valerie Berry's ROASTED CHICKEN WITH A SOUTH AMERICAN TWIST

'Caring and cooking for my two sisters during their cancer treatments was a real challenge. With reduced saliva, chewing and swallowing food was always a concern. In this recipe, the chicken and vegetables are basted for extra moisture and they are served with two very tasty and soothing sauces: guacamole and a caper-flavoured soured cream.' *Valerie Berry*

Serves 4

400g (14oz) onions, *cut into 8 wedges*
350g (12⅓oz) carrots, *cut into chunks*
200g (7oz) parsnips, *halved, cored and cut into chunks*
275g (9¾oz) red pepper, *cored, seeded and roughly chopped*
200g (7oz) celery, *roughly sliced*
350g (12⅓oz) butternut squash, *unpeeled, seeded, and cut into chunks*
300g (10½oz) baby potatoes
1 head of garlic, *halved, plus 5 unpeeled cloves*
100g (3½oz) pancetta, *roughly chopped*
½ teaspoon ground cinnamon
1 teaspoon cumin
Large pinch of chilli flakes
2 teaspoons dried oregano
2 tablespoons olive oil
1 large corn-fed chicken
10 cherry tomatoes
500ml (17fl oz) good-quality hot chicken stock, *kept warm on the hob*
3 avocados
1 lemon
Small handful of chopped coriander
300ml (10fl oz) soured cream
100g (3½oz) salted capers, *rinsed and soaked for 30 minutes*

Preheat the oven to 190°C/gas mark 5/375°F. Place the onions, carrots, parsnips, pepper, celery, squash, potatoes, the 5 garlic cloves and the pancetta in a large roasting tin. Season with the spices and oregano. Drizzle with 2 tablespoons of olive oil and toss well.

Tuck the halved garlic head inside the chicken and season well. Place the chicken on the vegetables, breast down (a trick that keeps the breast meat juicy) and roast for 45 minutes. After this time, turn the chicken over using two flat spatulas. Add the cherry tomatoes to the vegetables and roast for a further 45 minutes, basting the chicken with warm stock every 15 minutes and making sure the vegetables are roasting nicely without burning. Add a little stock if they are too dry. Check that the chicken is cooked by piercing the thickest part of a thigh: the juices should run clear. If they are still pinkish, cook for 10–15 minutes longer.

Remove the chicken from the oven, cover tightly with baking parchment and foil, and let it rest for 10 minutes before carving.

Drain the juices from the roasting tin into a saucepan and return the roasting tin with the vegetables to the oven. Skim the fat off the surface then taste the juices. Reduce over a high heat to concentrate the flavours if needed, then pour the juices back over the vegetables, toss and turn off the oven.

Carve the chicken and put back in the roasting tin on top of the vegetables. Keep warm in the turned-off oven.

Energy 816 kcal/3398 kJ
Protein 45g
Fat 54g
Sat. Fat 17.6g
Carbohydrate 38.7g
Fibre 13.6g

Halve and stone the avocados. Spoon the flesh into a bowl. Add the lemon juice and chopped coriander and mash with a fork until smooth. Adjust the seasoning. Pour the soured cream into a bowl and top with the capers.

Serve the chicken and vegetables with generous spoonfuls of guacamole and caper-flavoured soured cream. Steamed spring greens are a good complement.

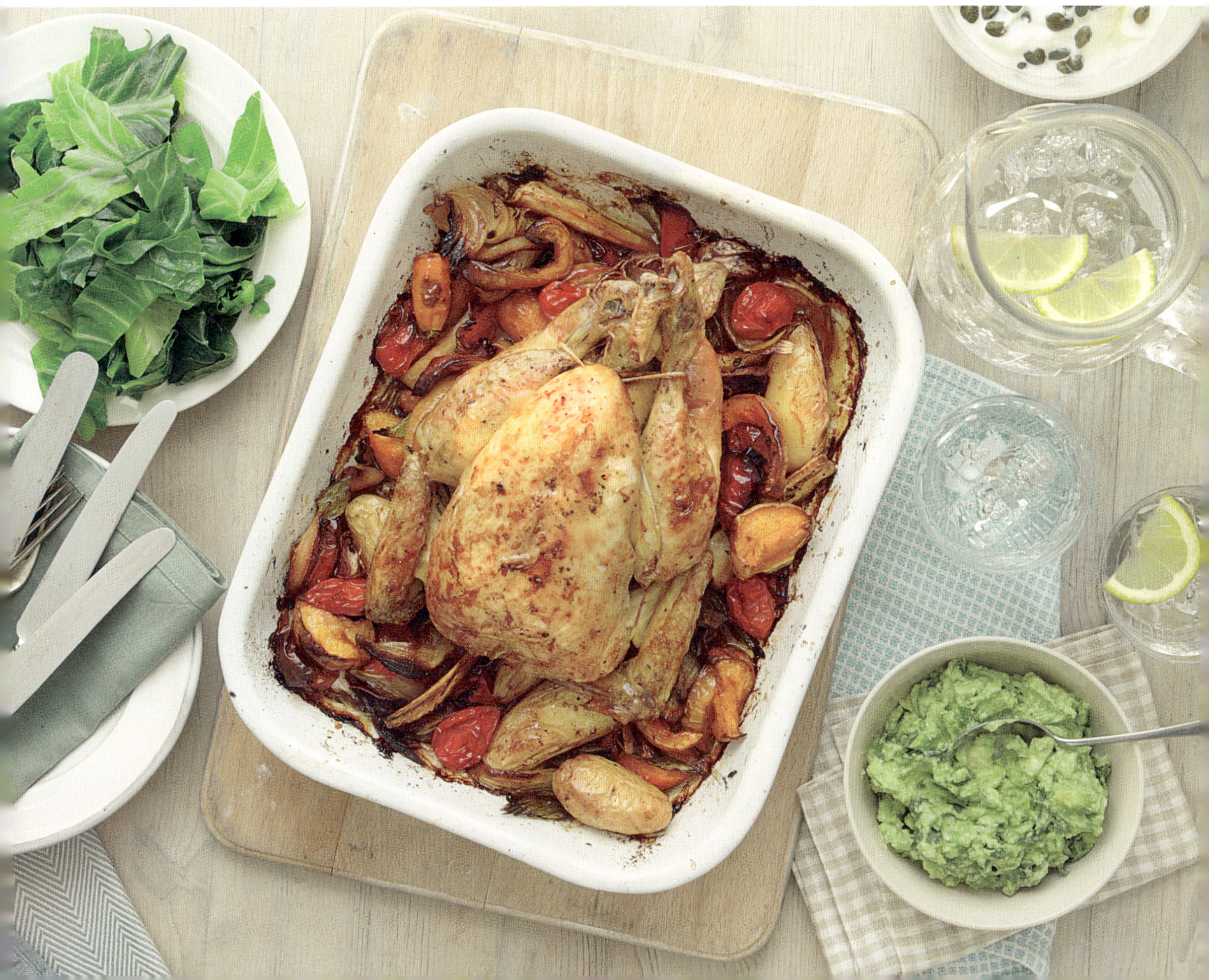

David Tanis'
HAM AND CHEESE BREAD PUDDING

'This is like a quiche but easier. Adding briefly cooked spinach or chard makes a lovely green version, or you can sprinkle in a handful of freshly chopped herbs with the spring onions.' *David Tanis*

Butter, *softened, for spreading*
½ day-old French baguette, *cut on the diagonal into 5mm slices*
50g (2oz) good-quality smoked ham, *diced*
75g (2⅗oz) Gruyère cheese, *grated*
200g (7oz) spinach or chard, *well washed, blanched and drained*
2 large free-range eggs
100ml (3½fl oz) single cream
150ml (5fl oz) milk
½ teaspoon salt
Freshly ground black pepper, to taste
Grated nutmeg
3 spring onions, *finely slivered*

Serves 4

Preheat the oven to 180°C/gas mark 4/350°F. Lightly butter a shallow 1-litre baking dish.

Lightly butter the baguette slices. Line the baking dish with half the baguette slices, butter-side down. Arrange the ham, half the cheese and the spinach or chard over the bread. Top with the remaining baguette slices, butter-side up, and sprinkle with the remaining cheese.

Beat together the eggs, cream and milk, adding the salt and pepper to taste.

Grate in a little nutmeg, add the spring onions, and beat again. Pour the egg mixture into the baking dish, pushing down to submerge the bread, if necessary. Bake for about 45 minutes, until the custard is set but still a bit jiggly and the top is nicely browned.

Energy 432 kcal/1808 kJ
Protein 21.0g
Fat 22.6g
Sat. Fat 12.0g
Carbohydrate 38.9g
Fibre 3.6g

TIP

- This is a good all-rounder providing protein, calcium, iron, beta-carotene and vitamin E. Serve with tomatoes or red peppers roasted with basil and olive oil for extra vitamins.

Royal Marsden's NUT ROAST

1 small onion
60g (2oz) leeks (½ small leek)
220g (8oz) carrots
40g (1½oz) ground almonds
40g (1½oz) mixed nuts, chopped
6g (⅕oz) garlic puree
2 teaspoons olive oil
1 teaspoon flat-leaf parsley, chopped
1 tablespoon marmite
150–200g (5–7oz) breadcrumbs
salt and pepper

Nutritional information
Energy 390 kcal/1628 kJ
Protein 11.2g
Fat 19g
Sat. Fat 2.5g
Carbohydrate 69g
Fibre 14.3g

This is a firm favourite for vegetarians. Serve with traditional roast potatoes, vegetables and onion gravy or prepare a tray of vegetables such as red onions, peppers, baby new potatoes and butternut squash to cook alongside the nut roast.

Serves 3–4

Preheat the oven to 180°C/gas mark 4/350°F.

Finely dice the onions and leeks, grate carrots and make the bread into breadcrumbs by grating, or in a food processor (can also buy ready made – but better to use fresh, not dehydrated ones!).

Lightly grease a bread tin or suitable container (will depend on the recipe volume).

Heat half the oil in a saucepan and sweat off the onions and leeks until soft. Then add in the nuts, breadcrumbs, herbs, marmite, grated carrots. Season with salt and pepper to taste. It should be a soft, paste like consistency – if it is too wet add more breadcrumbs and if it is too dry add a little water.

Take off the heat and press into the prepared tin and place in a preheated oven and cook for about 50 minutes.

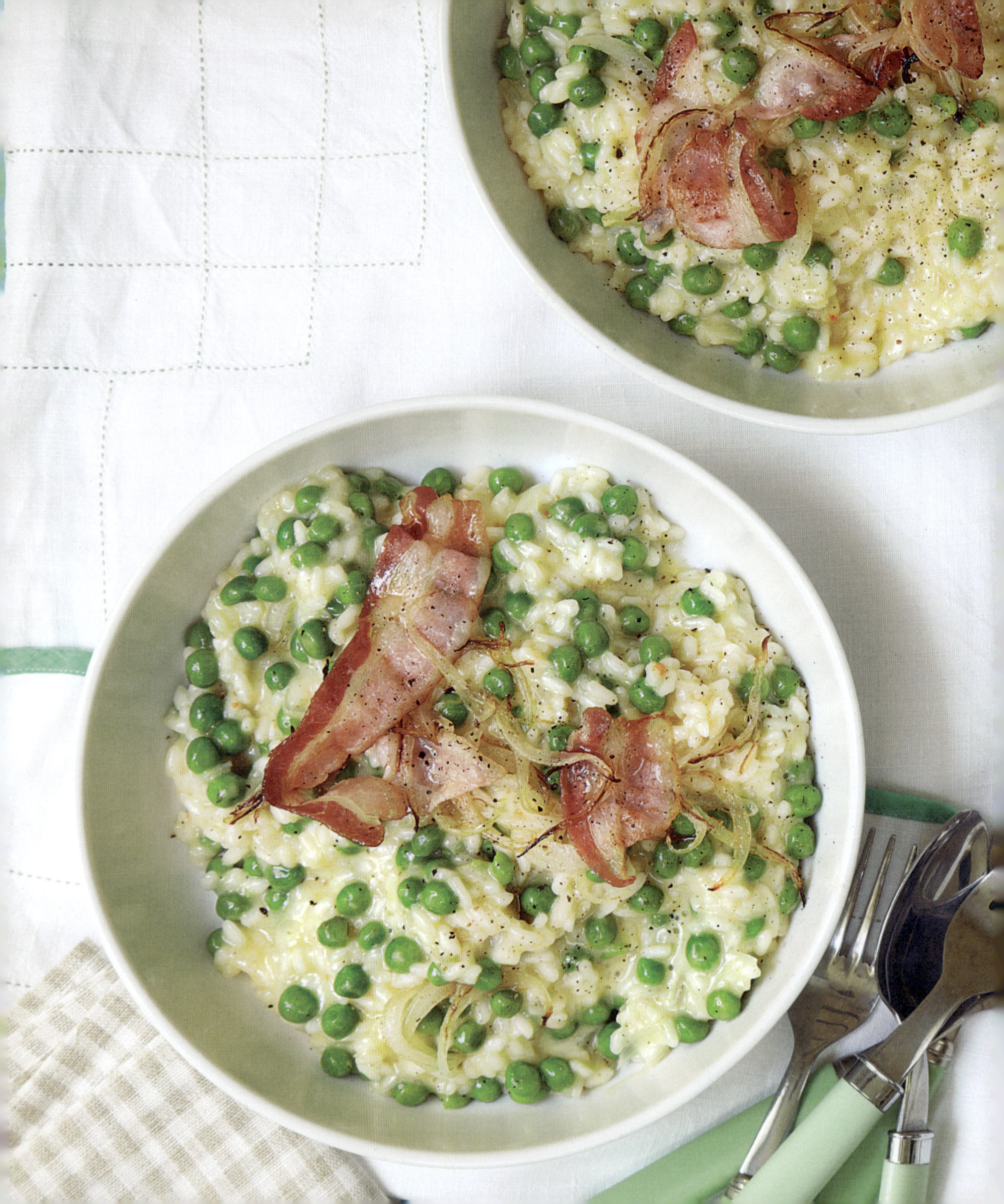

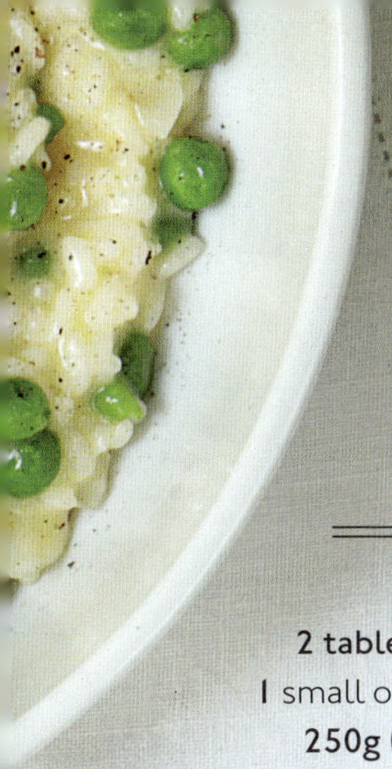

Angela Harnett's PEA AND PANCETTA RISOTTO

'I first used this pancetta garnish to enliven a pasta dish and then found it worked equally well as a finishing touch on risotto.' *Angela Harnett*

Serves 4

2 tablespoons olive oil
1 small onion, *finely chopped*
250g (9oz) risotto rice
200ml (7fl oz) white wine
800ml (27fl oz) (approx.) hot vegetable stock
400g (14oz) frozen peas
50–75g (2–2¾oz) cold unsalted butter, *diced*
50g (2oz) Parmesan cheese, *freshly grated, plus extra to serve*
Salt and freshly ground black pepper

For the garnish:
2 tablespoons oil
200g (7oz) pancetta, *chopped*
1 onion, *chopped*

Energy 569 kcal/2359 kJ
Protein 23.9g
Fat 37.6g
Sat. Fat 15.5g
Carbohydrate 27.7g
Fibre 8.9g

Heat the oil in a large pan over a medium heat. Add the onion and cook, stirring, until soft and translucent. Stir in the rice and cook for a further 2 minutes. Turn up the heat and add the wine – it should sizzle as it hits the pan. Cook for about 2 minutes to evaporate the alcohol.

Once the liquid has reduced, begin adding the hot stock, a ladleful at a time, over a medium heat, allowing each addition to be absorbed before adding the next, and stirring continuously. The rice should always be moist but not swimming in liquid. The process of adding and stirring should take about 18 minutes. Add the peas towards the end of the cooking time so that they warm through.

Meanwhile, make the garnish. Heat the olive oil in a separate pan and sauté the pancetta. Remove the pancetta from the pan. Add the onion and cook until a light golden brown. Mix it in the pancetta.

When the risotto is ready, remove from the heat and stir in the diced butter. Finish with the Parmesan, then season well and serve topped with the onion and pancetta mixture.

Grate over some extra Parmesan, if you like.

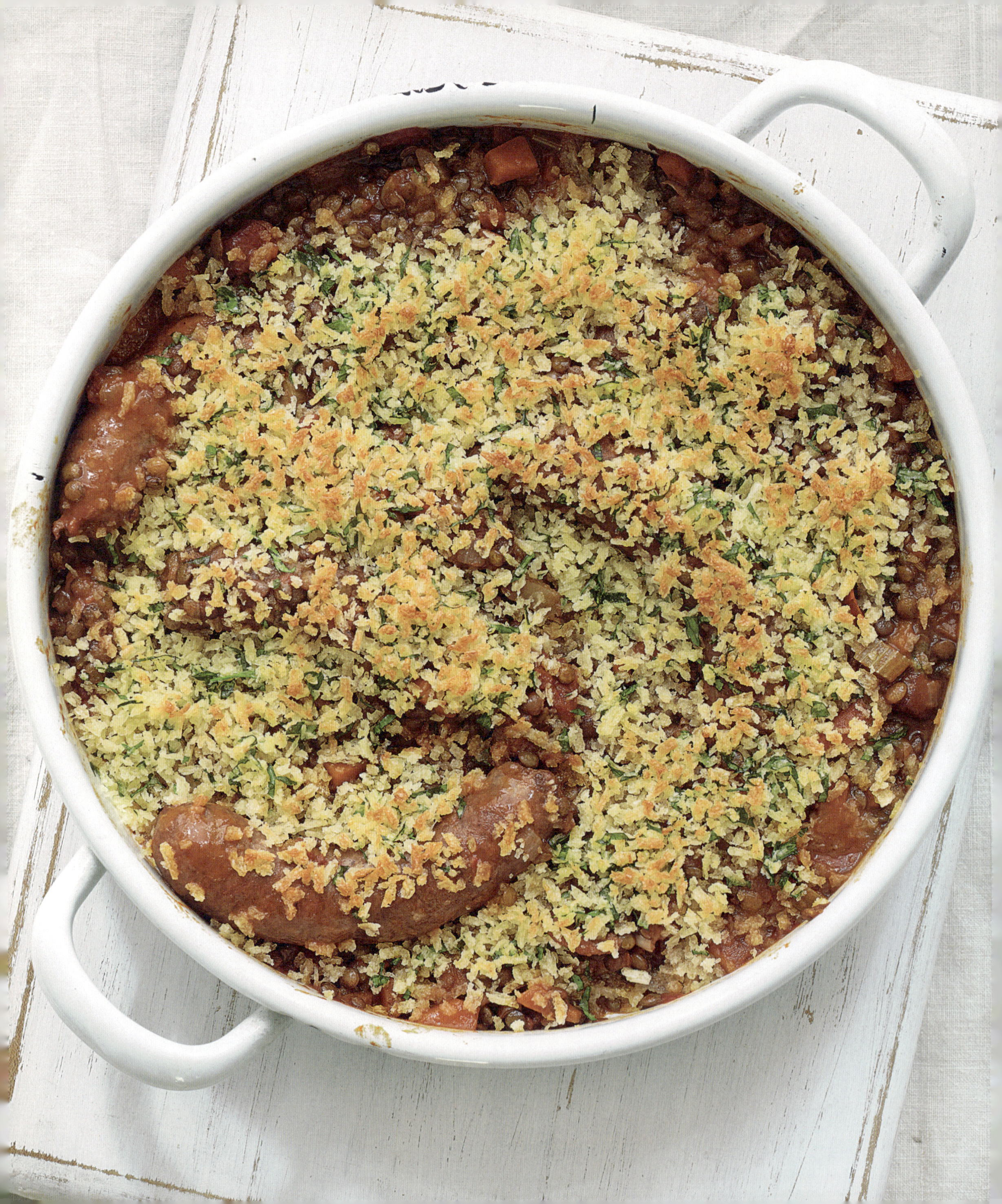

SAUSAGE AND PUY LENTIL CASSEROLE

This makes a nice change from sausage and mash, with the added benefit that it freezes brilliantly if you make it to the stage before you add the crust. The fennel seeds and tarragon add a bit of soothing sweetness here. The crust isn't essential, but will add a bit more texture to the final dish. If your appetite is small, start with a small portion of one sausage with the delicious sauce and crust. It is a very nutritious dish containing good amounts of protein, iron, zinc, B and E vitamins and beta-carotene. If you have a larger appetite, then serve with a baked sweet potato or potato, for some starchy carbohydrate.

Serves 4

1 teaspoon vegetable oil
8 sausages
100g (3½oz) smoked good-quality bacon lardons
1 onion, *finely diced*
1 carrot, *finely diced*
1 stick of celery, *finely diced*
2 garlic cloves, *finely chopped*
1 teaspoon fennel seeds
1 tarragon sprig
1 thyme sprig
200g (7oz) uncooked Puy, brown or green lentils
400g (4oz) can of chopped tomatoes
650ml (22fl oz) hot stock (chicken or vegetable)
Pinch of sugar

For the crust (optional):
50g (2oz) breadcrumbs
25g (¾oz) Parmesan cheese, *finely grated*
2 tablespoons chopped fresh flat-leaf parsley
25g (¾oz) unsalted butter, *melted*

Flat-leaf parsley leaves, *chopped or torn, to serve*

Heat the vegetable oil in a large casserole. Brown the sausages on all sides, then remove from the casserole. Add the bacon and fry until it is crisp and brown and the fat is starting to render out.

Turn down the heat and add the vegetables and garlic. Cook for about 5 minutes until starting to soften and brown around the edges. Add the fennel seeds, tarragon, thyme and lentils to the pan, then pour over the tomatoes, stock and sugar and let it bubble for a few minutes. Return the sausages to the casserole. You can cut them into chunks if you prefer.

Bring the casserole to the boil and leave for 5 minutes to get the lentils started, then turn down the heat to a gentle simmer, cover and cook for about 45 minutes, stirring regularly to make sure nothing catches on the bottom of the pan. Add more liquid if you feel it's getting too dry.

To make the crust, preheat the grill to high. Mix the breadcrumbs, Parmesan and parsley with the melted butter, and sprinkle this mixture over the lentils. Put under the grill until golden brown and bubbling.

Serve with a sprinkling of parsley.

TIP

- This is an excellent dish for batch cooking, as it will freeze very well in any number of portion sizes.

Energy 769 kcal/3212 kJ
Protein 38.6g
Fat 42.5g
Sat. Fat 17.1g
Carbohydrate 55.7g
Fibre 11.5g

Jeremy Lee's
WARM SALAD OF PORK BELLY, FENNEL AND HERBS

2 onions, *peeled and roughly chopped*
3 fennel bulbs, *chopped*
1 lemon, *sliced*
4 garlic cloves
1.5kg (52oz) pork belly, *in one piece*
1 tablespoon fennel seeds, *ground*
½ teaspoon black peppercorns, *ground*
6 tablespoons olive oil
6 tablespoons white wine (or chicken stock)

Couple of handfuls of boiled, peeled potatoes
A few bunches of watercress or a lovely green leaf

Energy 475 kcal/1973 kcal
Protein 29.8g
Fat 37.3g
Sat. Fat 11.9g
Carbohydrate 4.8g
Fibre 1.0g

'This dish is very fast in the preparation, long and very slow in the cooking, but don't worry – you can leave it in the oven all day if you like, or even overnight. It will also reheat beautifully. A thought: there is a happy moment when you can add lovely things that may suggest themselves from the garden, like herbs and any rogue vegetables such as beetroots, carrots, beans, mint and/or parsley.' *Jeremy Lee*

As this makes such a large quantity, it is a great dish for a family gathering or when friends come over. This is a wholesome recipe packed with protein, iron, zinc and B vitamins.

Serves 10

Preheat the oven to 240°C/gas mark 9/460°F.

Lay the onions, fennel, lemon and garlic in a roasting tin big enough to hold the piece of belly pork.

Score the skin of the belly. Mix the ground fennel and black peppercorns together, and rub into the skin of the belly pork. Sit the pork, skin-side up, on the vegetables. Pour over the olive oil and wine. Bake in the oven for 10 minutes or so until it darkens and the crackling begins to form. Cover the tray with tinfoil securely and lower the heat to about 120°C/gas mark ½/250°F and let cook gently. This can be overnight in an even gentler oven or for a minimum of 8 hours.

Come the time to serve, place the pork on a board and cut into coarse pieces. Decant the vegetables from the roasting tray onto a handsome dish. Strew the leaves around and then the potatoes, then tumble the pork over this, together with any crackling that may still be on the board. Spoon over any residual juices.

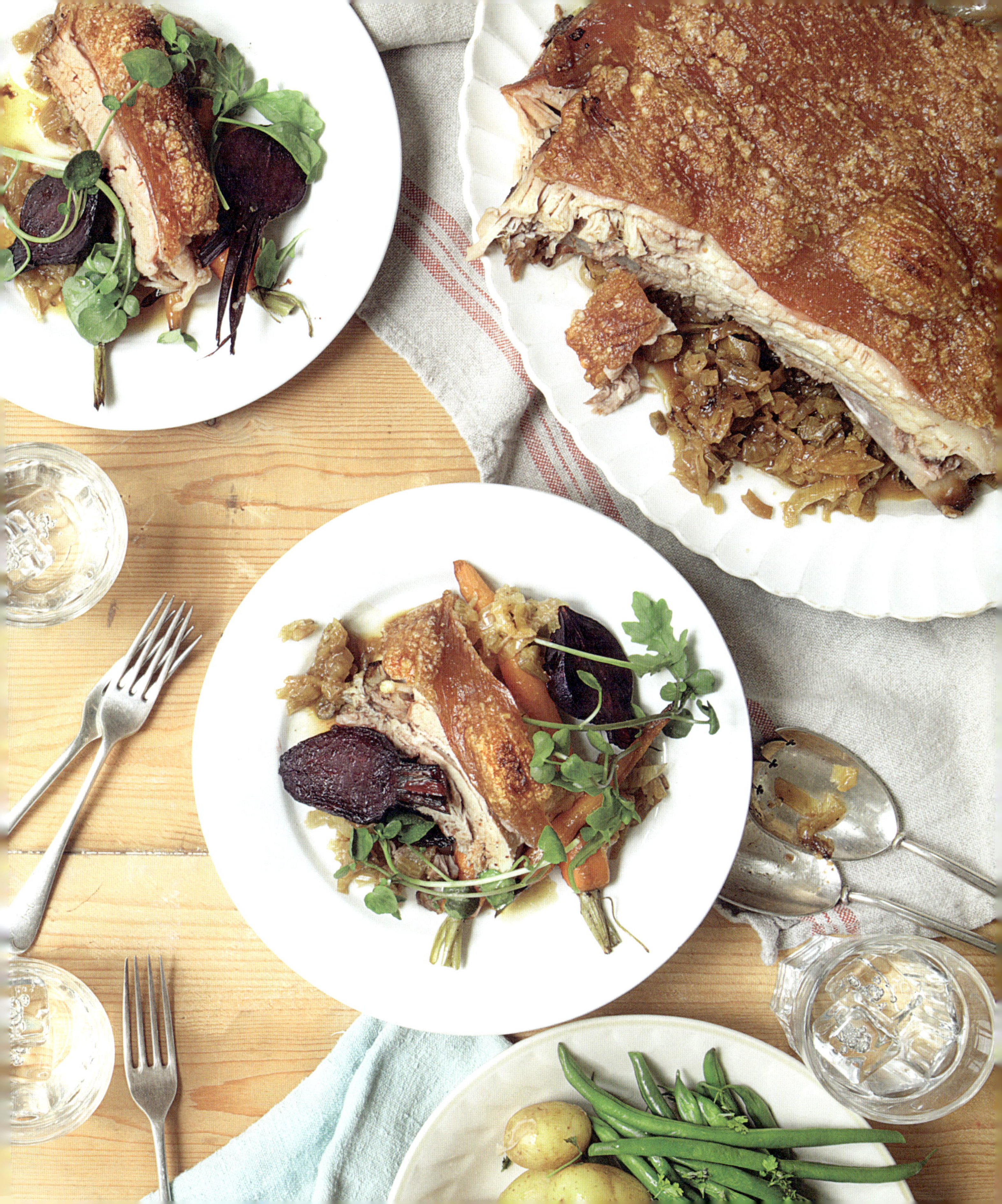

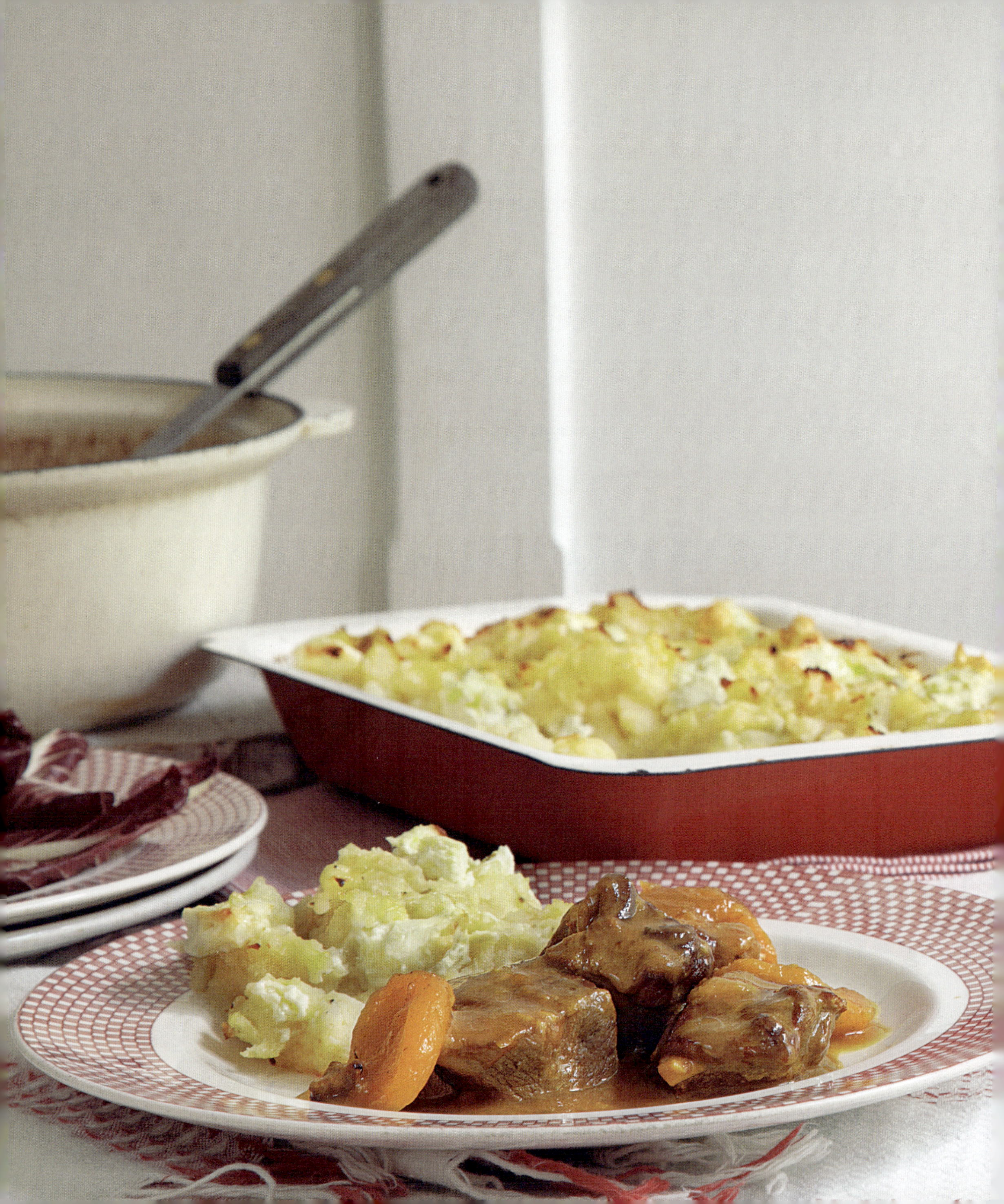

BRAISED LAMB

with Celeriac and Feta Bake

1kg (35oz) lamb neck fillet or shoulder, *cut into 5cm chunks*
2 tablespoons olive oil
1 large onion, *sliced into crescents*
4 garlic cloves, finely chopped
300ml (10fl oz) white wine *(optional – you can increase the amount of stock to 600ml or replace with water or apple juice)*
300ml (10fl oz) hot lamb or chicken stock
Pinch of saffron, *soaked in a little warm water*
¼ teaspoon ground cinnamon
1 teaspoon unwaxed lemon zest
2 large rosemary sprigs
100g (3½oz) dried apricots, *sliced crossways so still circular*
Handful of flat-leaf parsley
Salt and freshly ground black pepper

For the celeriac and feta bake:
1 large floury potato, *peeled and cut into chunks*
1 celeriac, *peeled and cut into chunks*
A few garlic cloves, *unpeeled*
Large knob of unsalted butter
1 tablespoon crème fraîche
100g (3½oz) feta cheese, *diced*

Energy 560 kcal/2332 kJ
Protein 38.3g
Fat 33.4g
Sat. Fat 15.1g
Carbohydrate 19.8g
Fibre 5.2g

This is a wonderful combination – Greek-style lamb with rich, creamy mash. Feta often has an astringency when raw, which can be unpleasant, especially when you have a sore mouth, but baking it with the celeriac mellows the flavour and takes away that harsh edge. I've kept tomatoes out of the braise, but you could add a tablespoon of tomato purée at the same time as the stock if you want. This meal is ideal for those trying to gain weight. It also has plenty of nutrients, including protein, iron, zinc and B vitamins, and a high energy content.

Serves 6 (or freeze half)

Season the lamb with salt and pepper. Heat the oil in a large casserole. Add the onion and cook for several minutes until softened. Add the garlic and fry for a further minute. Push the onion and garlic to the side and turn up the heat slightly. Add the lamb and brown on all sides. Pour over the white wine. Let it bubble fiercely and keep stirring to deglaze the base of the casserole. Add the stock, saffron and its soaking water, cinnamon, lemon zest, rosemary and apricots. Bring to the boil, then turn down the heat to a low simmer and cover. Simmer for about 1 hour or until the lamb is tender. Take the lid off the casserole and simmer for a further 15–20 minutes until the sauce has reduced a little and has a syrupy consistency.

For the celeriac and feta bake, preheat the oven to 200°C/gas mark 6/400°F. Put the potato, celeriac and garlic into a saucepan and cover with cold water. Bring to the boil, cover, then simmer until the potato and celeriac are tender – about 10 minutes. Drain the potato and celeriac into a colander, then transfer back to the saucepan. Remove the garlic cloves and squeeze out the flesh. Add this to the potato and celeriac, then season with salt and pepper. Add the butter and crème fraîche, and mash until smooth. Grease a shallow baking dish. Pile the mash into it, then take cubes of the feta and press them at intervals into the mash. Cover the cubes slightly with the mash, then dot butter all over. Bake for about 30 minutes until the bake is browning on top and the feta has softened. Serve the lamb and bake side by side.

TIP

- Both elements of this dish can be frozen, either separately or together. If making up complete meals, try to put the purée in one half of a foil container and the lamb in the other half, rather than on top of one another – that way, you can still bake it in the oven and get some browning on the purée.

Tim Hayward's BEEF COBBLER

For the stew:
1 tablespoon plain flour
500g (18oz) stewing beef, *cut into chunks*
2 tablespoons olive oil
2 onions, *finely chopped*
1 large carrot, *finely chopped*
1 stick of celery, *finely chopped*
1 leek, *finely chopped*
½ can stout or equivalent in red wine (about **250ml/8½fl oz**) *(optional, can instead use 500ml/17fl oz stock)*
250ml hot chicken stock
Pinch of dried thyme leaves or **1 teaspoon** of fresh
½ teaspoon smoked paprika
½ teaspoon balsamic vinegar
½ teaspoon mushroom ketchup
Salt and freshly ground black pepper

For the cobbler topping:
250g (9oz) self-raising flour
50g (2oz) cold unsalted butter
15g (½oz) horseradish sauce *(optional)*
150g (5⅓oz) whole milk

Energy 647 kcal/2715 kJ
Protein 38.0g
Fat 23.6g
Sat. Fat 10.3g
Carbohydrate 64.1g
Fibre 6.6g

'This is my go-to dish whenever I'm in need of steadying or calming. It makes good use of cheap stewing beef – ask your butcher for something with plenty of interesting texture to it – and I use a slightly odd technique to balance the flavours, though you can season just with pepper and salt if you prefer.' *Tim Hayward*

This dish is ideal if you are finding the taste of meat has changed during treatment and is an excellent source of all the nutrients that meat provides – protein, iron, zinc, B vitamins and with beta-carotene from the carrot.

Serves 4 (generous portions)

Put the plain flour in a polythene bag with some salt and pepper and add the beef. Give it a good shake until the beef is well coated. Heat 1 tablespoon of the olive oil in a large casserole. Brown the meat on all sides until it has developed a good brown crust. Don't crowd the pan as the meat will start to boil, rather than brown – you may have to do this in more than one batch. Remove the beef from the casserole and scrape up any brown bits that might be clinging to the base.

Heat the rest of the olive oil in the casserole. Add all the vegetables and cook over a low heat until softening around the edges and caramelising slightly. Turn up the heat and pour in the beer or red wine. This should bubble up fiercely and give off lovely smells. Keep it bubbling until it has almost completely boiled away, then add the stock. Once the liquid has come up to a gentle simmer, return the meat to the pan. Add the thyme. Cover, and simmer the casserole gently for about 1 hour until the meat is tender.

Preheat the oven to 200°C/gas mark 6/400°F. For the cobbler topping, combine the flour and butter in a bowl. Season with salt, then rub in until you have a mixture resembling fine breadcrumbs. Add the horseradish sauce if you fancy it. Add the milk gradually until you have a dough. Split the dough into four balls, then flatten them down to give a rough scone shape.

Taste the casserole gravy. Smoked paprika will add a bassy flavour, not really identifiable as smoke if you're sparing with it; the balsamic adds a hint of sharpness and perks everything up; mushroom ketchup adds woody depth. Use these three entirely according to how you want to flavour the gravy.

Drop the cobbler pieces on top of the casserole and allow to half sink. Put in the oven for 20 minutes until fluffy and well browned on top.

KEEMA PEAS

1 tablespoon olive oil
Knob of unsalted butter
1 onion, *finely chopped*
2 garlic cloves, *finely chopped*
2cm piece fresh ginger, *grated*
2 tablespoons finely chopped coriander stems
750g minced lamb
1 large or **2** smaller waxy or new potatoes, *peeled and diced*
½ teaspoon turmeric
1 cinnamon stick
2 cloves
4 green cardamom pods
1 teaspoon cumin seeds
1 teaspoon coriander seeds
1 teaspoon black peppercorns
1 bay leaf
300ml hot chicken stock
400g fresh or frozen peas
1 tablespoon tomato purée *(optional)*
Salt and freshly ground black pepper

To serve:
Handful of coriander leaves
2 mild green chillies, *finely sliced* *(optional)*
Greek yogurt

I've upped the quantities of this a bit, as it's such a useful dish to make a lot of; it freezes brilliantly, is very easy to eat and it's also one children will love because of its sweet, aromatic flavour. Don't be put off by the long list of spices – all you have to do with them is pop them in a little square of muslin. Or you can just use a favourite mild curry powder instead. It has a good balance of nutrients with plenty of protein, iron, zinc, B vitamins and some beta-carotene. This is best eaten with soft, fluffy flatbreads.

Serves 6

Heat the oil and butter in a large casserole or saucepan. Add the onion and cook until soft – about 5 minutes. Add the garlic, ginger, coriander stems and lamb. Cook until the lamb is well browned, then add the potato and turmeric. Cook for a further 2 minutes.

Put all the whole spices and bay leaf into a little square of muslin and tie into a bundle (think Dick Whittington). Bash the spices about a bit with a rolling pin or similar, just to help release their flavours. Add this to the casserole.

Pour over the chicken stock and season with salt and pepper. Add the peas and the tomato purée, if using. Bring to the boil, then turn the heat down, cover and simmer for about 30 minutes, until the flavour of the sauce has developed and the peas are soft and sweet.

Serve with coriander, green chillies, if you wish, and dollops of Greek yogurt.

Energy 295 kcal/1233 kJ **Protein** 20.5g **Fat** 15.7g
Sat. Fat 5.9g **Carbohydrate** 20.7g **Fibre** 5.9g

TIP

- This will freeze well, in individual portions.

DESSERTS and BAKING

Sweet foods can be a real treat for some and the ideas in this section are ideal as part of a meal or as a snack between meals. Many of these recipes are high in sugar and fat and would not always be considered as 'healthy eating' but for those who have lost weight or have a tiny appetite, the recipes may be ideal to help boost a poor food intake.

- Stewed, baked or canned fruit served with custard, cream, yogurt or ice cream
- Fruit crumble or flan served with cream, custard or ice cream
- Fresh fruit trifle
- Baked egg custard – use a ready-made pastry case to make a tart
- Greek yogurt swirled with fruit coulis or honey; add nuts or granola for extra flavour and texture
- Slice of cake, such as ginger or apple cake, served with home-made or ready-made custard or ice cream
- Rice pudding – add jam, stewed fruit or dried fruit
- Fruit sundae made from soft fruit such as raspberries or strawberries: layer with whipped cream and ice cream – add crushed meringue nests for extra crunch (Eton Mess)
- Quick-fried bananas: cut the banana into 1 cm-thick slices, on the diagonal; melt some butter in a frying pan and wait for it to foam; add the banana and cook for a minute or two on each side; sprinkle with cinnamon; mix honey or maple syrup with 1 or 2 tablespoons of water and another of lime juice; pour this over the banana and simmer for a couple of minutes – excellent with cream or ice cream for added energy.

Ching He Huang's COCONUT MILK PUDDINGS WITH NUT & SESAME SEED TOPPING

1 litre (34fl oz) coconut milk drink
coconut cream from a **400g (14oz)** can coconut milk (chill the can in the fridge overnight to separate the cream and milk, then scoop out the cream from the top of the can)
3 teaspoons agar agar powder
3 tablspoons caster sugar

To serve:
handful roasted salted peanuts
handful roasted cashews
3 tablespoons toasted sesame seeds
2 tablespoons toasted dried coconut flakes
2 tablspoons golden caster sugar
condensed coconut milk
9 rose petals or other edible flowers

Energy 312 kcal/1305 kJ
Protein 4.8g
Fat 15g
Sat. Fat 1.75g
Carbohydrate 18g
Fibre 2.5g

These little puddings are like plant-based, wobbly panna cotta. They are a great make ahead dessert, perfect for when you want something quick and easy straight from the fridge.

Makes 9

Place the coconut milk drink in a wok over a medium heat. Warm through, then add the coconut cream and stir to combine. Add the agar agar and stir to dissolve, then add the sugar and, again, stir to dissolve.

Pass the mixture through a sieve and divide it between 9 small circular ramekins (5cm/2in deep and 5cm/2in wide). Transfer to the refrigerator and chill for 1 hour to set. Meanwhile, grind the peanuts and cashews in a pestle and mortar. Stir in the toasted sesame seeds, coconut flakes and sugar. Set aside.

To serve, remove the puddings from the refrigerator. Place the ramekins in a tray of hot water to loosen, then tip each pudding on to a serving plate. Drizzle with condensed milk and sprinkle over the ground nut mixture. Top with a rose petal or edible flower.

Prue Leith's MUSCOVADO HEAVEN

200–250g (7–9oz) fruit
100ml (3½fl oz) double cream
100ml (3½fl oz) Greek yogurt
4 tablespoons muscovado sugar

Energy 530 kcal/2212 kJ
Protein 4.5g
Fat 32.2g
Sat. Fat 20.2g
Carbohydrate 59.0g
Fibre 4.8g

This is possibly the easiest dessert you will ever make. You can use any fresh fruit or compôte, or even canned fruit, which takes even less preparation. Prue says it is particularly delicious with fresh mango or passionfruit, but use whatever takes your fancy. If you want to serve this with a biscuit, a gingery one would work very well.

Serves 2

Divide the fruit between two glass dishes or large ramekins.

Mix together the double cream and Greek yogurt, until well combined, thick, but not set. Spoon this over the fruit.

Sprinkle the sugar over the cream and yogurt. You will need to do this in a very thick layer. Put in the fridge to chill for around 30 minutes. The sugar will dissolve into a dark lake. To introduce a little crunch, sprinkle over a little more sugar or eat with a thin, sweet biscuit.

A USEFUL APPLE SAUCE

500g (18oz) cooking apples, *peeled and diced*
2 tablespoons runny honey
Juice of ½ lemon *(optional)*
Small knob of unsalted butter

Nutritional information for ¼:
Energy 83 kcal/356 kJ
Protein 0.4g
Fat 0.7g
Sat. Fat 0.3g
Carbohydrate 20.3g
Fibre 2.7g

This apple sauce can be used as the basis for all kinds of things. Mix it with equal quantities of lightly whipped cream for a fool, stir it into yogurt or custard, dollop it on ice cream or pancakes, or turn it into mini trifles with moistened sponge fingers, custard and cream. The lemon juice here is purely to stop the apples from turning brown – if you don't mind this and can't cope with lemon juice, miss it out. It will store well in the fridge and freezer, so it's worth making a large batch of the sauce and freezing individual portions

Makes about 500ml (17fl oz) (4 portions)

Put the apples in a saucepan, drizzle over the honey and add a splash of water along with the lemon juice, if using, just so the base of the pan is coated. Add the butter and simmer slowly until the apples have completely collapsed into a sauce – there shouldn't be any need to purée this. Chill and use as needed.

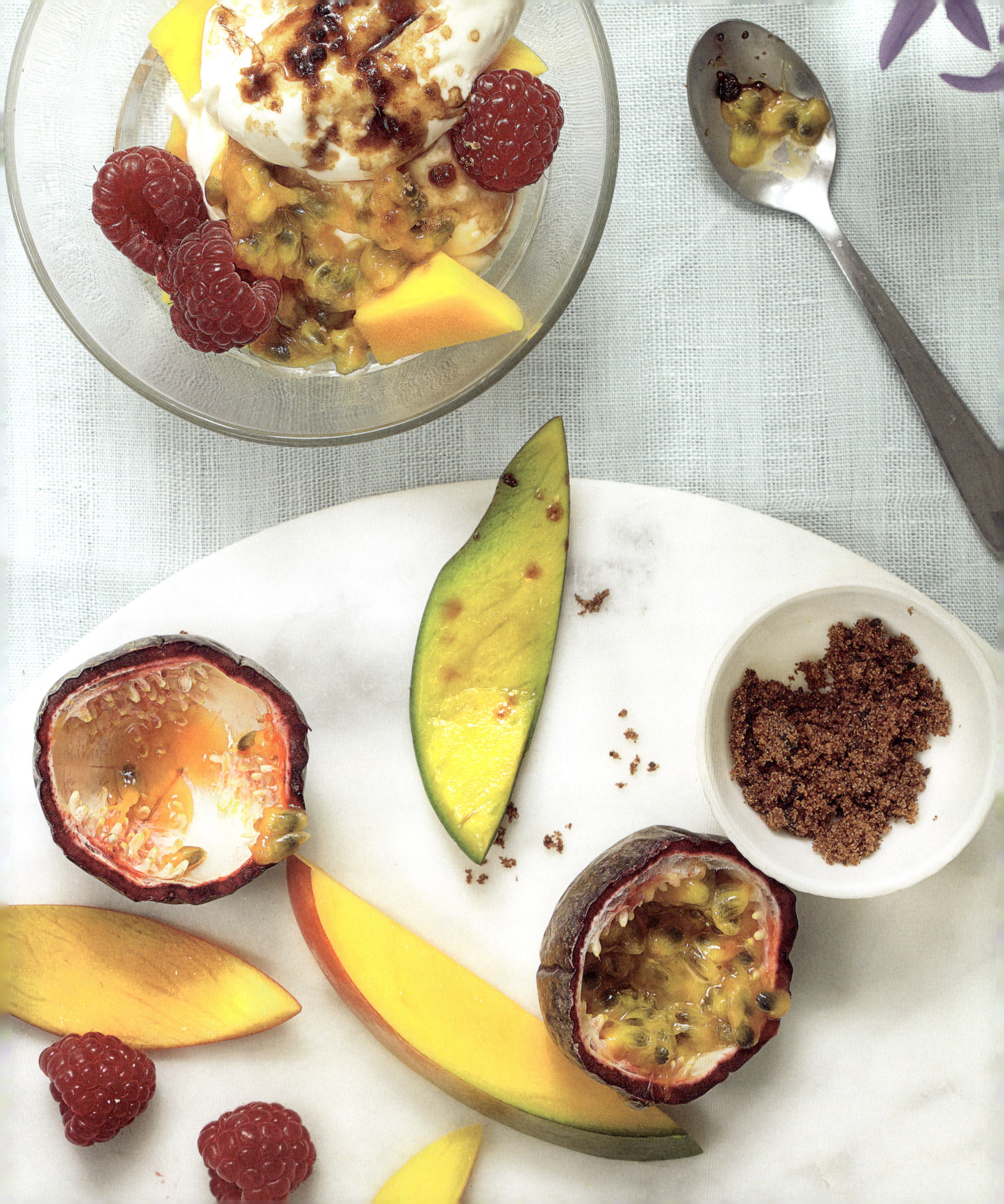

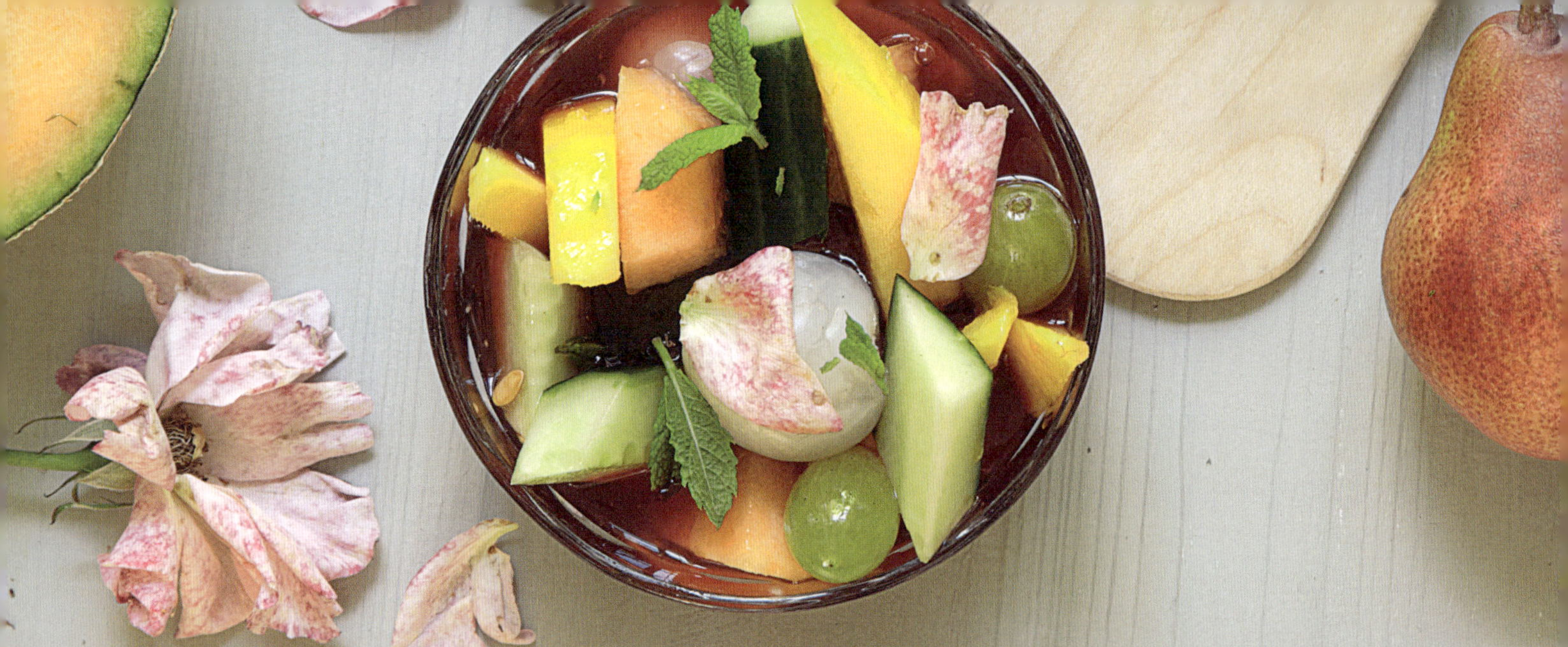

SOOTHING FRUIT SALAD

with a Rosewater, Pomegranate and Cardamom Syrup

For the syrup:
50ml (1¾fl oz) pomegranate juice or the seeds from ½ pomegranate
2 cardamom pods, *lightly crushed*
50g (2oz) runny honey
1 teaspoon rosewater

To serve:
Ice cream, crème fraîche or yogurt

To decorate:
A few mint leaves and/or rose petals and/or pistachio nibs

Nutritional information for the fruits suggested with the syrup:
Energy 129 kcal/551 kJ
Protein 1.2g
Fat 0.2g
Sat. Fat 0g
Carbohydrate 32.9g
Fibre 2.5g

This fruit salad is designed to include fruits that hopefully won't aggravate any problems with a sore mouth. The other thing about some of these fruits – the melon and grapes especially – is that their high sugar content means they freeze easily and can be munched straight from frozen. So do consider open-freezing a few portions if you want to really cool the mouth. The number of servings depends on how much fruit you use. The syrup will cover enough fruit for four though.

Serves 4

A selection of fruit including: chunks of all kinds of melon, grapes, lychees (canned are good), pears (also good canned, if not, peeled, cored and tossed in lime juice to stop them browning), mango, and even peeled and deseeded cucumber.

Put all the syrup ingredients, along with 100ml (3½fl oz) cold water, in a saucepan and simmer gently until the honey has melted. If you are using pomegranate seeds instead of the juice, lightly crush them with the back of a spoon so they release some of their colour. Taste, and adjust the sweetness and flavours with more honey and or rosewater if necessary. Strain.

Pour the syrup over the prepared fruits and chill. Serve with any of the finishing touches mentioned, and dollops of ice cream, crème fraîche or yogurt to boost the energy, protein and calcium.

Tom Aikens' CARAMELISED CARDAMOM PLUMS

12 ripe plums, *halved and stoned*
2 tablespoons muscovado sugar
Large pinch of mixed spice
Large pinch of ground ginger
Large pinch of five-spice powder
Small pinch of ground cloves
Seeds from **1** cardamom pod, *finely crushed*
Zest of **2** unwaxed oranges
3 tablespoons unsalted butter, *softened, plus extra for greasing*
1 tablespoon brioche crumbs

For the spiced crème fraîche:
300g (10½oz) crème fraîche
Seeds from **½** vanilla pod
80g (3oz) caster sugar
½ teaspoon ground cinnamon

Nutritional information for the plums
Energy 155 kcal/648 kJ
Protein 1.4g
Fat 9.9g
Sat. Fat 5.9g
Carbohydrate 17.9g
Fibre 2.0g

There are lots of spices here, but they combine to make a lovely sweet topping, which is delicious with these plums. The topping is also really good spread on toast and will keep well in the fridge, so consider making double the amount. Cooking the fruit and serving the spiced crème fraîche takes away some of the sharpness of the fruit. These lovely flavours provide a high-energy dessert that is both easy to eat and delicious.

Serves 4

Preheat the oven to 200°C/gas mark 6/400°F or heat the grill to its highest setting. Grease a large roasting tin with butter.

Arrange the plums, cut-side up, in the roasting tin. Mix together all the spices, orange zest, butter and brioche crumbs. Spread a little of this mixture in the pit of each plum – you should have enough for a scant half teaspoon per half plum. Bake in the preheated oven for 15 minutes. Alternatively, put under a hot grill until they start to caramelise.

For the spiced cream, put the crème fraîche in a bowl. Split the vanilla pod lengthways down the middle and scrape out the seeds with the tip of a sharp knife. Add this to the crème fraîche with the caster sugar and cinnamon. Beat together using an electric whisk for a minute until light and fluffy. Alternatively, beat for 3–4 minutes using a wooden spoon.

Serve the plums with the spiced crème fraîche.

Nutritional information for the spiced crème fraîche:
Energy 364 kcal/1523 kJ **Protein** 1.7g **Fat** 30.0g
Sat. Fat 20.3g **Carbohydrate** 22.9g **Fibre** 0g

FENNEL PANNA COTTA WITH CHERRY COMPÔTE

300ml (10½oz) double cream
1 tablespoon fennel seeds
Vegetable oil, *for brushing*
100ml (3½fl oz) full-fat milk
50ml (1¾fl oz) buttermilk (or add **½ teaspoon** lemon juice to **100ml (3½fl oz)** milk and let it stand for a few minutes)
75g (2¾oz) honey
2 gelatine leaves

Energy 451 kcal/1864 kJ
Protein 4.0g
Fat 41.9g
Sat. Fat 25.7g
Carbohydrate 17.3g
Fibre 0g

These are very elegant little desserts, quite rich, but silky smooth. They are very easy to eat, so if your mouth is sore, then try the panna cotta on its own. They are high in energy, so ideal for those wishing to gain weight. You could have one as a dessert or as a snack between meals.

Serves 4

Put the cream in a small saucepan. Crush the fennel seeds very lightly with a pestle and mortar and add to the cream. Heat slowly, until almost at simmering point, then remove from the heat and leave for a while to infuse – at least until the cream is at room temperature again.

Prepare four ramekins or moulds by brushing with a little vegetable oil and lightly wiping over with some kitchen paper.

Add the milk, buttermilk and honey to the saucepan, and warm through. Soak the gelatine leaves in some cold water until soft, then squeeze out the water and add the leaves to the cream mixture, making sure that the liquid is warm and nowhere close to boiling point. Stir until the gelatine has dissolved, then strain into a jug.

Pour the mixture into the prepared ramekins. Allow to cool, then chill for at least 4 hours, by which time it should have set.

Remove from the fridge just before serving. To turn out, dip the sides of each ramekin into some just-boiled water for a few seconds, then invert onto a plate.

Spoon around some of the cherry compôte.

TIP

- If you are nervous about turning them out, you can always make them in slightly bigger ramekins and spoon some of the compôte on top.

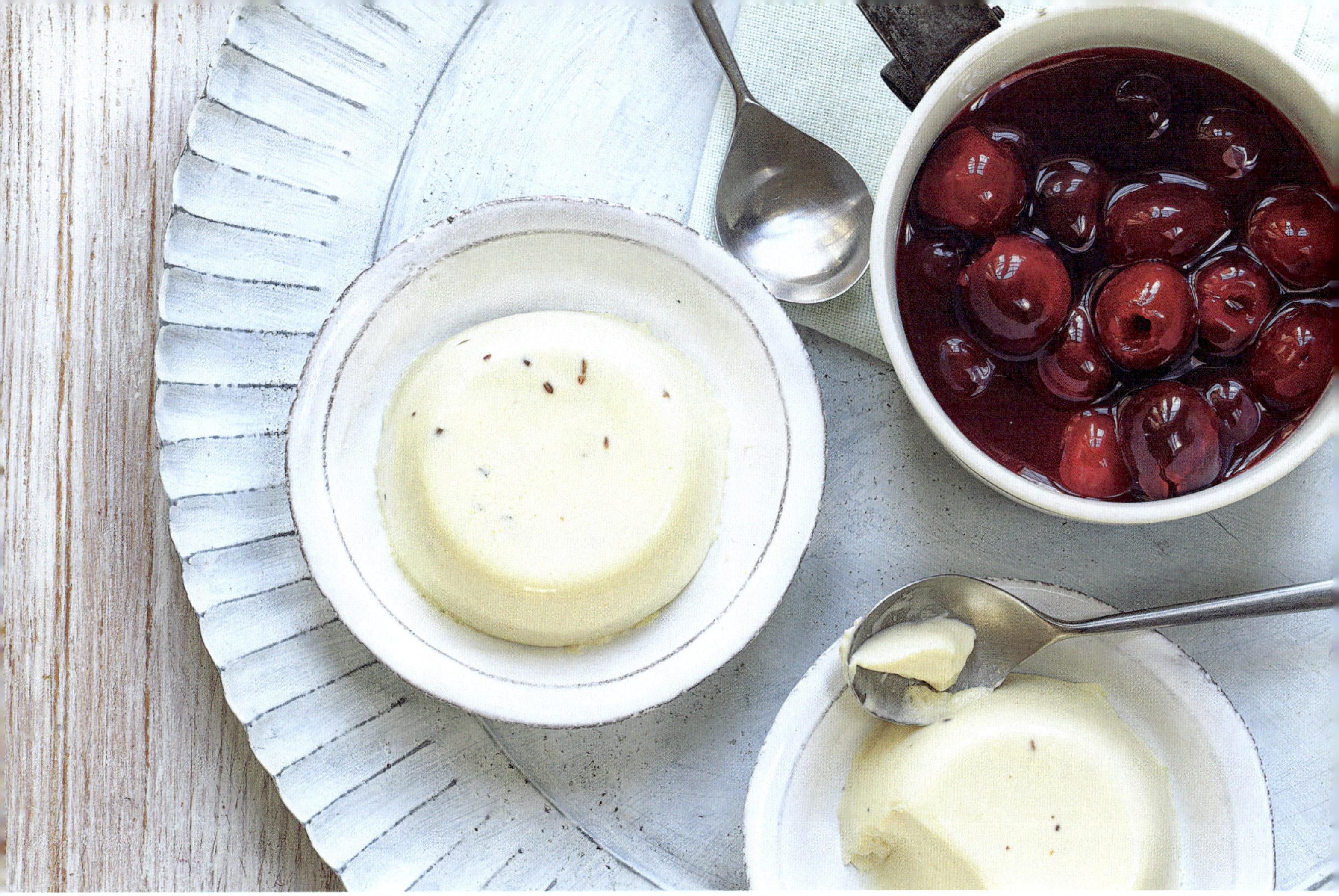

CHERRY COMPÔTE

400g (14oz) cherries, *pitted*
2 heaped **tablespoons** honey
Juice of ½ lemon
1 tablespoon cornflour *(optional)*

This makes slightly more cherry compôte than you need, but it will keep for a few days in the fridge and is a very useful thing to have around. Try it with Greek yogurt, swirled into rice pudding or spooned over ice cream.

Put the cherries in a saucepan with the honey and lemon juice, and just cover with water. Heat slowly, stirring until the honey has dissolved, then simmer until the cherries are soft. The cherries should be sitting in a fairly thin syrup. If you prefer this a little thicker, mix the cornflour with some cold water and stir into the cherries until the compôte has thickened.

Energy 143 kcal/609 kJ
Protein 1.0g
Fat 0.2g
Sat. Fat 0.0g
Carbohydrate 36.6g
Fibre 1.2g

TIP

- If you don't think you will use up the compôte all at once, it will freeze well.

PLUM AND STAR ANISE CRUMBLE

For the fruit:
2 cinnamon sticks
1 star anise
75g (2¾oz) sugar or honey
200ml (7fl oz) water or wine
1kg (35oz) firm but ripe plums, *halved and stoned*

For the topping:
175g (6oz) plain, spelt or wholemeal flour
75g (2¾oz) unsalted butter
25g (¾oz) porridge oats
25g (¾oz) flaked almonds
50g (2oz) demerara sugar

Energy 283 kcal/1193 kJ
Protein 4.0g
Fat 10.1g
Sat. Fat 5.1g
Carbohydrate 46.9g
Fibre 3.9g

You can make a crumble without precooking the plums, but the skins can be a bit tannic, so I thought best to remove them here. As with the cobbler, you can make individual portions of these in ramekins and freeze them. You can also use the plums as a compôte and even use the leftover syrup as a cordial. The fruit and nut combination provides a good balance of nutrients, including beta-carotene and vitamin E, with a generous amount of dietary fibre.

Serves 8 (small portions)

Preheat the oven to 180°C/gas mark 4/350°F.

Put the spices in a saucepan with the sugar or honey and the liquid. Put over a low heat and bring up to a gentle simmer, and cook for a few minutes to allow the flavours to develop. Add the plums and simmer until they are soft enough for the skins to slip off. Remove from the heat, strain, reserving the liquor, and remove the skins. Put in a pudding dish.

To make the topping. put the flour in a bowl. Add the butter and rub in with your hands until the mixture resembles breadcrumbs. Stir in the porridge oats, almonds and half the sugar. Spoon this over the plums – don't smooth it down. Sprinkle over the remaining sugar.

Bake for about 30–35 minutes until the crumble is golden brown and the juice from the plums is seeping through. If you make individual crumbles, bake for 20 minutes.

TIP

- For the filling, you could use bramley apples mixed with cinnamon and ginger, or gooseberries, when they are in season.

PEACH AND BLUEBERRY COBBLER

This is a very light pudding, thanks to the buttermilk in the cobbler topping, but it's pure comfort all the same. You can make it in a large ovenproof dish, but it will also make eight small individual puddings. So it's really worth dividing the mixture between eight buttered ramekins, cooking the lot, then freezing them. They will reheat beautifully in the microwave or, if you let them defrost naturally, in the oven or steamer. They're also quite good cold! It's also a really lovely store cupboard pudding. You don't even need to buy buttermilk specially – simply add 1 teaspoon of lemon juice to 100ml milk and let it stand for a few minutes and you have a thickened milk which will work in exactly the same way. This is a delicious way to use both fresh and canned fruit, providing some vitamins including beta-carotene and other antioxidants. Increase the energy and protein by serving with custard or yogurt.

Serves 8

For the topping:
225g (8oz) self-raising flour
2 teaspoons baking powder
100g (3½oz) caster sugar
75g (2¾oz) cold unsalted butter, *diced, plus extra for greasing*
100ml (3½fl oz) buttermilk (or **100ml (3½fl oz)** milk with **1 teaspoon** of lemon juice)
1 free-range egg, *beaten*

For the filling:
400g (14oz) can of peaches, drained, or
4 fresh peaches, *peeled and stoned*
100g (3½oz) blueberries
1 tablespoon soft, light brown sugar

Energy 261 kcal/1103 kJ
Protein 4.6g
Fat 9.0g
Sat. Fat 5.2g
Carbohydrate 43.5g
Fibre 2.6g

Preheat the oven to 190°C/gas mark 5/375°F. Butter a large pudding dish or eight individual ramekins.

To make the topping, put the self-raising flour, baking powder and caster sugar in a bowl or food-processor and add the butter. Mix until the mixture resembles fine breadcrumbs. (Or you can do this by hand.)

Mix the buttermilk and egg together, then lightly stir this into the flour mixture until you have a soft, sticky dough.

To make a single large pudding, put the peaches in the bottom of the dish and sprinkle over the blueberries and sugar. Take dessertspoon-sized pieces of dough and space them over the peaches and blueberries – don't worry about gaps between them, as they will spread during baking time and you want some of the juice from the fruit to bubble up through. Bake for about 30–35 minutes.

To make individual servings, cut the peaches into cubes. Divide these and the blueberries between the ramekins and sprinkle over the sugar. Put 1 heaped dessertspoon of the dough on top of each and bake for 20 minutes.

Lucy Young's
SUMMER FRUITS AND LEMON PAVLOVA

The key to a perfect pavlova or meringue is to whisk the egg whites and add the sugar slowly, otherwise the sugar will sink to the bottom and the pavlova will collapse. Be patient and do not add the sugar too soon! The cornflour and vinegar give the gooey middle.

Serves 8

For the pavlova:
120g (4½oz) pasteurised egg whites
175g (6oz) caster sugar
1 teaspoon cornflour
1 teaspoon white wine vinegar

For the filling:
150ml (5fl oz) double cream, *whipped*
200ml (7fl oz) half-fat crème fraîche
3 good tablespoons luxury lemon curd
100g (3½oz) fresh raspberries
100g (3½oz) fresh blueberries
100g (3½oz) fresh strawberries, *quartered*
Mint leaves, *to decorate*

Preheat the oven to 120°C/gas mark ½/250°F. Line a large baking sheet with greaseproof paper.

To make the pavlova, whisk the egg whites until very stiff. Gradually add the sugar, a teaspoon at a time, whisking the whole time, until stiff and glossy. It is easiest to do this with a stand mixer or electric whisk. Mix the cornflour and vinegar together and stir into the meringue mixture. Spoon the meringue onto a baking sheet in a circle around 23cm (9in) in diameter. Using a spoon, push up the side so there is a dip in the middle (like a nest), ready for the filling. Bake in the oven for about 1 hour. Turn the oven off and leave the pavlova inside until it is stone cold.

Mix the whipped cream and crème fraîche together, and stir in the lemon curd and half the fresh fruits. Spoon into the centre of the pavlova nest. Decorate with the remaining fruits and mint leaves.

Energy 247 kcal/1033 kJ
Protein 2.5g
Fat 14.1g
Sat. Fat 8.9g
Carbohydrate 29.3g
Fibre 1.0g

TIPS

- Any leftover meringue can be stored in an airtight container or frozen – it is then good crumbled up over yogurt, cream, ice cream or compôte, or a combination of all of the above!
- If you don't want to make a pavlova but have meringue on hand, you can break it up and use it to make lots of individual Eton messes as well, using the same ingredients or anything else you have to hand.

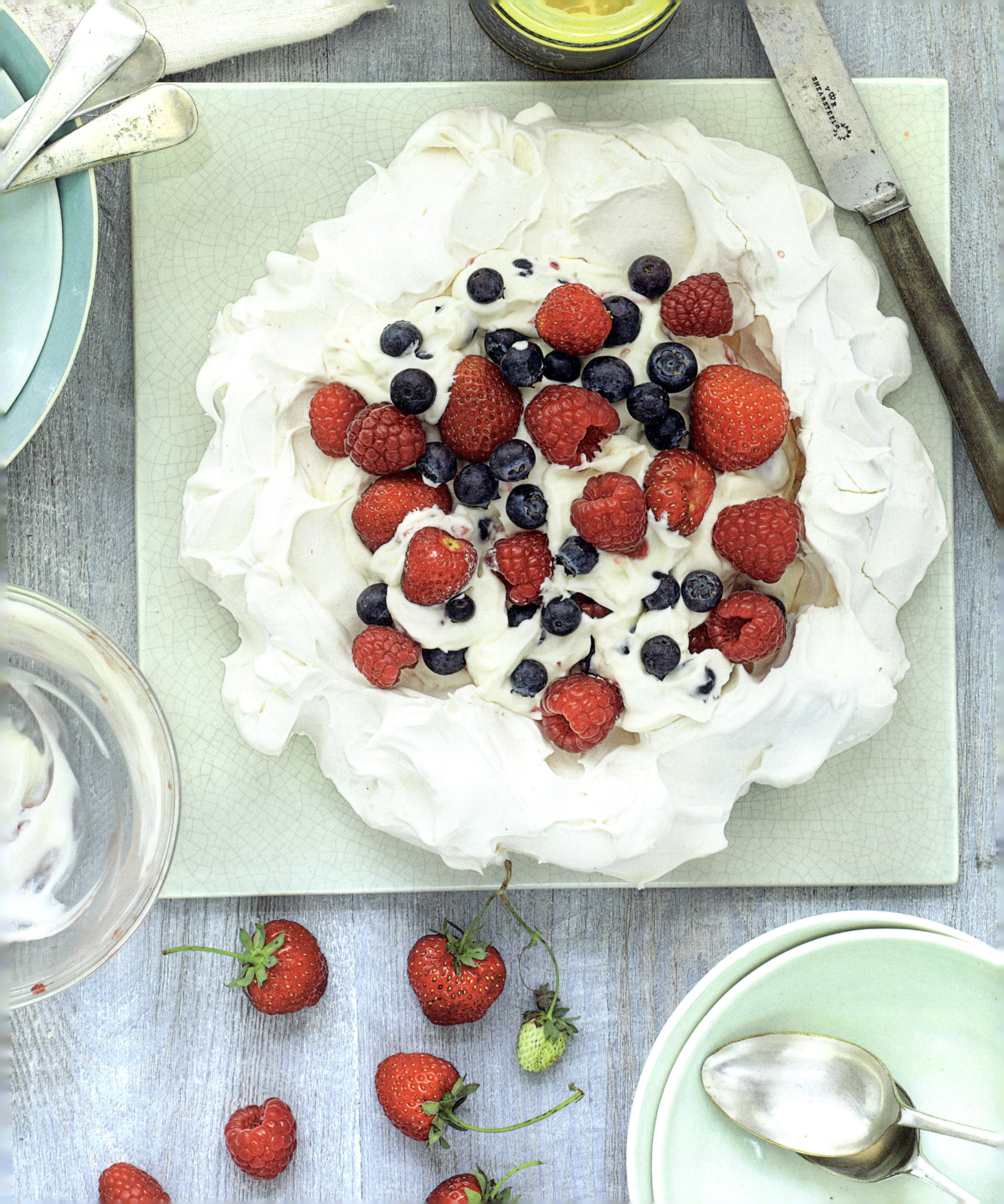

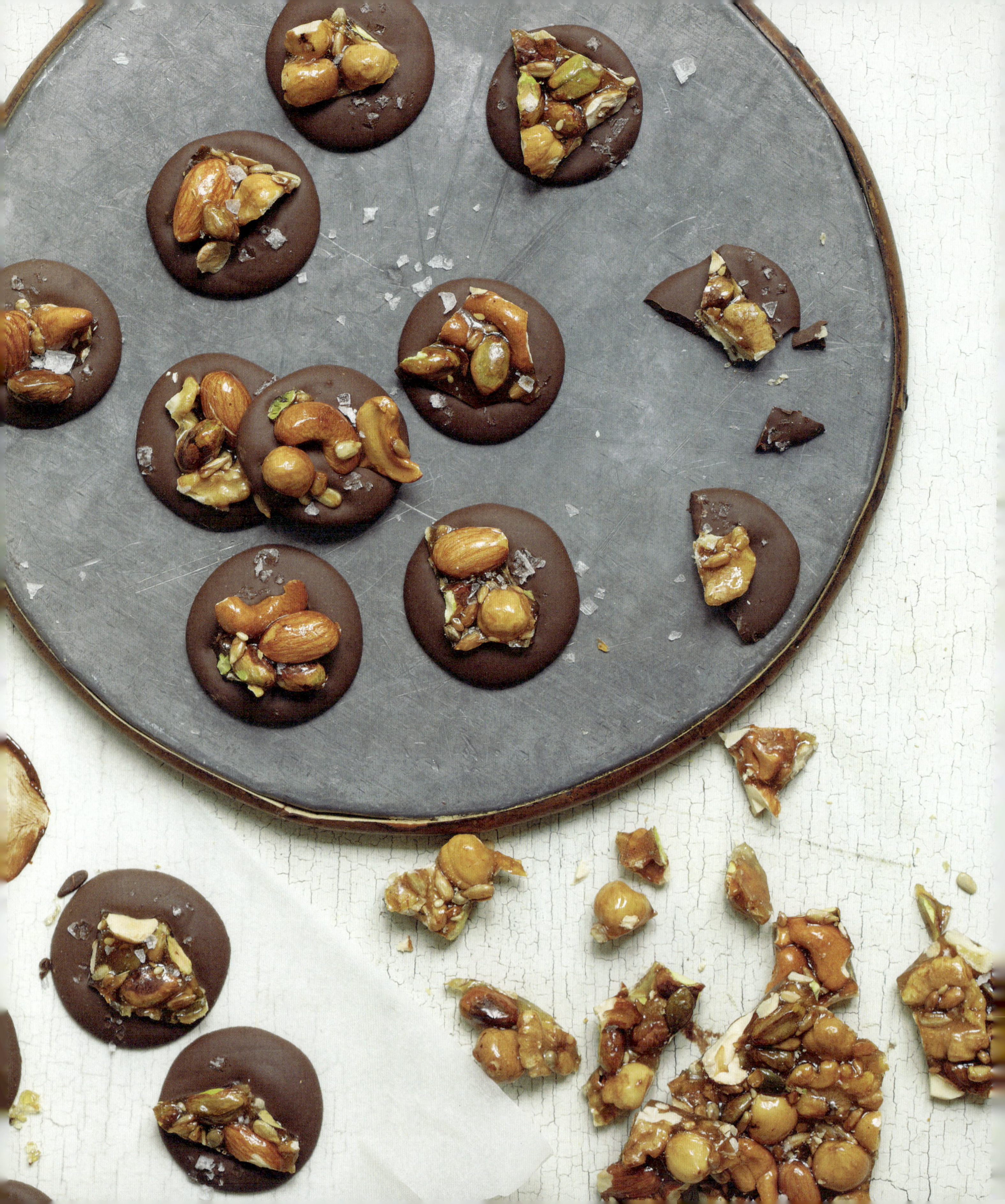

Georgia Glynn Smith's CHOCOLATE DROPS

80g (3oz) mixed nuts and seeds
- often sold in small bags, choose more seeded or nutty to taste
100g (3½oz) glucose syrup – *comes in an easy-squeeze tube*
200g (7oz) Green and Black's Maya Gold Chocolate, *or any dark chocolate that takes your fancy*
½ teaspoon ground cinnamon
Maldon sea salt flakes

Nutritional information per drop:
Energy 45 kcal/189 kJ
Protein 0.7g
Fat 2.4g
Sat. Fat 1.0g
Carbohydrate 5.5g
Fibre 0.2g

'These little delights are wanted at any stage in your life, whatever age and probably whatever location. They are simple to make, divine to eat and always make you smile. If you make the crunchy nut topping first, you can eat some as you melt the chocolate, as long as you don't eat it all! Perfect as a gift to take to a friend, or to make with children for a well-needed moment of distraction, or quite simply perfect to make for one's own moment of self indulgence.' *Georgia Glynn Smith*

Makes around 40 drops

Toast the nuts and seeds in a frying pan over a medium heat until golden brown. Add the glucose syrup to the pan and cook until caramelised. This will take about 5 minutes. Leave, shaking occasionally, until it starts to bubble and turn brown.

Pour the caramelised nuts onto a nonstick or parchment-lined baking sheet and leave to cool completely. Don't be tempted to check them for a while – they'll burn your fingers.

Break the chocolate into a heatproof bowl and set over a pan of simmering water, ensuring the base of the bowl doesn't touch the water. Add the cinnamon and gently stir until completely melted.

Break the caramelised nuts into small, irregular shapes, about 1–2cm (⅜–¾in).

Place teaspoons of melted chocolate onto another nonstick or lined baking sheet. Top them with shards of the caramelised nuts and seeds. For a vital finishing touch, sprinkle over a delicate flake or two of Maldon sea salt.

TIP

- Stored in an airtight container, somewhere cool, these will keep almost indefinitely.

CHOCOLATE POTS

I swear these will be the easiest chocolate pots you will ever make. They are also very adaptable, depending on what kind of chocolate you use (think of all the flavours out there). These pots are creamier than most. If you want a more chocolatey version, just reduce the amount of cream – you can lose as much as half.

100g (3½oz) dark chocolate
1 teaspoon vanilla extract
150ml (5fl oz) whipping cream

Makes 6 espresso-sized portions, which will keep for a week in the fridge

Bring a small saucepan of water to the boil. Break the chocolate into a bowl that will fit snugly on top of the saucepan. Make sure the bowl does not touch the boiling water. Turn the heat down and melt the chocolate, stirring until is completely liquid and smooth. Remove from the heat.

Add 50ml (1¾fl oz) just-boiled water to the chocolate very gradually. Gently mix in the vanilla and whipping cream.

Pour into small espresso cups or glasses and leave to set. Serve at room temperature as they will harden up if chilled.

Nutritional information for the basic chocolate pot recipe:
Energy 182 kcal/754 kJ
Protein 1.3g
Fat 14.7g
Sat. Fat 9.1g
Carbohydrate 11.3g
Fibre 0.6g

Variations:

Add 1 teaspoon of instant espresso powder to the boiling water before pouring onto the chocolate. Try this with a pinch of ground cardamom, as these flavours work very well together.

Add pinches of spices to the chocolate – try ground ginger, cinnamon, fennel or cardamom.

Put fruit in the bottom of the pots before pouring over the chocolate.

Finely chop some stem ginger and stir this through.

Stephanie Alexander's
DATE SCONES

'Scones are the perfect choice for morning tea – quick and simple to make and lovely fresh from the oven.' *Stephanie Alexander*

250g (9oz) self-raising flour
½ teaspoon grated nutmeg
Pinch of salt
20g (¾oz) unsalted butter, *plus extra for greasing*
2 tablespoons caster sugar
150g (5½oz) dates, *stoned and chopped*
60ml (3fl oz) milk

Energy 134 kcal/569 kJ
Protein 2.6g
Fat 2.2g
Sat. Fat 1.3g
Carbohydrate 27.8g
Fibre 1.4g

Makes 10

Preheat the oven to 210°C/gas mark 7/425°F and grease a baking tray.

Sift the flour, nutmeg and salt together in a large bowl, then rub in the butter. Add the sugar and dates. In a jug, mix the milk with 60ml (2fl oz) water, then pour this into the flour mixture and combine until it becomes a soft, but firm, dough. Add a little more milk if it seems dry.

Quickly knead the dough on a floured work surface, then press the dough flat and cut into 10 squares.

Place the squares on the baking tray and bake for 7 minutes. Reduce the oven temperature to 180°C/gas mark 4/350°F, then bake for a further 8 minutes until golden. Remove the tray from the oven allow the scones to cool on a wire rack.

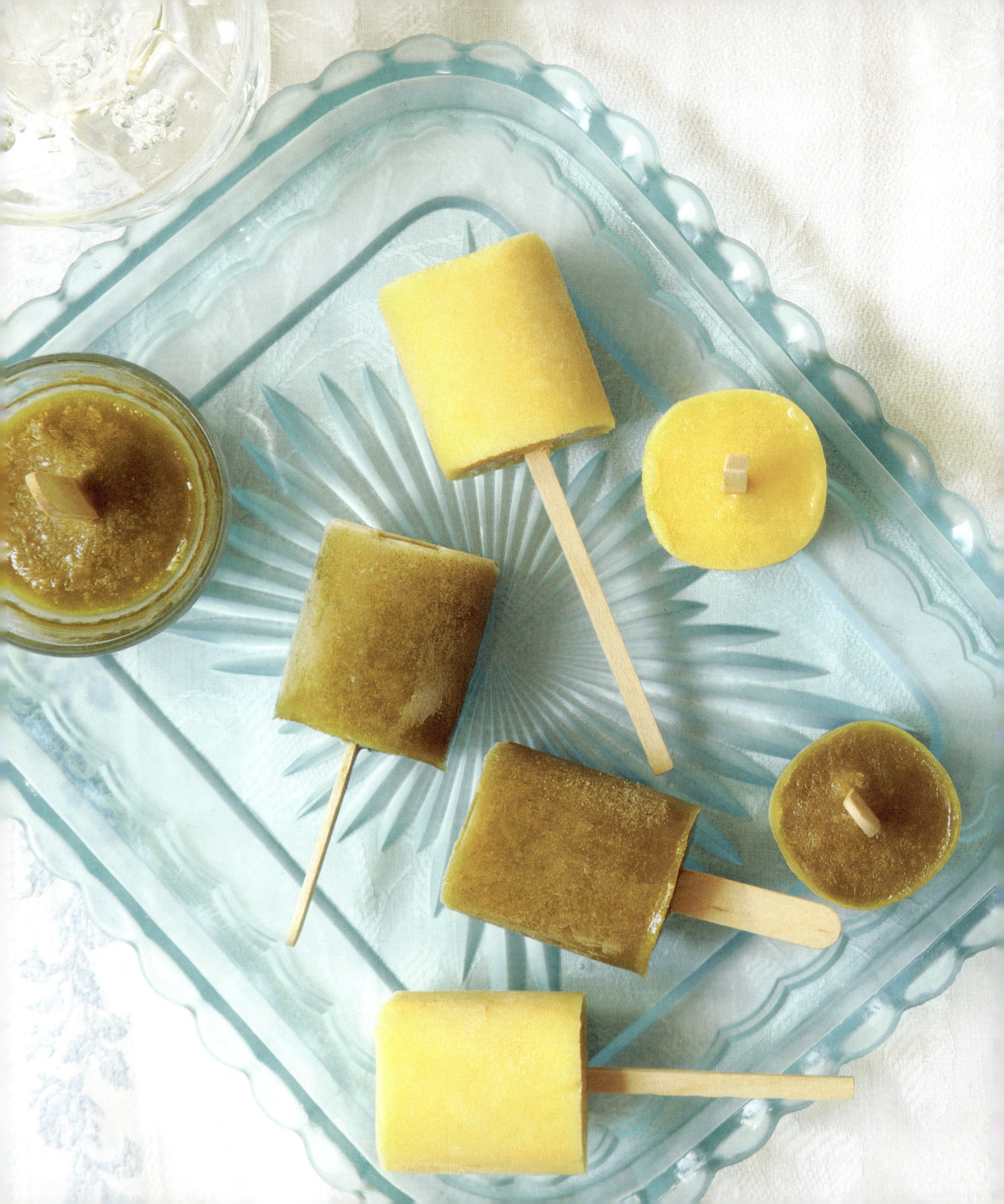

ICE LOLLIES

Both these recipes have deliberately been made quite soothing, so should hopefully be useful if you are dealing with a sore mouth. If you don't have ice lolly moulds, you can use small paper cups and spear them with lollipop sticks. You can also freeze them in small ice-cube trays or bags to eat smaller quantities more regularly.

Green Tea (Matcha) and Peach

This recipe uses the cold infusion method of tea making, which results in a much more gentle, less bitter flavour. Matcha is supposedly to be particularly high in antioxidants known as flavonoids. If you don't have Matcha you could use black, white or jasmine tea in its place.

1 teaspoon Matcha tea (or contents of 1 tea bag)
150g (5½oz) peaches – *canned are fine*
2 tablespoons runny honey

Makes 6 × 50ml (2fl oz) ice lollies

Pour 150ml (5fl oz) hot water over the tea and leave to infuse for several hours. Strain this into a blender along with the peaches and honey. Blitz and pour into moulds. Freeze until firm. To unmould, dip into hot water for a few moments.

Energy 31 kcal/134 kJ **Protein** 0.3g **Fat** 0g
Sat. Fat 0g **Carbohydrate** 8g **Fibre** 0.5g

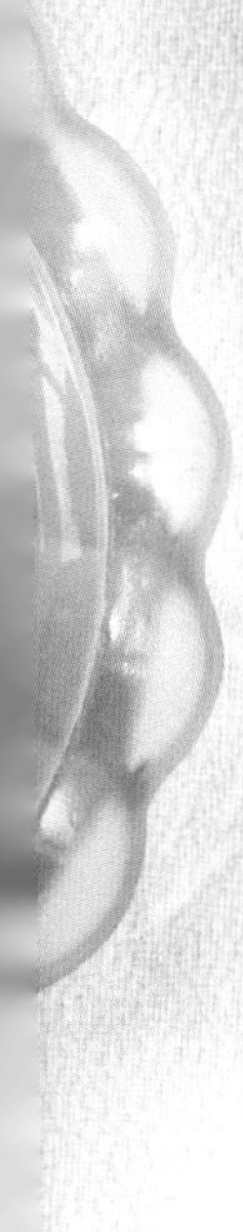

Melon, Coconut and Mint

All varieties of melon are very cooling and soothing, so you can use any in this recipe – just make sure it is very ripe.

4 tablespoons honey
½ teaspoon grated fresh ginger *(optional)*
A few sprigs of mint, *bashed*
150g melon, *deseeded and chopped*
100ml coconut milk or yogurt
Squeeze of lime *(optional)*

Makes 6 × 50ml (2fl oz) ice lollies

Put the honey in a very small saucepan with 1 tablespoon water, the ginger, if using, and the mint. Heat gently until the honey has melted, then remove from the heat and leave to infuse for a few minutes.

Put the melon and coconut milk in a blender and squeeze over some lime juice, if using. Strain the honey syrup through a sieve into the blender. Blitz until smooth, then pour into moulds. Freeze until firm. To unmould, dip into hot water for a few moments.

Energy 56 kcal/239 kJ **Protein** 0.3g **Fat** 0.1g
Sat. Fat 0g **Carbohydrate** 14.5g **Fibre** 0.2g

ICE CREAMS

It's good to always have some ice cream in the freezer. Ice cream is very easy to eat if you have a sore mouth or poor appetite. Homemade will taste fresher, but many are made with partially cooked eggs which should be avoided when your immune system is at a low ebb, such as when you are on chemotherapy. These, however, are all egg-free and are as quick as can be to make. They combine the nourishment of fruit, milk and cream. If you don't have an ice-cream maker, simply put into a freezerproof container and, while it is setting, whisk it up at regular intervals – the trick is to get air into it.

BANANA ICE CREAM

This ice cream is lovely as it is, but is also a good flavour carrier – try adding pinches of cinnamon, nutmeg or cardamom.

3 large very ripe bananas *(with skins starting to blacken)*
Juice of ½ large lime
200g (7oz) soft, light brown sugar
250ml (8½fl oz) full-fat milk, *chilled*
250ml (8½fl oz) double cream, *chilled*

Makes round 1 litre (34fl oz) of ice cream / Serves 8

Peel the bananas and whizz them in a food-processor with the lime juice and sugar until perfectly smooth. Add the milk and whizz again, then gently stir in the double cream until completely combined.

Pour into an ice-cream maker and freeze-churn until thick, smooth and aerated. Transfer to the freezer.

Nutritional value for 1/8th of the recipe (134g):
Energy 309 kcal/1292 kJ
Protein 2.1g
Fat 18.1g
Sat. Fat 11.3g
Carbohydrate 37.7g

MANGO KULFI

425g (15oz) can of mangoes or other fruit, approx. **250g (9oz)** drained weight
100g (3½oz) sugar or honey
125ml (4fl oz) evaporated milk
125ml (4fl oz) double cream

Nutritional value for ⅛th of the recipe (75g)
Energy 165 kcal/688 kJ
Protein 1.7g
Fat 9.9g
Sat. Fat 6.2g
Carbohydrate 18.2g
Fibre 1.2g

This is the perfect storecupboard ice cream – you could just as easily use canned peaches, apricots and even pears. Don't worry about kulfi moulds. You can use ice-lolly moulds, ice-cube trays or simply freeze as a tub of ice cream. This is even easier than the banana ice cream recipe above as you don't need to churn it. Again, you can add spices to this one – cardamom or saffron both work very well, as does a drop of rosewater.

Makes a 600g (21oz) tub / Serves 8

Purée the fruit with the sugar or honey until it is smooth. Add the evaporated milk and blitz again. Lightly whip the cream and stir it into the fruit purée. Pour into moulds or whatever receptacle you choose to use. Transfer from the freezer to the fridge a few minutes before serving.

Divya Sharma's STRAWBERRY AND PISTACHIO FROZEN YOGURT

720g (1lb 9oz) full-fat Greek yogurt (or your non-dairy yogurt of choice)
280g (10oz) frozen strawberries
2 tsp vanilla extract
4 tbsp maple syrup (optional)
100g (3½oz) pistachios, crushed

Energy 387 kcal/1619 kJ
Protein 12.8g
Fat 22.5g
Sat. Fat 9.4g
Carbohydrate 37.7.g
Fibre 4.5g

Serves 4

Spoon the yogurt into an ice-cube tray (or mini muffin pan) and freeze for 8 hours or overnight. Put the yogurt ice cubes in a blender with the frozen strawberries, vanilla and maple syrup, if using, until creamy. Stir in the crushed pistachios. Serve immediately or store in the freezer until ready to serve.

TIP

- If you're using a non-dairy yogurt, opt for a higher fat one like coconut, otherwise the frozen yogurt will come out icy

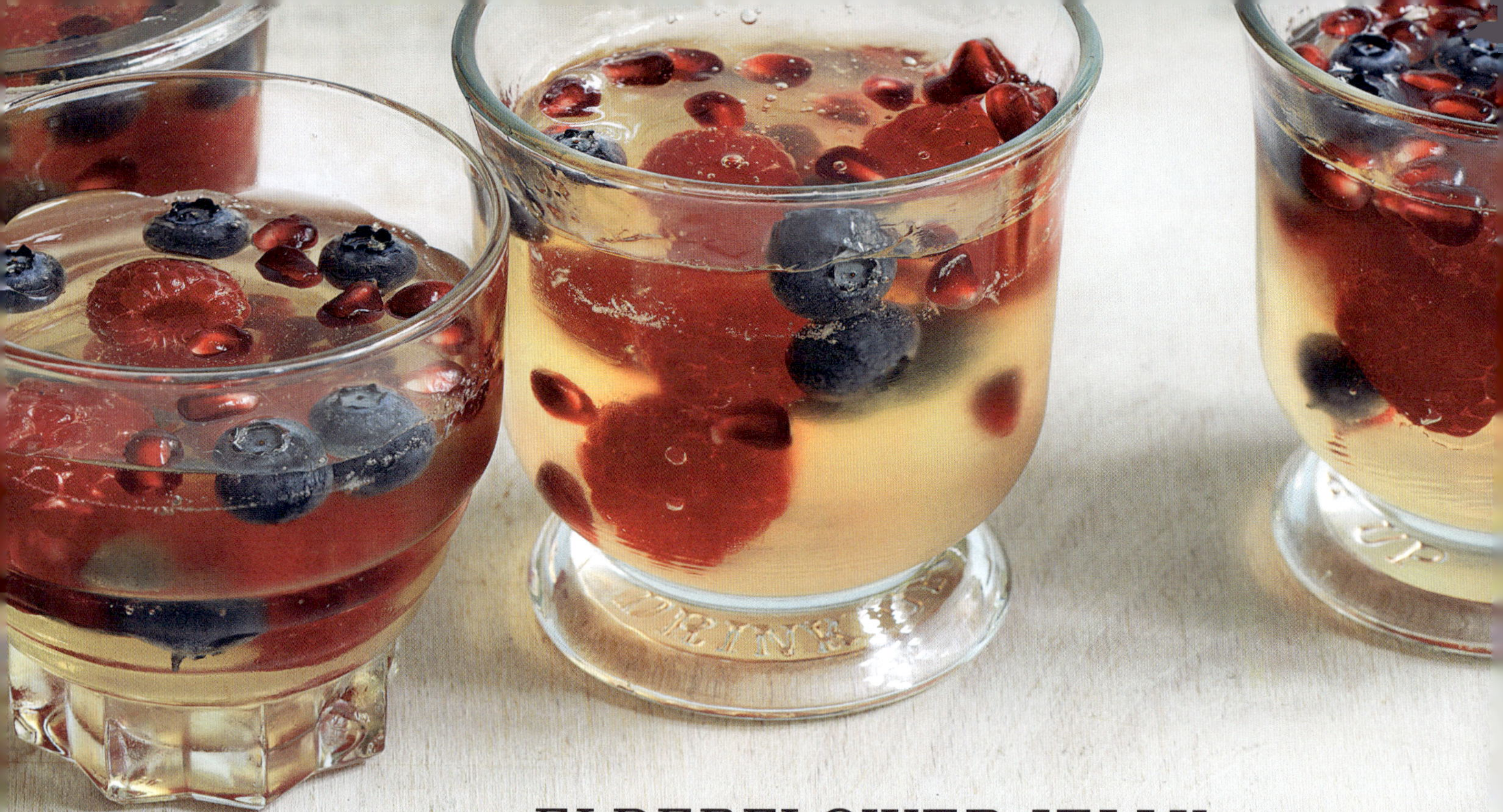

ELDERFLOWER JELLY

5 gelatine leaves
200ml (7fl oz) elderflower cordial
300ml (10fl oz) water or wine
50g (2oz) honey

Fruit of your choice *(optional)*

Nutritional content for 4 portions:
Energy 102 kcal/432 kJ
Protein 2.2g
Fat 0.2g
Sat. Fat 0.2g
Carbohydrate 21.6g
Fibre 0g

You can make jellies out of all kinds of fruit and they will be much better flavours than the packet varieties. Try any of your favourite fruit juices and suspend fruit in them if you like. Just follow the method below and remember that five leaves of gelatine will set around 500ml (17fl oz) liquid. Jelly is lovely to eat if you are feeling a little queasy or have a sore mouth. Remember it is not particularly high in nourishment, so choose other foods when you are able to do so. This version is very quick to make, using cordial. You can suspend any fruit in it you like – raspberries or blueberries look very pretty.

Makes 500ml (17fl oz) jelly, enough for 4–6 portions depending on size

Soak the gelatine leaves in a little cold water.

Put the cordial, water or wine and honey in a saucepan, and gently heat until the honey has melted. Wring out the softened gelatine and add the leaves to the saucepan. Stir until the gelatine has dissolved, making sure you don't let the mixture boil, as this will affect the gelatine's ability to set.

If you are using fruit, put these in a jelly mould or individual glasses. Strain the jelly through a sieve into the mould or glasses and stir. When the jelly is at room temperature transfer to the fridge. Stir every few minutes until starting to set to evenly distribute the fruit if you don't want it all collecting at the top.

PUMPKIN COOKIES

200g (7oz) unsalted butter, *softened*
100ml (3½fl oz) maple syrup
100g (3½oz) wholemeal spelt flour
1 teaspoon baking powder
½ teaspoon ground ginger
½ teaspoon ground cinnamon
½ teaspoon mixed spice
1 free-range egg, *beaten*
150g (5½oz) porridge oats
50g (2oz) puréed pumpkin
100g (3½oz) chocolate chips (or dried fruit)

Nutritional content per cookie:
Energy 91 kcal/381 kJ
Protein 1.3g
Fat 6.0g
Sat. Fat 3.5g
Carbohydrate 8.4g
Fibre 0.8g

There is enough mixture for 36 cookies here, which will fill three baking trays. Either cook in batches or perhaps freeze half the dough for another time – it will keep well in the freezer. You don't have to add chocolate chips to these – any dried fruit or nuts would work just as well. These make an excellent snack between meals – they not only provide extra energy, but a little added beta-carotene from the pumpkin.

Makes 36 cookies

In a large bowl, cream the butter and maple syrup together until light and fluffy. In a separate bowl, sift the flour with the baking powder and spices. Add 1 tablespoon of this to the creamed butter, alternating with the beaten egg, then gradually mix in the rest of the flour and the oats. Fold in the pumpkin, then stir in the chocolate chips.

Chill the cookie dough for at least 1 hour. You can freeze all or part of it at this stage if you don't want too many cookies all at once.

Preheat the oven to 180°C/gas mark 4/350°F. Line a baking tray with baking parchment. Spoon walnut-sized pieces of dough onto the baking tray and press them down lightly with a fork. Bake for 15-20 minutes until golden brown. Remove from the oven and allow to cool and firm up on the tray before transferring to an airtight container.

TIP

- The cookies can be stored for up to a week in an airtight container or in the freezer – just refresh for a couple of minutes in a hot oven to give them a new lease of life.

Mary Berry's SUNDAY ORANGE SPICE CAKE

For the cake:
1 small thin-skinned orange
275g (9¾oz) self-raising flour
3 level teaspoons baking powder
275g (9¾oz) caster sugar
225g (9¾oz) unsalted butter, softened, *plus extra for greasing*
4 free-range eggs
1 teaspoon ground cinnamon
1 teaspoon mixed spice

For the filling:
50g (2oz) unsalted butter, softened
175g (6oz) icing sugar, sifted, *plus a little extra for dusting*
2 level tablespoons orange pulp, *reserved from the cake*

Energy 429 kcal/1801 kJ
Protein 4.9g
Fat 21.4g
Sat. Fat 12.6g
Carbohydrate 58g
Fibre 1.2g

'A fresh, spiced orange cake. You could use just under half the orange filling to sandwich the cakes together, and spread the rest on top.'
Mary Berry

Makes 1 × 20cm (8in) cake / Serves 12

Preheat the oven to 180°C/gas mark 4/350°F. Grease and base line two deep 20cm (8in) sandwich tins.

Place the whole orange in a small saucepan, cover with boiling water and simmer until soft, about 20 minutes. Set aside to cool.

When the orange is cool enough to handle, cut in half and remove any pips. Transfer the whole orange, skin included, to a food-processor and process until medium chunky. Remove and reserve 2 level tablespoons of the orange pulp for the icing. Add the remaining cake ingredients to the processor and blend until just smooth. Divide the mixture evenly between the two tins.

Bake in the preheated oven for 25–30 minutes. When the cake is shrinking away from the sides and is springy to touch, remove from the oven. Leave to cool in the tins for a few moments, then turn out onto a cooling rack and peel off the paper.

To make the orange filling, cream the soft butter, then add the sifted icing sugar and reserved orange pulp. Sandwich the cakes together with the icing, and sift icing sugar over the top of the cake.

This is best eaten freshly made but it will store in an airtight container for 2–3 days. You could also freeze the filled cake for up to 2 months. Thaw for 2–3 hours at room temperature.

TIP

- Thin-skinned oranges are usually smaller – avoid using Jaffa oranges as they have a very thick pith.

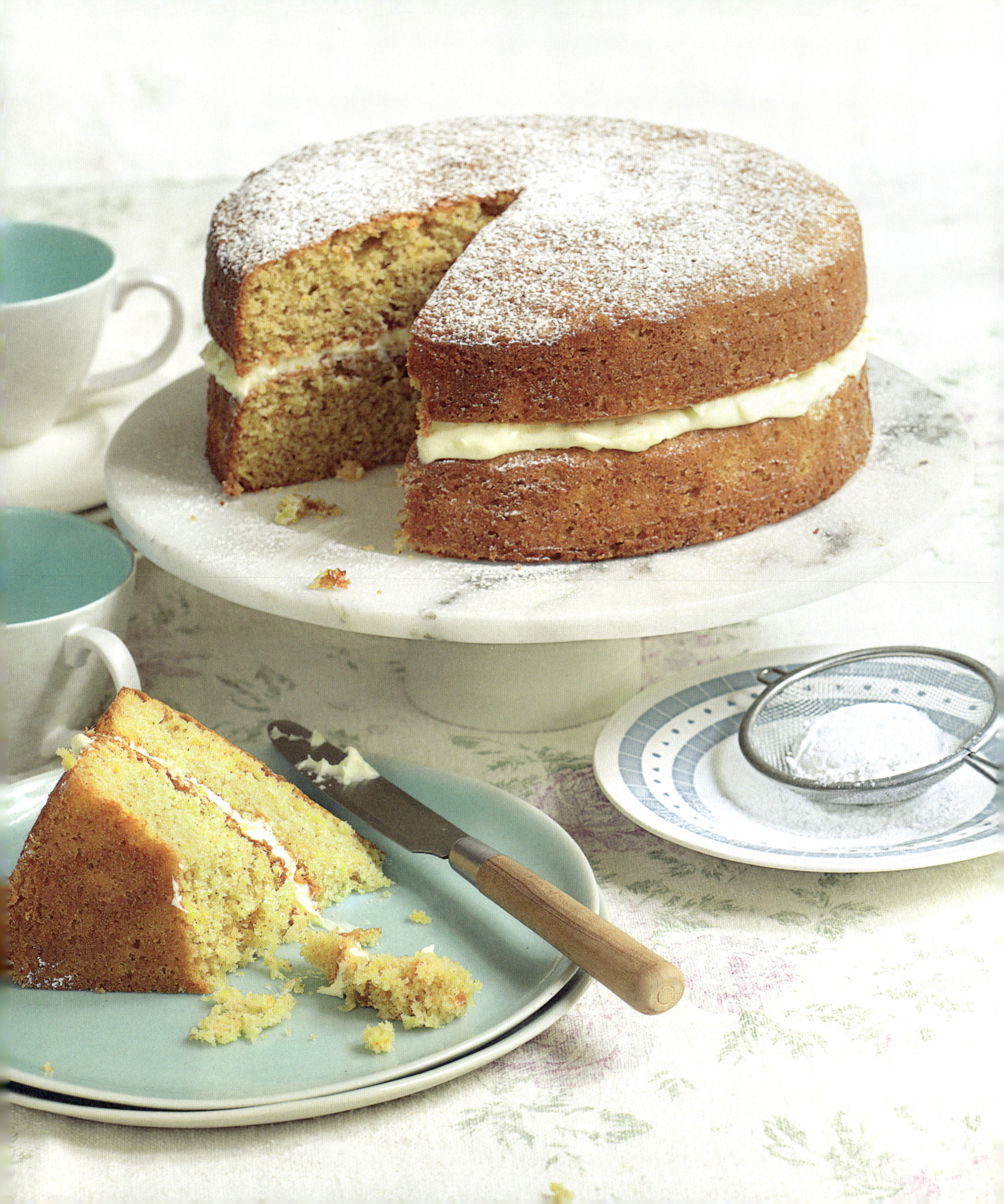

Richard Bertinet's GINGERBREAD

100ml (3½fl oz) double cream
100g (3½oz) caster sugar
250g (9oz) honey
½ teaspoon mixed spice
2 teaspoons ground ginger
125g (4½oz) plain flour
50g (2oz) buckwheat flour
200g (7oz) rye flour
1 teaspoon baking powder
3 free-range eggs
Knob of unsalted butter, *for greasing*
Pinch of salt

1 additional egg for eggwashing the bread

Energy 399 kcal/1687 kJ
Protein 7.1g
Fat 10.3g
Sat. Fat 5.1g
Carbohydrate 73.7g
Fibre 4.5g

This is a wonderfully dense, sticky gingerbread – the flavour of the honey pairs beautifully with the rye flour. If you can't find buckwheat, use 250g rye flour instead. The preparation for this recipe seems lengthy, but there's actually very little work involved, just patience!

Makes 1 × 400g (14oz) loaf / Serves 8

Put the cream in a heavy-based saucepan. Add the sugar, honey, mixed spice and ginger. Place over the heat and heat gently until it just starts to quiver, then turn off the heat and leave to cool. Once it has cooled, transfer it to a bowl or jug, cover and place in the fridge to infuse overnight.

The following day, place the flours and the baking powder in a bowl. Remove the cold cream from the fridge and beat in 3 whole eggs. Gradually mix all of the liquid into the flour until it comes together and combines to make a thick batter. There is no need to work it too much, just make sure that all of the ingredients are properly combined.

Place in a bowl, cover with a cloth or clingfilm and leave to rest for 2 hours.

Preheat the oven to 190°C/gas mark 5/375°F. Grease a 400g (14oz) loaf tin with the knob of butter.

Transfer the dough to the greased tin. Beat the remaining egg with a pinch of salt and then brush the egg wash over the top of the dough.

Put the loaf tin into the oven for 10 minutes, then turn the heat down to 150°C/gas mark 2/300°F. Bake for a further 45–50 minutes until a skewer comes cleanly out of the middle. Remove from the tin and transfer to a cooling rack. Store wrapped in greaseproof paper.

Serve in slices with lots of butter!

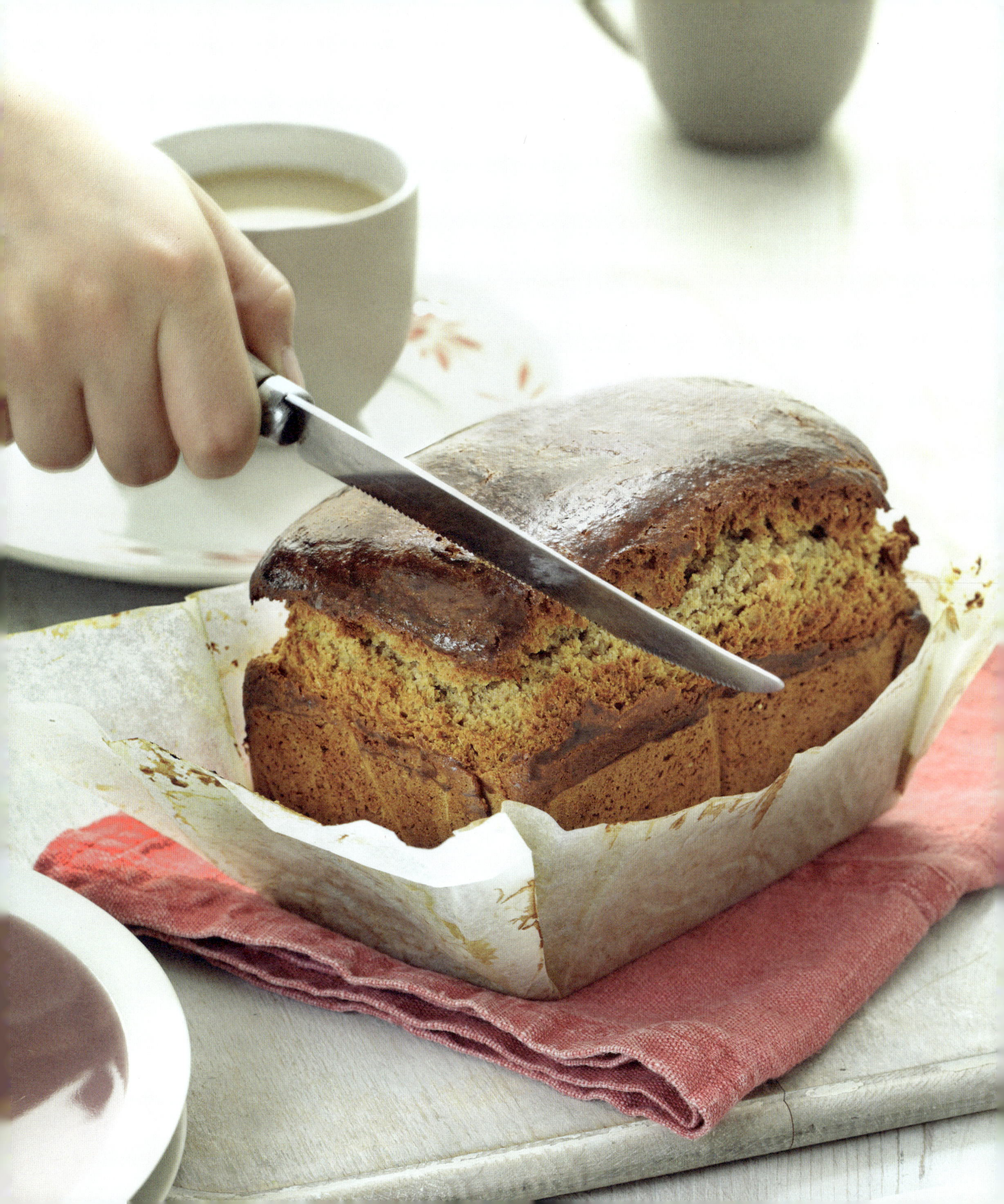

SNACKS and DRINKS

Snacks can be a really important way to increase intake of protein, energy, vitamins and minerals. They are especially important if you need to gain weight or struggle to eat normal sized portions at mealtimes. Take between meals on a regular basis or occasionally, if intake at a mealtime has been particularly low. Try some of the ideas below:

- Nuts – choose salted or unsalted according to taste buds
- Crisps – potato and vegetable
- Crackers or toast with cheese, including cream cheese, hummus, fish pate, smoked salmon, nut butter
- Cold sausages or sausage rolls
- Samosas, pakoras or bhagis
- Chunks of cheese with fruit, e.g. apple, pineapple, grapes
- Tortilla chips or nachos with salsa, guacamole, soured cream or cheese dips
- Oven or microwave chips
- Dim sum (meat or vegetarian)
- Mini spring rolls or sesame toast
- Satay
- Poppadoms with chutney
- Prawn or vegetable crackers with sweet chilli sauce
- Fried dumplings/bakes with ackee and saltfish or fried plantain
- Tamarind balls
- Breadsticks
- Doubles
- Muffins or crumpets (sweet or savoury)
- Small bowl of cereal
- Fruit buns
- Coconut drops
- Toasted teacake or scone
- Home made drinks – milky coffee, malted milk drink, milky hot chocolate, milkshake, smoothie, lassi, peanut punch

BAGNA CAUDA

2 heads of garlic, *broken into cloves, unpeeled*
Milk, *to cover*
200ml (7fl oz) olive oil
50g (2oz) can anchovy fillets, *drained* (about **30g (1oz)** drained weight)
50g (2oz) unsalted butter

Energy 412 kcal/1698 kJ
Protein 4.5 g
Fat 41.1g
Sat. Fat 9.4g
Carbohydrate 6.5g
Fibre 2.1g

Another Mediterranean-inspired dish, perfect when contrasted with crisp, cool vegetables such as radishes, carrots and cucumber, but use any you like. It's also wonderful with steamed or grilled asparagus or sprouting broccoli. Don't worry about the amount of garlic – it is poached, which will get rid of any harsh astringency and leave it sweet and mellow.

This is a high-fat snack, so eat sparingly. It is ideal if you are trying to gain weight, as extra energy is provided by the olive oil, a monounsaturated fat. The raw vegetables add vitamins and minerals to create a better balance, or serve on cooked vegetables as suggested in the tip below.

Serves 6 with the crudites

Put the unpeeled garlic in a small saucepan and cover with milk. Simmer gently for about 20 minutes until the garlic is tender. Drain the cloves from the milk and, when cool enough to handle, squeeze out the flesh and discard the skins.

Heat the olive oil in a saucepan. Add the garlic flesh and anchovies. Keeping over a very low heat, mash the anchovies until they have completely dissolved into the oil and garlic. Whisk the butter into the sauce, a small knob at a time, until the sauce is well combined.

Serve with a selection of crudités.

TIPS

- This sauce will keep well in the fridge. You can also reheat it or simply stir it into some pasta with lots of fresh herbs for a quick supper dish.
- It's also very good drizzled over steamed vegetables such as tenderstem broccoli or griddled endive.

Xanthe Clay's MINI MEZZE

Serves 2, with extra hummus for another day

'A collection of little dishes to tempt your palate. Eat with chargilled slices of rustic, open-textured white bread, or else pitta bread – warmed but untoasted if you prefer a soft texture.' *Xanthe Clay*

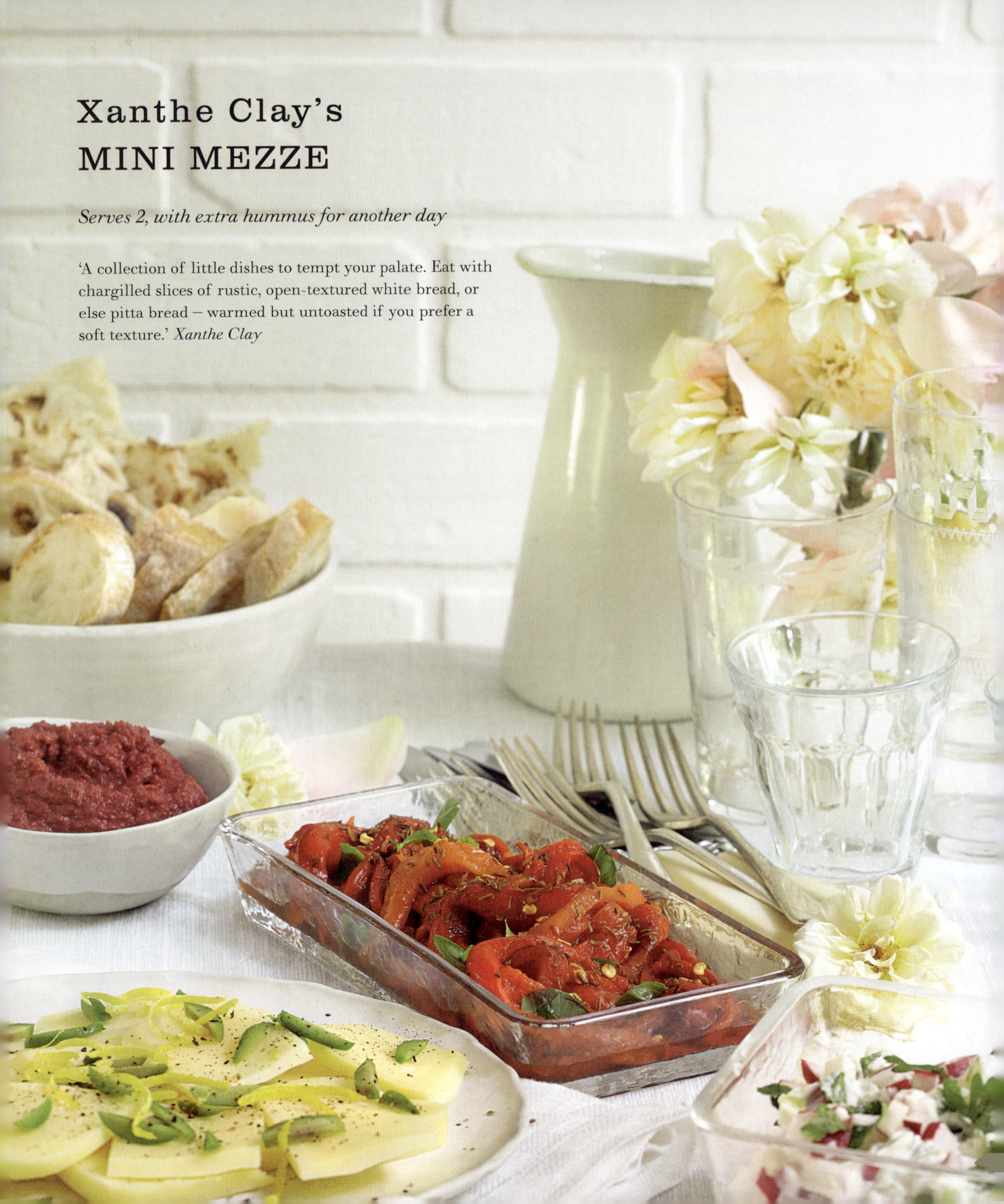

5cm (2in) piece of cucumber
3–4 radishes
3–4 tablespoons Greek yogurt
¼ garlic clove, crushed
A few sprigs of coriander, chopped
Fat pinch of sumac *(optional)*
Salt and freshly ground black pepper

Radish Tzatziki

Cut the cucumber in half lengthways and scoop out the seeds. Chop the flesh into pea-sized cubes. Do the same with the radishes. Mix with yogurt, garlic and salt and pepper. Scatter with coriander and sumac, if you have it.

Energy 124 kcal/513 kJ **Protein** 5.5g **Fat** 9.3g
Sat. Fat 6.1g **Carbohydrate** 5.0g **Fibre** 0.3g

A few slices of peynir or feta cheese
Grated zest of ½ lemon
Green olives
Olive oil
Freshly ground black pepper

Peynir (or Feta) with Lemon and Olives

'I love the creamy, salty Turkish cheese called peynir that comes in tall cans – many ethnic shops stock it. But feta cheese works here too.'

Scatter the cheese with lemon zest and olives (chop them if you prefer). Drizzle over a little olive oil and grind on some pepper.

Energy 151 kcal/627 kJ **Protein** 8.0g **Fat** 13.0g
Sat. Fat 7.3g **Carbohydrate** 0.8g **Fibre** 0.5g

2 cooked beetroot
400g (14oz) can chickpeas, drained
½–1 garlic clove, crushed
2 tablespoons olive oil
Juice of **1** lemon
3 tablespoons tahini
½ teaspoon smoked paprika, *plus extra to garnish*
Salt
Basil, marjoram or oregano leaves, *to serve*
Nigella seeds, *to serve*

Beetroot Hummus

This makes more that you need, but it's hard to get a good, smooth texture with less than a can of chickpeas. It keeps for several days in the fridge.

Whizz all the ingredients in a food-processor or (for a really smooth texture) a liquidizer, adding enough water to make a creamy, magenta-coloured dip. Season with salt. Spread on a plate and drizzle with olive oil, plus more smoked paprika. Scatter with basil, marjoram or oregano, and/or some nigella seeds.

Nutritional value for ¼ of recipe **Energy** 436 kcal/1814 kJ **Protein** 15.8g
Fat 33.7g **Sat. Fat** 4.7g **Carbohydrate** 18.8g **Fibre** 10.6g

2 red peppers, deseeded and halved
1 tablespoon olive oil
1–2 teaspoons pomegranate molasses, or **a few** drops of wine or sherry vinegar
A few mint or basil leaves, torn
A pinch of chilli flakes
1 teaspoon cumin seeds, *toasted in a dry frying pan and roughly crushed*
Salt

Grilled Peppers with Cumin and Chilli

If you have pomegranate molasses it's well worth using in this recipe as it is naturally sweet and less astringent than using vinegar.

Grill the peppers, skin-side up, until they are black and blistered. Pop them in a plastic bag and leave to cool, then strip away the skin. Cut the pepper flesh into strips. Toss in the olive oil and pomegranate molasses or vinegar, and season with salt and the chilli flakes. Sprinkle over the torn mint or basil leaves. Sprinkle the cumin over the peppers and mint.

Energy 114 kcal/472 kJ **Protein** 1.9g **Fat** 6.4g
Sat. Fat 1.0g **Carbohydrate** 12.7g **Fibre** 3.9g

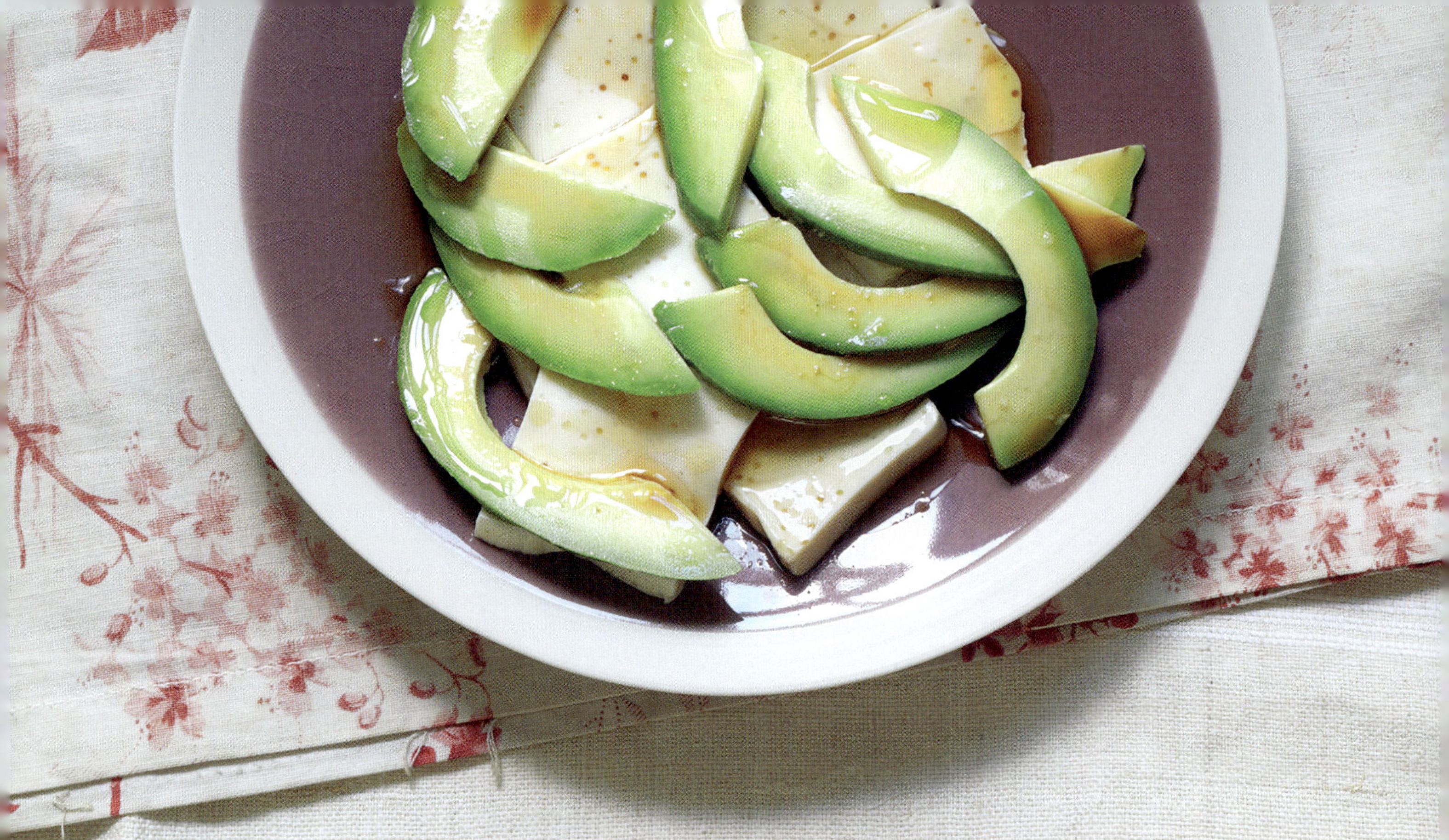

Fuchsia Dunlop's SILKEN TOFU WITH AVOCADO

200g (7oz) silken tofu
2 tablespoons light or tamari soy sauce, diluted with
1 tablespoon water
Hint of wasabi paste *(optional)*
½ teaspoon sesame oil
½ perfectly ripe avocado, *sliced*

Energy 134 kcal/555 kJ
Protein 9.0g
Fat 9.8g
Sat. Fat 1.6g
Carbohydrate 2.4g
Fibre 1.1g

This has a surprising flavour – Fuchsia says there is a 'delicate sympathy between the tender tofu and the ripe, buttery avocado'. The result is a perfect combination of refreshing and soothing. This is good for protein and vitamin E.

Serves 2 (generous portions)

Turn the block of silken tofu out onto a serving dish. Cut the block into ½–1 cm slices, then push down gently so the slices lean towards one end of the dish.

Pour over the diluted soy sauce (with wasabi stirred in, if you wish) and sesame oil. Top with the avocado and serve immediately.

Jekka McVicar's PANNA

300g (10½oz) spinach leaves, *washed*
1 onion, *finely chopped*
2 sprigs of tarragon, *leaves removed and chopped*
1 bunch of flat-leaf parsley, *finely chopped*
2 hard-boiled eggs, *peeled and quartered*
1 can sardines in olive oil **(88g (3oz)** drained weight)
1 can anchovy fillets in olive oil **(30g (1oz)** drained weight)
60g (2oz) unsalted butter
Freshly grated nutmeg

Energy 251 kcal/1040 kJ
Protein 13.5g
Fat 20.3g
Sat. Fat 9.8g
Carbohydrate 4.4g
Fibre 2.8g

'My mother inherited this dish from her mother Ruth Lowinsky who passed it onto me. Until I wrote this down I have never followed a particular recipe; it is one of those dishes that once you have the main ingredients – fish, spinach, egg and French tarragon – you can adapt to suit your palate or to work with what's in your cupboards.' *Jekka McVicar*

This dish is highly nutritious, providing good sources of beta-carotene, calcium and vitamins D and E.

Serves 4 (generous portions), served on toast

Put the spinach in a large saucepan over a medium heat. Gently stir until it has wilted and collapsed down. Strain the spinach into a colander and press out as much of the excess moisture as you can.

Put all the remaining ingredients, except the nutmeg, in a food-processor, then add the still-warm spinach. Pulse a few times. Make sure you don't over-process it, the texture is better if not too fine.

Grate in the nutmeg to taste, stir well, then put into a small dish. Cover and keep in the fridge until needed.

POTTED CHEESE

200g (7oz) hard cheese, *grated*
100g (3½oz) unsalted butter
2 tablespoons sherry, wine, cider or beer (anything you like, basically)
Grating of nutmeg
Freshly ground black pepper

Energy 359 kcal/1484 kJ
Protein 12.7g
Fat 33.6g
Sat. Fat 21.2g
Carbohydrate 0.3g
Fibre 0g

This is a very old recipe, useful if you have odd bits of cheese hanging around. It will keep for several weeks in the fridge and can be eaten cold, spread straight from the fridge, but also makes a good cheese on toast. Cheese is a good source of protein and calcium, with extra energy from the butter.

Serves 4 (generous portions)

Put the cheese, 75g (2½oz) of the butter and your alcohol of choice in a blender and blitz until smooth – you can also do this by pounding in a bowl. Season with pepper and a grating of nutmeg, then pile into an earthenware pot or similar.

Melt the remaining butter in a saucepan and strain off the solids. Pour over the cheese mixture and chill.

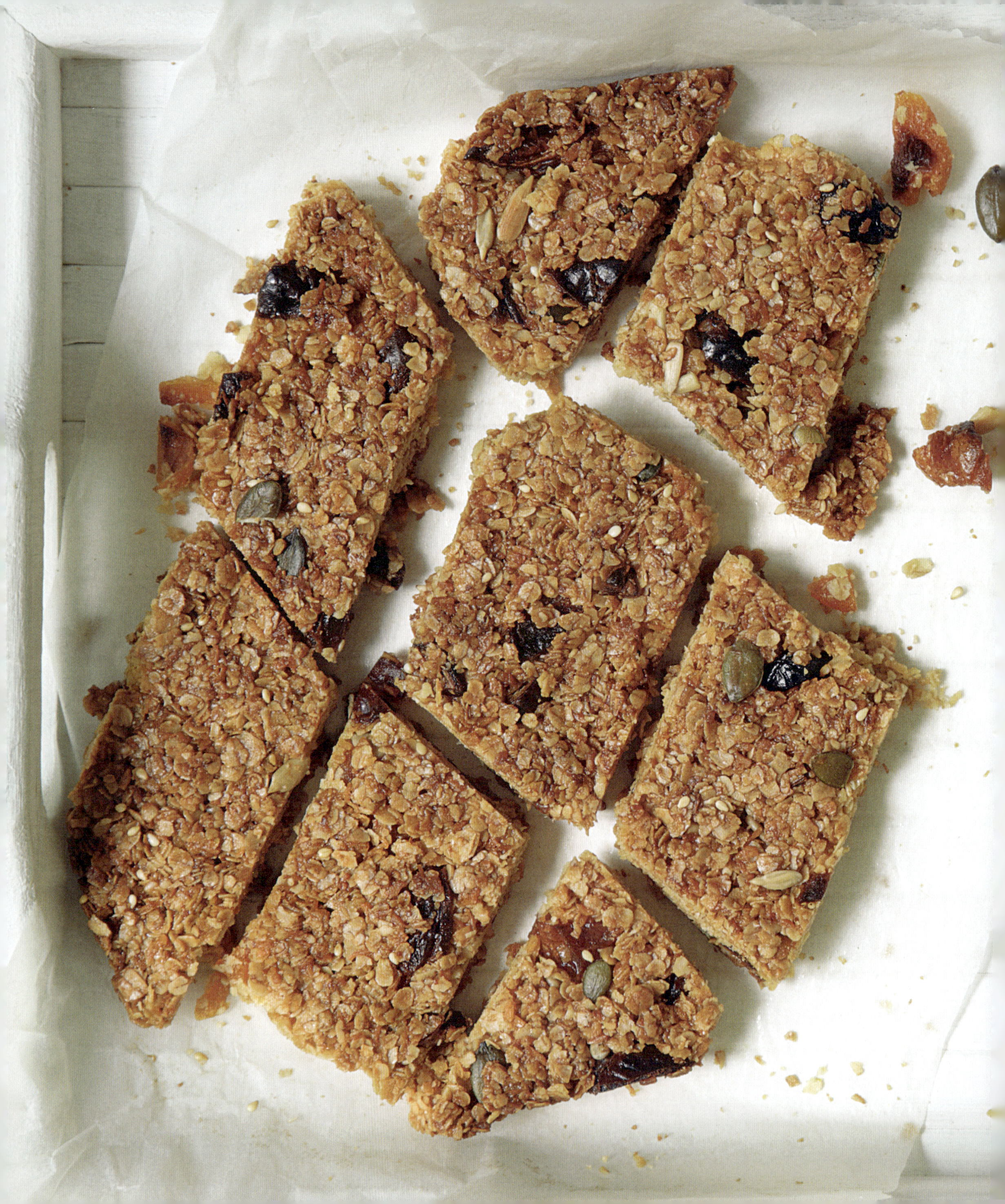

DATE AND MAPLE SYRUP FLAPJACKS

200g (7oz) unsalted butter
200g (7oz) honey or maple syrup
200g (7oz) pitted dates
450g (16oz) porridge oats
50g (2oz) desiccated coconut

Energy 184 kcal/772 kJ
Protein 2.6g
Fat 9.8g
Sat. Fat 5.5g
Carbohydrate 22.8g
Fibre 2.3g

This makes quite a soft flapjack, hopefully with no sharp edges. You can add different kinds of dried fruit or seeds, such as pumpkin, sunflower or sesame if you want to. An ideal snack for extra energy and some dietary fibre. The addition of seeds is an excellent way to add vitamin E.

Makes 24 small squares

Preheat the oven to 180°C/gas mark 4/350°F. Line a baking tin (about 20 x 30cm/ 8 x 11¾in) with baking parchment.

Put the butter in a saucepan with the honey or maple syrup and dates. Melt together, smashing the dates into the butter and honey with the back of a wooden spoon. Stir in the porridge oats and coconut.

Pile the mixture into the tin and press down firmly. Bake in the oven for 20–25 minutes. Remove from the oven and after a few minutes, cut into squares. Leave to cool in the tin until firm, then transfer to a cooling rack. Store in an airtight container.

TIP

- Flapjacks can be frozen – refresh after defrosting by putting in a hot oven for a couple of minutes, then when completely cool, store in an airtight container for up to a week.

MILKSHAKES

A lot of people have a nostalgic fondness for milkshakes but rarely make them, which is a shame because they're a cinch to make and the kids love them too. These are about indulgence – for really healthy, fruitier drinks, look to some of the smoothies and lassis on pages 62–63.

The first few recipes are high-energy, high-protein drinks and are an excellent way to supplement meals, especially if you find it difficult to eat. Nutritionally, they are the equivalent of a small meal but the best way to take these is to drink them between meals to boost intake and help weight gain (if that is what you need). They all contain protein, vitamins and minerals, particularly calcium.

The method for all of these is exactly the same – put in the blender and blitz. You can vary the amount of milk depending on how thick you want the milkshake to be. All recipes serve 1.

Malted Milkshake

1 large scoop of vanilla ice cream
1 heaped **teaspoon** malt extract
250ml (8½fl oz) full-fat milk

A jar of malt extract is good to have in the storecupboard, not least because eating a teaspoon of it at intervals is a sweet but nutritious pick-me-up. Here it's combined with vanilla, but you could use chocolate instead.

Energy 271 kcal/1130 kJ **Protein** 10.4g **Fat** 15.6g
Sat. Fat 9.9g **Carbohydrate** 23g **Fibre** 0g

Banana and Maple Milkshake

1 large scoop of vanilla ice cream
2 tablespoons maple syrup
1 ripe banana, *peeled*
250ml (8½fl oz) full-fat milk

This milkshake is almost banoffee-ish. You could use the banana ice-cream recipe on page 152 for this milkshake instead of using vanilla ice cream and a ripe banana.

Energy 445 kcal/1861 kJ **Protein** 11.6g **Fat** 16.0g
Sat. Fat 10.0g **Carbohydrate** 66.5g **Fibre** 1.5g

Chocolate and Peanut Butter Milkshake

1 large scoop of chocolate ice cream
2 tablespoons smooth peanut butter
250ml (8½fl oz) full-fat milk

A delicious combination that provides an excellent high energy shake.

Energy 453 kcal/1884 kJ **Protein** 17.2g **Fat** 31.2g
Sat. Fat 13.8g **Carbohydrate** 27.1g **Fibre** 1.6g

ICED TEA, TWO WAYS

Some teas can be a bit harsh on the taste buds because of the tannins they contain. In summer, if you want a refreshing drink this is a lovely way to infuse any kind of tea, which will pretty much eliminate the harshness.

Take a clean bottle. Put in it a pinch of your favourite tea – alternatively, you can just use a teabag. Cover with approx. 1 litre (34fl oz) of cold water. Leave in the fridge for a few hours or overnight to infuse. The flavour will be light and refreshing, with no need to sweeten.

You can also do this with coffee – using a coarsely ground coffee – but you will need to strain it.

Traditional Iced Tea

To make a sweetened iced tea, make a jugful of your favourite tea by pouring freshly boiled water over your tea or teabag of choice. Leave to steep until it is as strong as you like it. You can also add citrus zest and herbs such as mint at this stage, too. Add your desired amount of sugar or honey when the tea is still hot so it will dissolve easily. Chill in the fridge and serve over ice.

Fruity Iced Tea

For a lovely summer drink, you can blend iced tea with fruit juice. Popular combinations include cranberry juice, cherry juice or peach. Use equal quantities of tea and juice.

Energy 75 kcal/317 kJ **Protein** 3.5g **Fat** 1.0g
Sat. Fat 0.1g **Carbohydrate** 13.8g **Fibre** 0g

A SOPORIFIC HOT DRINK

This is an excellent bedtime drink, being fortified hot milk. Simply add a heaped teaspoon of honey, a pinch of turmeric and a pinch of cinnamon to a cup of milk. Heat gently until the honey has dissolved and the milk is almost boiling. Add a nip of whisky or rum if you like, but always check first that you are able to take alcohol.

Energy 188 kcal/783 kJ **Protein** 8.5g **Fat** 10g
Sat. Fat 6.3g **Carbohydrate** 17.4g **Fibre** 0g

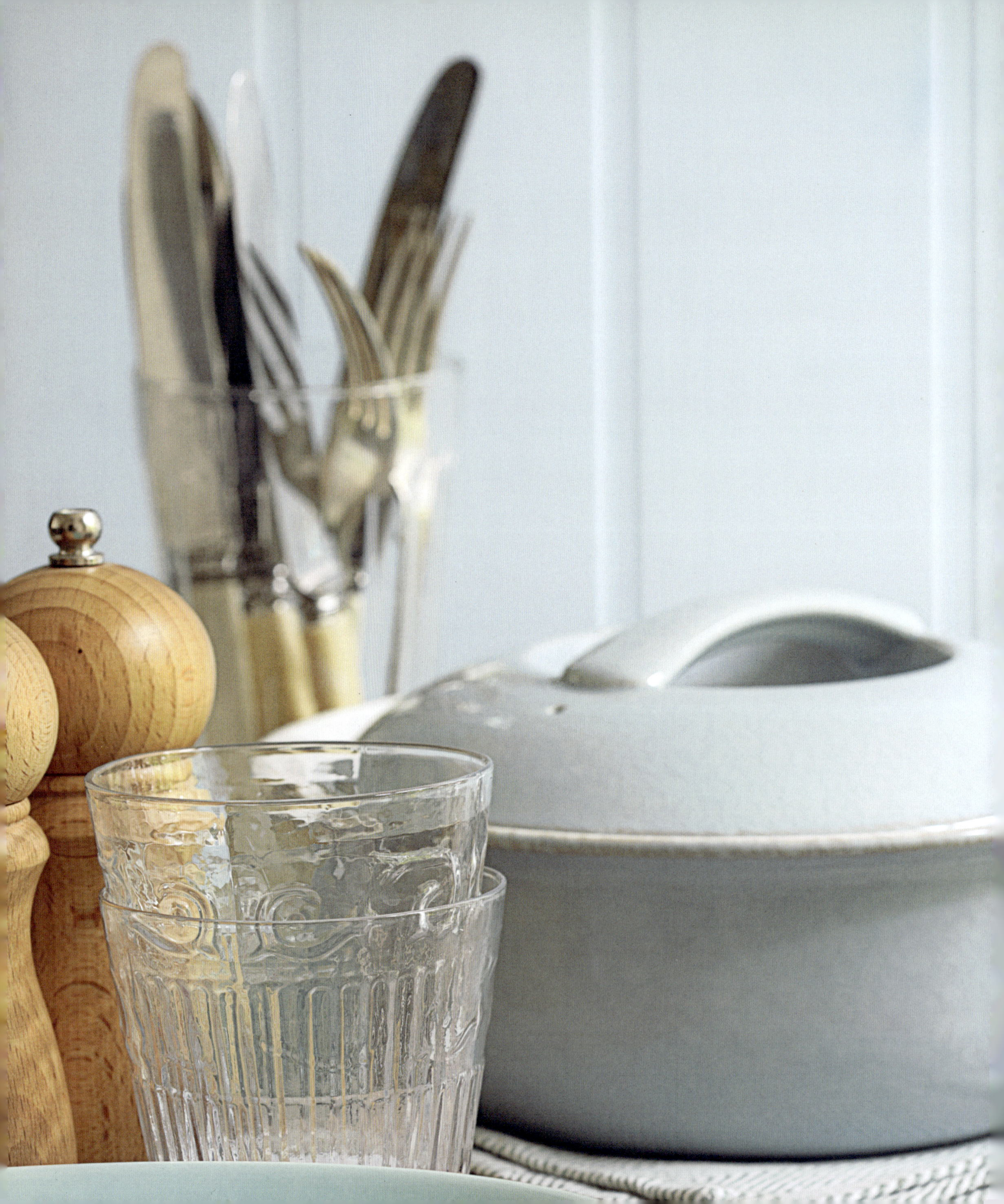

AFTER TREATMENT RECIPES

These recipes are aimed at those who are eating well, trying to lose weight or don't want to gain extra weight. These recipes can be eaten by friends and family too, as healthy eating should be encouraged for everyone!

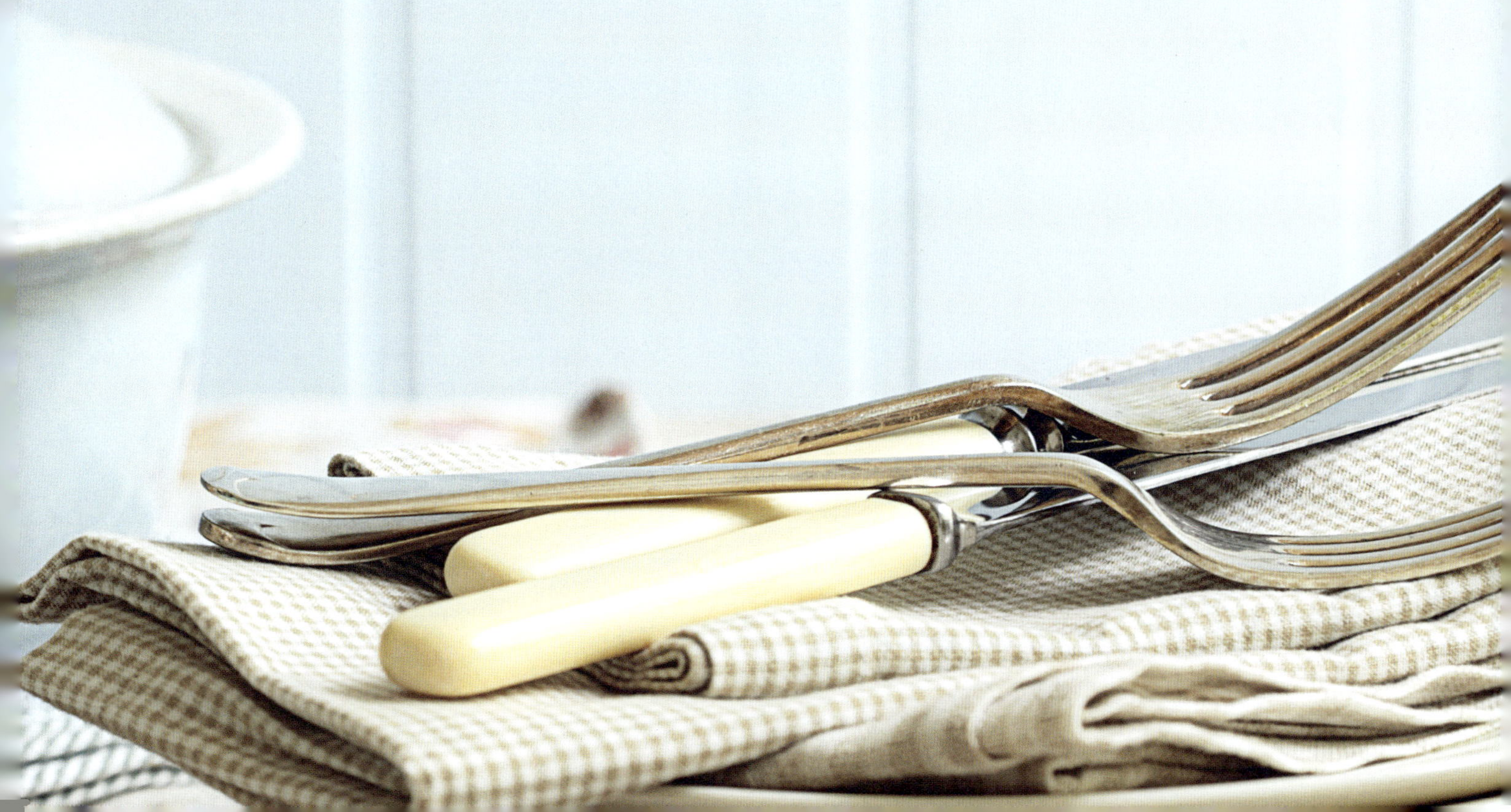

BREAKFASTS

Having a good breakfast is an ideal way to set yourself up for the day. Start the day with some fruit or fruit juice. Here are some ideas:

- Wholegrain cereals served with skimmed or semi-skimmed milk, or low fat yogurt
- Porridge made with oats or congee (rice) – add fresh fruit such as berries and bananas or dried fruit, such as raisins, apricots and pears
- Dried fruit compôte flavoured with cinnamon sticks
- Fresh fruit salad
- Fresh fruit compôte served with low-fat yogurt or fromage frais – add a sprinkling of granola, nuts or seeds

If you fancy a cooked breakfast, then choose one portion of cooked meat or egg and serve with vegetables such as grilled or baked tomatoes, baked mushrooms (toss in a small amount of olive oil before baking in a hot oven for about 15 minutes), baked beans or spiced cooked vegetables (Indian style) for a tasty, lower fat choice.

Poached or boiled eggs served with wholemeal bread.

Scrambled egg made in a non-stick pan with a small amount of butter or oil.

Bircher muesli (see opposite) – make in bulk and store in the fridge for an easy nutritious breakfast. Before serving add cream or full-fat Greek yogurt, as well as fresh or dried fruit such as blueberries, mangoes or bananas. Always use fresh milk or yogurt and make a fresh batch every 2–3 days.

BIRCHER MUESLI

125g (4½oz) porridge oats
2 tablespoons wheatgerm
Large pinch of ground cinnamon
50g (2oz) dried fruit, *roughly chopped – dates, apricots, prunes or anything you like*
250ml (8½fl oz) apple juice
2 eating apples, *peeled or unpeeled and cored*
100ml (3½fl oz) yogurt *(full-fat or low-fat)*

To serve
Handful of chopped nuts or seeds *(optional)*
Drizzle of runny honey or maple syrup

Nutritional information for recipe made with full-fat yogurt
Energy 422 kcal/1788 kJ
Protein 15.4g
Fat 11.6g
Sat. Fat 1.7g
Carbohydrate 68.6g
Fibre 9.4g

Bircher muesli was invented by Dr Bircher-Benner, a Swiss doctor, as a suitable breakfast for his patients. Over a hundred years later this dish is still recognised as a highly nutritious start to the day and would also be ideal as a snack. The oats have a low glycaemic index (GI) due to the presence of soluble fibre, so the starchy carbohydrate is absorbed slowly. The mix of fruit and nuts provides folate and iron, and the wheatgerm provides more than double the recommended amount of vitamin E in just one serving. Many people find apple skin difficult to digest – if you are one of them, peel the apples before grating them.

Serves 3

Put the oats, wheatgerm, cinnamon and dried fruit in a bowl and pour over the apple juice. Mix well and cover. Refrigerate overnight, or for a few hours if you aren't eating this first thing.

When you are ready to eat, grate in the apples and stir in the yogurt. Sprinkle with nuts or seeds, if using, and drizzle with either honey or maple syrup.

A Tropical Variation

Add some fresh grated coconut or 2 tablespoons of desiccated coconut along with the oats instead of the wheatgerm and use dried dates and/or sticky, semi-dried bananas. Grate in some nutmeg instead of cinnamon. You can still serve with grated apples or pears, but you could also finely dice some pineapple or mango instead. This is good with coconut yogurt, too.

HOMEMADE GRANOLA

250g (9oz) jumbo oats
50g (2oz) desiccated coconut
100g (3½oz) nuts, *lightly crushed*
Pinch of salt
2 tablespoons coconut oil
150g (5½oz) runny honey
1 free-range egg white
200g (7oz) mixed dried fruit – *raisins, sultanas, chopped dates, apricots or anything you like*

Nutritional information for granola:
Energy 255 kcal/1074 kJ
Protein 5.4g
Fat 10.4g
Sat. Fat 4.5g
Carbohydrate 37.3g
Fibre 3.1g

Nutritional information per granola bar:
Energy 286 kcal/1201 kJ
Protein 5.5g
Fat 13.8g
Sat. Fat 6.6g
Carbohydrate 37.3g
Fibre 3.1g

This recipe can be a springboard for endless variations, as it is entirely up to you what kind of fruit or nuts you use. I especially like almonds and pecans and always include dried dates – but you can try anything, including some of the more tropical dried fruits, such as mango, papaya and pineapple. Just make sure whatever you use is cut into small pieces, roughly the size of a large raisin. You can use any kind of oil here, but coconut oil has a great flavour. Eat as a breakfast cereal with milk or yogurt, or eat dry handfuls as a snack.

Makes around 800g (29oz) / Serves 12

Preheat the oven to 150°C/gas mark 2/300°F. Line a large baking tray with baking parchment.

Mix the oats, coconut, nuts and salt together in a large bowl. Put the coconut oil and honey in a saucepan and whisk over a gentle heat until liquid and combined. Pour this over the oat mixture and stir thoroughly, trying to make sure everything is coated – it should resemble raw flapjack mix.

Whisk the egg white until slightly aerated but still very liquid. Pour this over the other ingredients and stir to coat. Spread the mixture over the baking tray in an even layer. Bake for about 30–35 minutes. Check halfway through and turn the tray round if necessary. The granola will be done when it is a light golden brown and dry to the touch.

Remove from the oven and leave in the baking tray to cool. Break up into pieces – you will find some of the mixture will crumble, but it should all be crisp. Add the dried fruit and store in an airtight container.

To turn into a granola bar:

Preheat the oven to 180°C/gas mark 4/350°F. Line a straight-sided baking tin (approx. 20 x 30cm / 8 x 11¾in) with baking parchment.

Follow the above recipe, but either double the amount of oil or add 50g (2oz) butter. Mix thoroughly and pile into the baking tin. Spread out evenly and press down firmly. Bake for about 20–25 minutes until golden brown. Remove the tin from the oven. After 3–4 minutes, while the mixture is still soft, score into bars. When it is completely cold, follow the scored lines to cut into bars. Store in an airtight container.

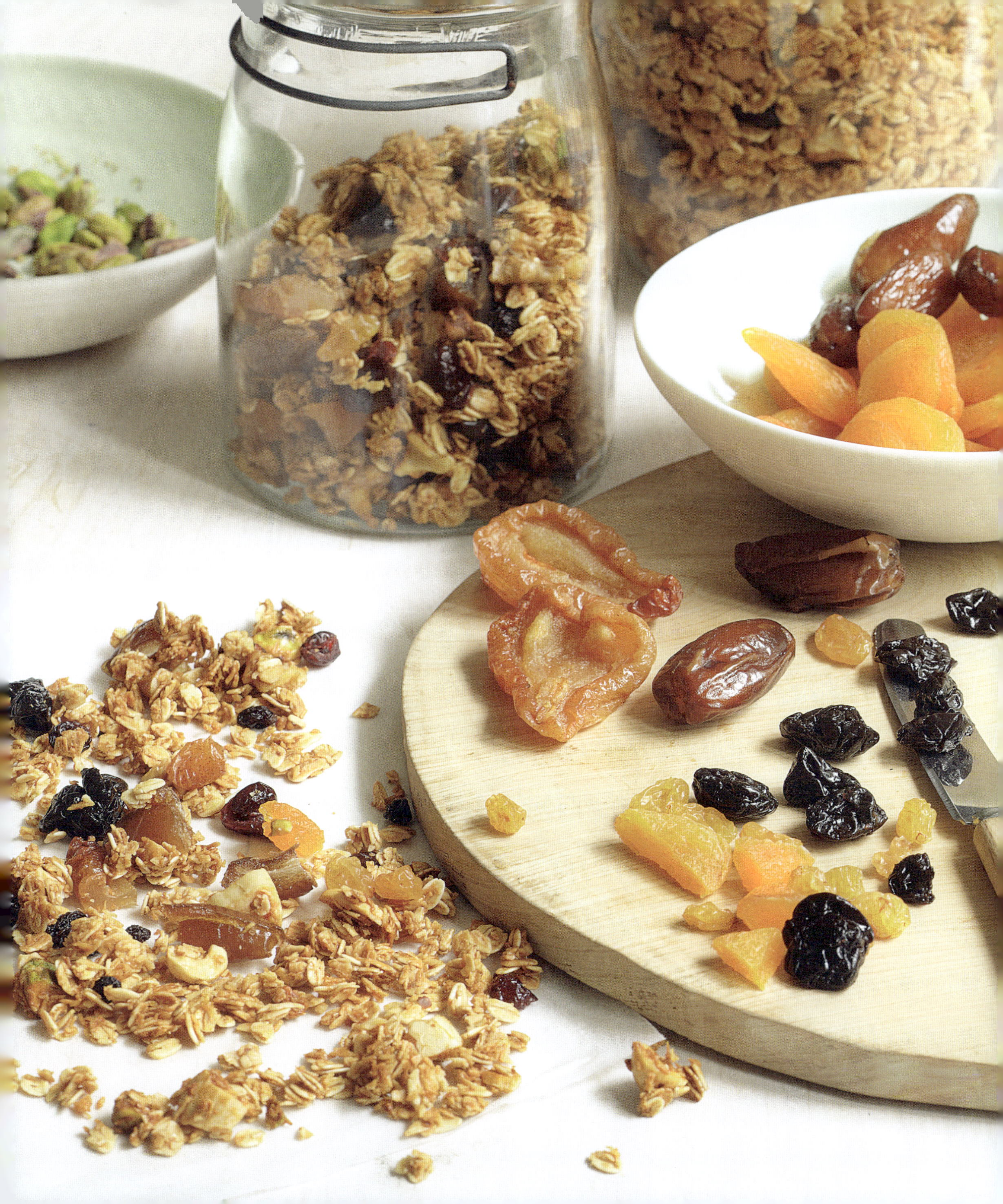

MULTIGRAIN SEEDED BREAD

500g (17⅔oz) multigrain flour
100g (3½oz) seed mix *(sunflower, flax, sesame, etc.)*
1 tablespoon malt extract
7g (¼oz) sachet fast-action yeast
1 teaspoon salt

Nutritional information for ⅛ of recipe:
Energy 262 kcal/1110 kJ
Protein 9.7g
Fat 7.2g
Sat. Fat 1.1g
Carbohydrate 47.9g
Fibre 3.3g

For this bread, use either the quantities given below or 600g (21oz) of a seeded multigrain flour – there are several available. You also don't have to use a seed mix for this, you can tailor-make your own. I think some of the smaller seeds work best, such as sunflower, sesame, poppy and flax. Adding seeds into bread does increase the fat content due to the oil contained within the seeds, but they are an excellent source of vitamins, especially vitamin E. Iron, zinc and calcium are also provided in good amounts.

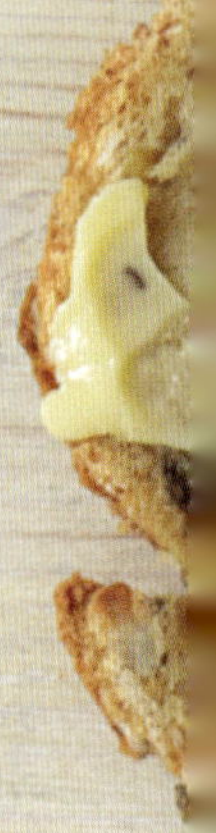

Put the flour and seed mix in a large bowl or stand mixer. Dissolve the malt extract into 300ml (10fl oz) warm water. Sprinkle the yeast into the flour, give it quick stir so it is well coated, then add the salt.

Either make a well in the flour, or start the motor of the stand mixer. Gradually stir in the water and malt extract and combine into a fairly soft, sticky dough. If it seems too dry and stiff, add more water, a very little at a time.

Cover the dough with a damp tea towel or lightly oiled cling film and leave to rest for half an hour. Knead the dough until smooth, elastic and no longer sticky. This will take around 5 minutes with a dough hook, double the time if kneading by hand. Put the dough in a bowl and cover with oiled clingfilm or a damp tea towel again. If possible, leave somewhere warm to rise until it is double the volume. This will take up to about 2 hours, longer if it is kept quite cool.

Turn the bread out onto a lightly floured work surface and knead lightly into an oblong loaf shape if using a tin, or into a round if baking on a tray. Put into a 1kg loaf tin or a lightly floured tray. Cover with the clingfilm or tea towel.

Leave the bread to prove for around 30 minutes, then preheat the oven to 250°C/gas mark 8/475°F. When the bread is well risen again, put it in the oven and immediately lower the temperature to 220°C/gas mark 7/425°F. Bake for 30–35 minutes, until the bread has a good brown crust and is well risen. To make sure it is cooked through, tap on the bottom – it should sound hollow. Leave to cool on a rack.

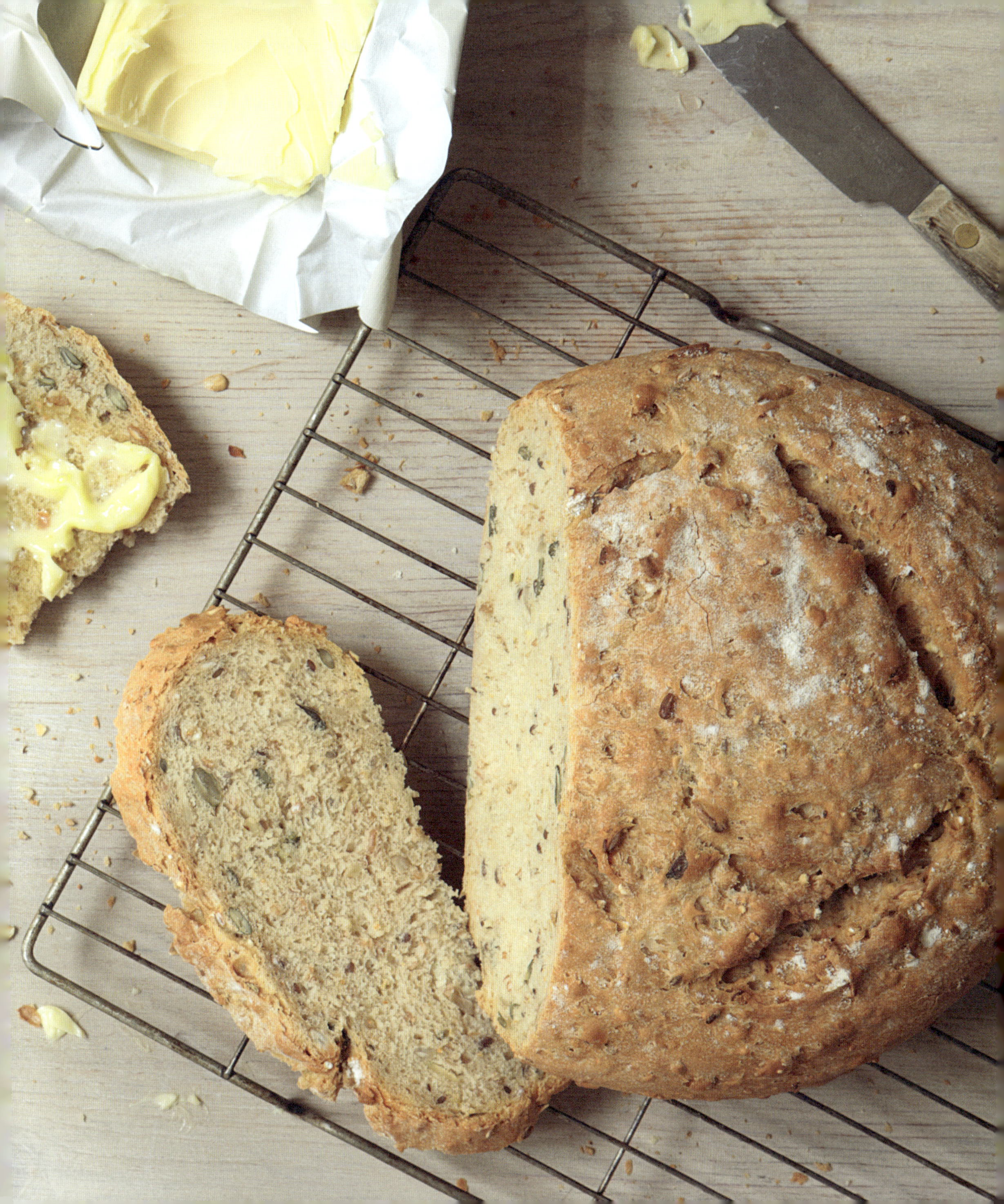

TURKISH EGGS

1 small garlic clove, *crushed*
75–100ml (2½–3½fl oz) low-fat Greek-style yogurt
2 very fresh free-range eggs
Large knob of unsalted butter
1 teaspoon cumin seeds
½ teaspoon paprika
¼ teaspoon chilli flakes
Handful of mint, dill or parsley leaves
Salt and freshly ground black pepper

Energy 290 kcal/1209 kJ
Protein 21.3g
Fat 19.4g
Sat. Fat 7.1g
Carbohydrate 9.1g
Fibre 0.8g

This is good served with flatbreads, especially the light ones on page 87. The quantities serve 1, but you can easily increase the proportions to serve as many as you like.

Mix the garlic with the yogurt and put in a shallow serving bowl. Bring a pan of water to the boil and stir it to make a whirlpool. Drop your eggs into it, turn down the heat and simmer for about 3 minutes. Drain thoroughly and place on top of the yogurt.

Melt the butter in a small frying pan. When it foams, remove from the heat, then sprinkle in the cumin seeds, paprika and chilli flakes.

Drizzle the spiced butter over the eggs and season with salt and pepper. Sprinkle over the herbs and serve immediately.

MASALA OMELETTE

1 teaspoon vegetable oil
2 spring onions, *sliced into rounds*
1 small piece ginger, *finely chopped*
1 garlic clove, *finely chopped*
1 mild red chilli, *finely chopped*
1 teaspoon cumin
½ teaspoon ground coriander
¼ teaspoon turmeric
Pinch of cinnamon
4 free-range eggs
Salt and freshly ground black pepper
Mint or coriander leaves, torn, *to serve*

This omelette is an excellent way to start the day as it contains lots of zingy ingredients to wake up the taste buds. You could swap the spices for garam masala or curry powder, if you wish; it's also the kind of recipe to which you could add any other cooked vegetables. Try a tablespoon of frozen peas, or some cooked and diced butternut squash. The eggs are a great high-protein food, providing good amounts of iron, selenium and vitamin D.

Serves 2, but you can easily double it up as required

Preheat the grill. Heat the vegetable oil in an omelette pan or fairly small frying pan. Add the spring onions, ginger, garlic and chilli. Sauté for a few minutes over a medium heat until softened. Sprinkle over the spices and cook for a further minute or two.

Beat the eggs in a bowl and season with salt and pepper. Pour them over the contents of the frying pan and swirl the pan around so that the eggs evenly coat the base of the pan. Cook for a couple of minutes until they have set and turned golden brown underneath, then put under the hot grill to brown the top. Serve immediately, sprinkled with herbs.

Energy 205 kcal/853 kJ **Protein** 16.2g **Fat** 15.4g
Sat. Fat 4.0g **Carbohydrate** 1.6g **Fibre** 0.4g

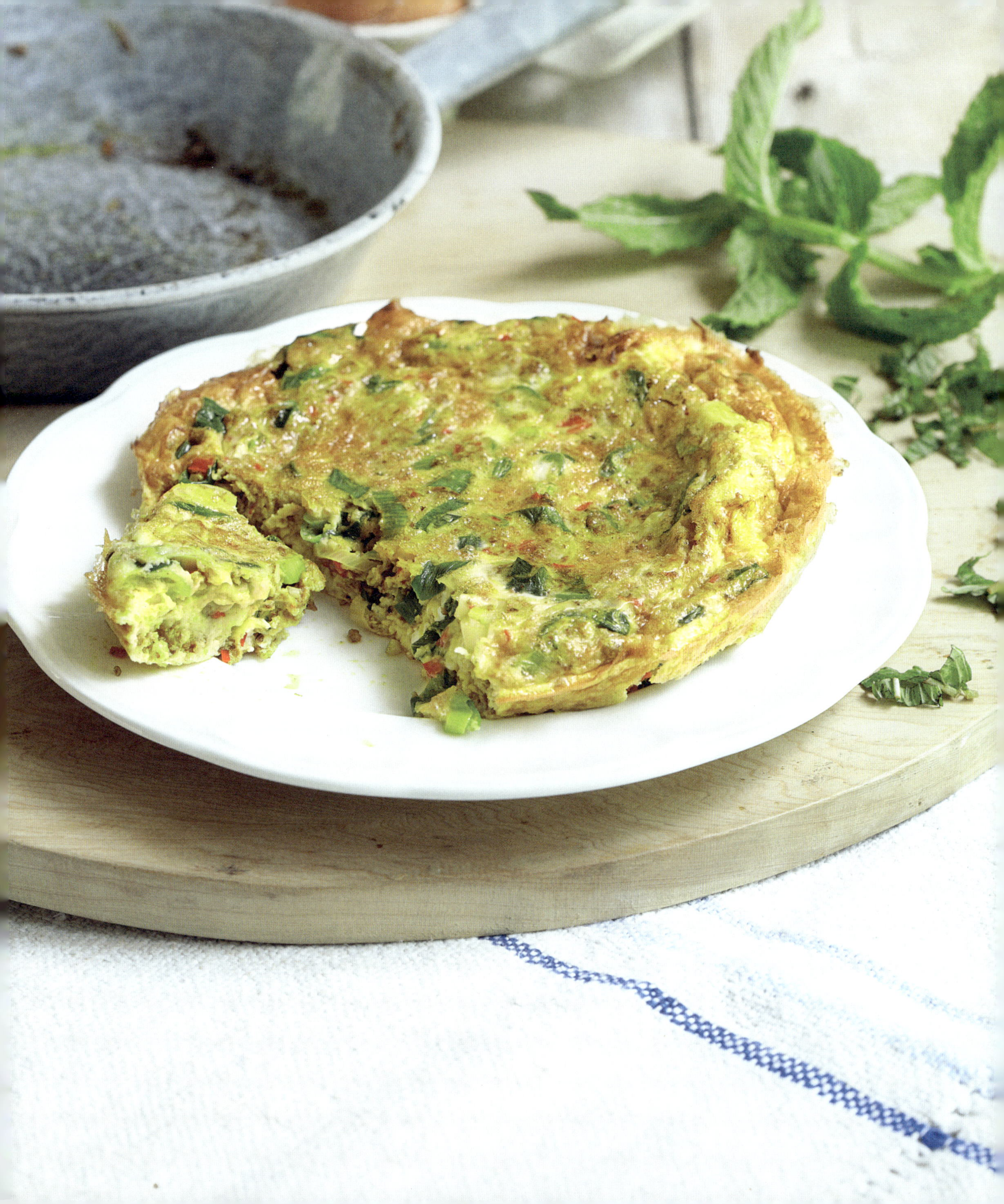

LIGHT MEALS

This is a great opportunity to eat vegetables or salad as part of your overall daily intake. There are lots of ideas for light meals in the treatment section, too (see page 66) – just choose lean meat, oily fish and lower fat cheeses or watch the portion size to adapt these recipes for healthy eating. Pulses are a good choice – think of baked beans or mixed bean salads. If you are trying to lose weight then limit dressings, pickles and sauces, as these can be high in fat.

Quick and easy salads – serve with fresh bread, jacket potatoes, brown rice, pasta, quinoa or couscous. Use a variety of salad leaves to add different flavours and textures. Add roasted sunflower seeds or pine kernels. Use balsamic vinegar, other flavoured vinegars and lemon juice to add flavour. These are ideal for a packed lunch, if you have a fridge to store them.

- Mozzarella with cherry tomatoes, olive oil and basil leaves – serve with leaves or rocket
- Feta cheese with tomato and cucumber
- Smoked mackerel or smoked salmon
- Salad Niçoise (tuna, tomatoes, beans, hard-boiled eggs, cooked new potatoes and salad leaves) – serve with an olive oil and white wine vinegar, add Dijon mustard for extra flavour
- Poached salmon or prawns
- Avocado with tomatoes and leaves
- Caesar salad
- Mixed beans – used canned beans and rinse well before use
- Roasted butternut squash with edamame beans
- Slow-roasted tomatoes with rocket and goat's cheese
- Grilled halloumi cheese with pesto or an olive oil, lime and coriander dressing
- Oven-roasted vegetables

Snacks on toast, with pitta bread or sandwiches. Choose different types of bread, such as sourdough or rye. Choose wholemeal bread, if possible, for extra vitamins and flavour. Salad ingredients provide extra colour and vitamins. For a packed lunch it may be better to carry salad ingredients separately and add them to the sandwich at the last minute.

- Chicken and salad
- Salmon, tuna or prawns with salad
- Lean meat, such as beef or pork, with salad
- Hummus or tzatziki with crunchy vegetables
- Brie, Edam or Gouda with salad
- Hard-boiled egg sliced with tomatoes or cucumber

Stir-fried vegetables. Add chicken, pork, fish, prawns or roasted cashew nuts as a source of protein. Use a combination of the following to add flavour: garlic, grated root ginger, sesame seeds, sesame oil, soy sauce, lemon and chilli. Serve with noodles or rice.

Baked potato or sweet potato with butter and a variety of easy toppings, such as baked beans, a small portion of cheese, tuna (canned in spring water), ratatouille and tuna and sweetcorn with a small portion of mayonnaise.

CREAM OF TOMATO WITH LENTILS AND VEGETABLES

1 tablespoon olive oil
1 onion, *diced*
2 sticks of celery, *diced*
2 large carrots, *diced*
1 leek, *diced*
1 large sweet potato, or **300g (10½oz)** butternut squash, *peeled and diced*
½ a small celeriac, *peeled and diced* (about **200g (7oz)** weight)
2 teaspoons fennel seeds, *ground*
½ teaspoon turmeric
Pinch of ground cinnamon
2 garlic cloves, *finely chopped*
50g (2oz) red lentils
1.2 litres (40fl oz) hot vegetable or chicken stock
400g (14oz) can chopped tomatoes
Handful of basil leaves, *shredded*
Salt and freshly ground black pepper

Energy 216 kcal/912 kJ
Protein 8.0g
Fat 4.6g
Sat. Fat 0.6g

The cream of tomato soup that comes in a can is a great standby, obviously, but if you want something a bit more nutritious, try this. Despite the title, if you can't handle tomatoes miss them out, or, even better, replace them with greens – spinach, chard and even peas! You will still have a lovely creamy, easy-to-eat lentil and vegetable soup. This is exceptionally high in beta-carotene and a good source of folate and lycopene. Serve with a slice of fresh wholemeal bread for extra fibre and B vitamins.

Serves 4

Heat the olive oil in a large saucepan. Add the onion, celery, carrots, leek, sweet potato or squash and celeriac, and sauté over a high heat, stirring regularly, until the vegetables start to brown slightly around the edges and give off a sweet aroma.

Add the spices and garlic, and sauté for a further 2 minutes. Add the red lentils and pour over the stock. Season with salt and pepper. Simmer for 10 minutes.

Add the tomatoes, if using, and simmer for a further 15–20 minutes until the vegetables and red lentils are completely soft. Add the basil and let it wilt into the soup. Remove from the heat. Purée the soup until smooth. Taste for seasoning and adjust if necessary.

TIP

- This recipe will freeze well – a good one for batch cooking.

Raymond Blanc's VEGETABLE AND CHERVIL SOUP

'Façon Maman Blanc'

1 tablespoon unsalted butter
1 medium onion, *finely chopped*
1 garlic clove, *finely chopped*
2 large carrots, *finely sliced*
2 medium leeks, *outer leaves removed, cut into 1cm slices*
3 sticks of celery, *sliced into 5mm lengths*
1 large courgette, *cut in half lengthways and into 5mm slices*
2 ripe tomatoes, *cut into quarters and roughly chopped*
1 tablespoon unsalted butter, *(or soured cream)*
Large handful of chervil, *finely chopped*
Salt and freshly ground white pepper

Nutritional information for soup before butter or soured cream added:
Energy 95 kcal/397 kJ
Protein 3.7g
Fat 4.1g
Sat. Fat 2.2g
Carbohydrate 11.6g
Fibre 5.8g

'A small tribute to "Maman Blanc", and I should say to "Papa Blanc" too, as most of the vegetables would come from his garden. This soup offers a multitude of flavours, varying according to the seasons. The choice of vegetables and herbs is completely yours. Chervil is one of my favourite herbs; it is very popular in French cuisine yet is little-known and little-used in Great Britain. You can also blend the soup for that delightful texture – a spoon of crème fraîche would always be welcome.' *Raymond Blanc*

Serves 4

Heat the butter in a large saucepan over a medium heat and add the onion, garlic, carrots, leeks and celery. Sweat for 5 minutes until soft and translucent. Season with salt and freshly ground white pepper.

Add 1 litre (34fl oz) of just-boiled water, the courgette and tomatoes, and boil for
5 minutes.

Whisk in the butter or soured cream (or even both!) and add the chervil. Taste and correct the seasoning if necessary. Serve to your guests.

TIP

- This will freeze but works better if blended, which means you could have two soups in one: a textured soup to start with, then blend and freeze the leftovers.

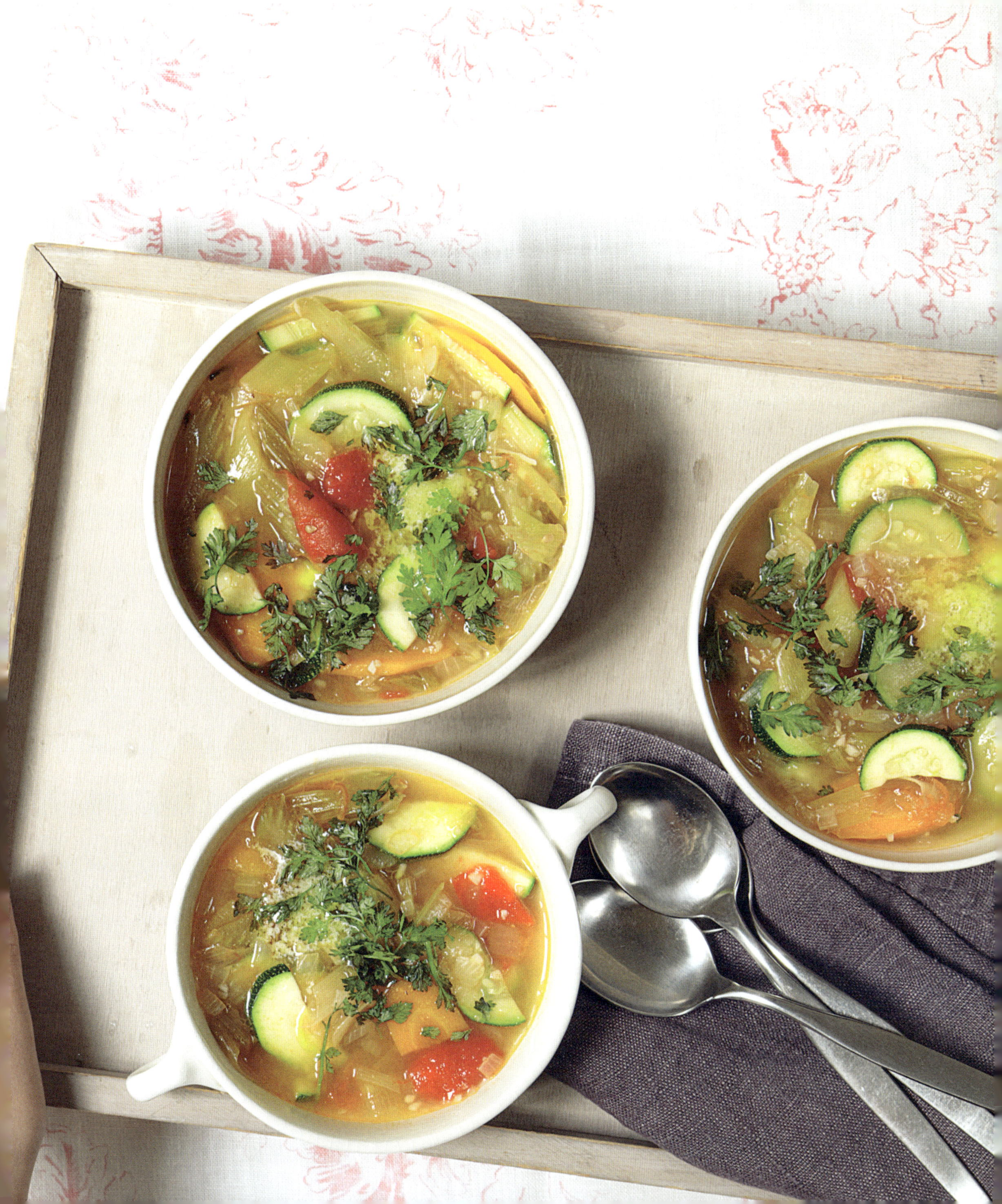

Mary McCartney's QUINOA, KALE AND BEAN SOUP

'A meal in a bowl, packed full of nutrition and very satisfying.'
Mary McCartney

This is an excellent, filling soup. The beans are low GI, so are absorbed slowly. The kale and carrots mean that this soup is packed with beta-carotene and vitamin E. Serve with wholemeal bread for extra B vitamins.

Serves 6

2 tablespoons olive oil
1 onion, *finely chopped*
3 shallots, *finely chopped*
2 large carrots, *finely diced*
2 celery sticks, *finely diced*
400g (14oz) can cannellini or other white beans (**240g (8½oz)** drained weight)
1 teaspoon dried mixed herbs
1 bay leaf
400g (14oz) can chopped tomatoes
1.5 litres (50fl oz) hot vegetable stock
50g (2oz) kale, *shredded*
60g (2½oz) quinoa, *well rinsed*
25g (¾oz) basil leaves
Salt and freshly ground black pepper

Heat the oil in a large saucepan. Add the onion, shallots, carrots and celery, and sauté over a medium heat for 5 minutes. Add the beans and cook for a further 2 minutes.

Add the herbs and tomatoes, then pour in the vegetable stock. Season with salt and pepper. Simmer for 20 minutes. Finally, add the kale and quinoa, and cook for a further 12–15 minutes until the quinoa is cooked through. Stir in the basil and serve immediately.

TIP

- This freezes very well, even with the kale. Omit the basil leaves and add after defrosting. Or simply add more basil leaves as a garnish once reheated.

Energy 227 kcal/958 kJ
Protein 12.1g
Fat 5.5g
Sat. Fat 0.8g
Carbohydrate 34.3g
Fibre 12.4g

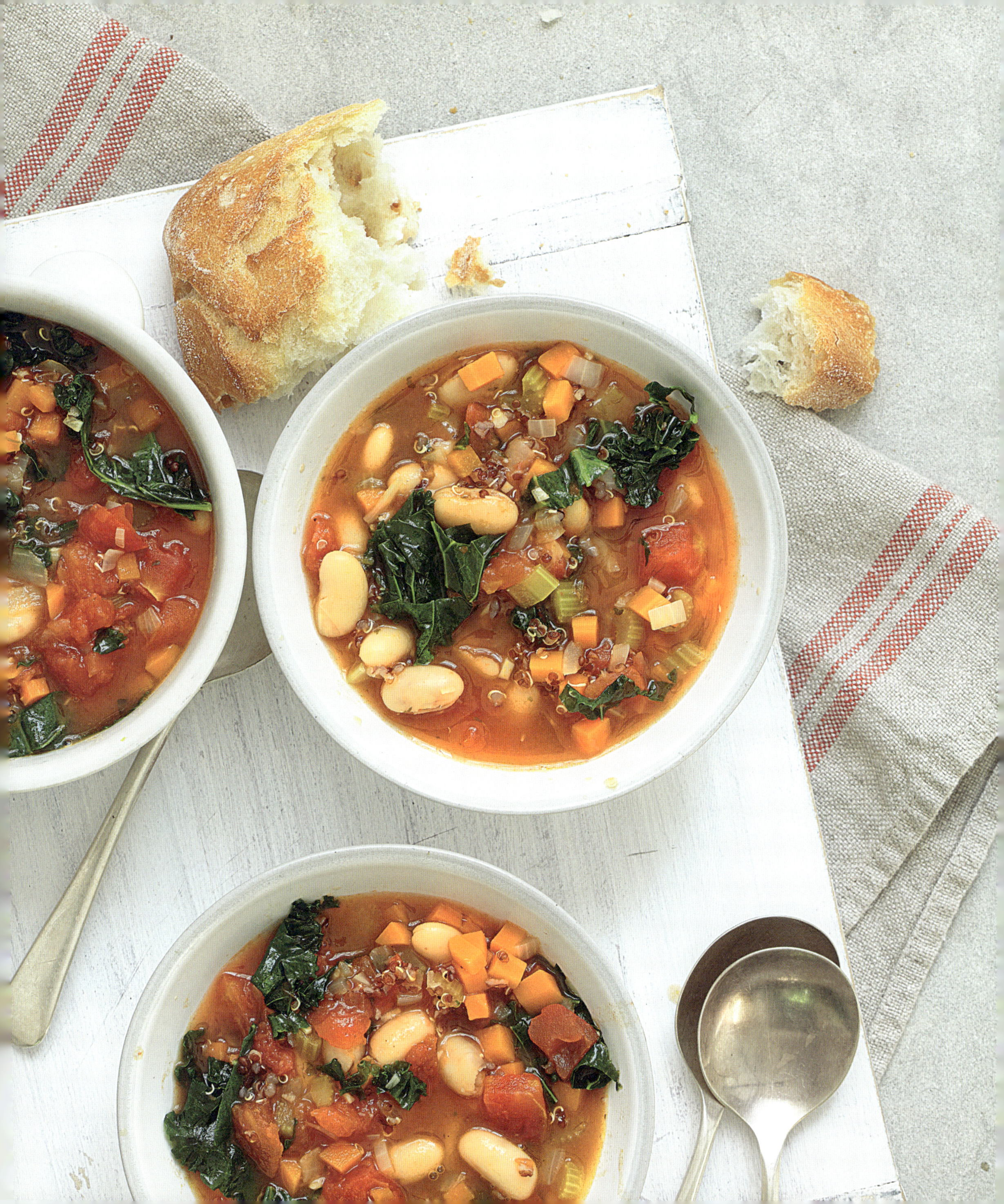

Sam Gates'

PEA AND PRAWN WONTONS IN A TASTY BROTH

20–25 wonton wrappers, *defrosted and covered with a damp tea towel*

For the wonton filling:
100g (3½oz) frozen petits pois, *defrosted*
180g (6⅓oz) raw king prawns, *chopped*
1 tablespoon finely chopped fresh chives
1 garlic clove, *crushed*
1 tablespoon dry sherry
1 tablespoon soy sauce
1 teaspoon fish sauce
1 teaspoon sesame oil

For the broth:
1.5 litres (50fl oz) good-quality hot chicken stock
3cm (1¼in) piece of fresh ginger, *peeled and finely chopped*
¼ fresh red chilli, *deseeded and finely chopped (optional)*
1 teaspoon brown sugar
200g (7oz) young green vegetables, *preferably a mixture of fine beans, mangetout or sugar snaps, all destringed and cut into bite-sized pieces*
1 tablespoon soy sauce
1 teaspoon sesame oil
1 tablespoon chopped fresh chives

'This soup is perfect for those trying times when you need external help to get things back on track. Not only does it look and smell gorgeous, all steamy, fragrant and rammed with fresh emerald-green veggies, but when the time comes to tuck in, the combination of soft parcels packed with peas and velvety prawns and feisty, rich broth is the perfect antidote to so-so days. Clear, chicken stock-based soups can taste a little bland, so this recipe uses ginger and chilli to add warmth and flavour. Most people relish the chilli content, but if you're dealing with more delicate tummies, you can happily leave it out without compromising on flavour. The ingredients list might seem long, but once you have prepared the filling, cooking time is less than 10 minutes. Make sure you lay out plenty of napkins – there will be a whole lot of slurping going on.' *Sam Gates*

Serves 4

Mash the defrosted peas with a potato masher so they break down but still have texture – you want a lumpy mush but not a purée. Mix with the other filling ingredients.

Pour a little cold water into a bowl.

Take a wonton wrapper and lay it out flat. Wet a finger from the bowl and trace the four edges of the wrapper. You need a thin, wet line all the way round to help to seal the wonton. Place 1 tablespoon of the filling in the centre, then take one corner of the wrapper and take it across to meet the opposite corner. Gently press the sides together so that you end up with a bulging triangle. Make sure there are no holes or the filling will leak out when it is cooking. Set the filled wonton aside and make the next one. Repeat with the rest of the wrappers, until you have used all of the filling mixture.

To make the broth, put the stock, ginger, chilli and sugar in a wide saucepan and bring to the boil. Turn the heat down to a good simmer, and very carefully slide the filled wontons into the stock, taking care to make sure they don't stick together. The best way is to gently drop them in a circle, separating them as you go. When they are all in, wave stock over the top of the dumplings so they don't dry out.

Energy 239 kcal/1003 kJ
Protein 17.8g
Fat 2.5g
Sat. Fat 0.3g
Carbohydrate 37.6g
Fibre 3.0g

Allow the pan to simmer for a further 2 minutes, and don't be alarmed if they blow up like balloons – they will deflate and tuck themselves nicely around the filling when you finish the cooking process.

Add the chopped vegetables and simmer for a further 2–3 minutes until they are cooked but still crunchy. Turn off the heat, stir through the soy sauce and sesame oil, sprinkle with chopped chives and serve in big bowls.

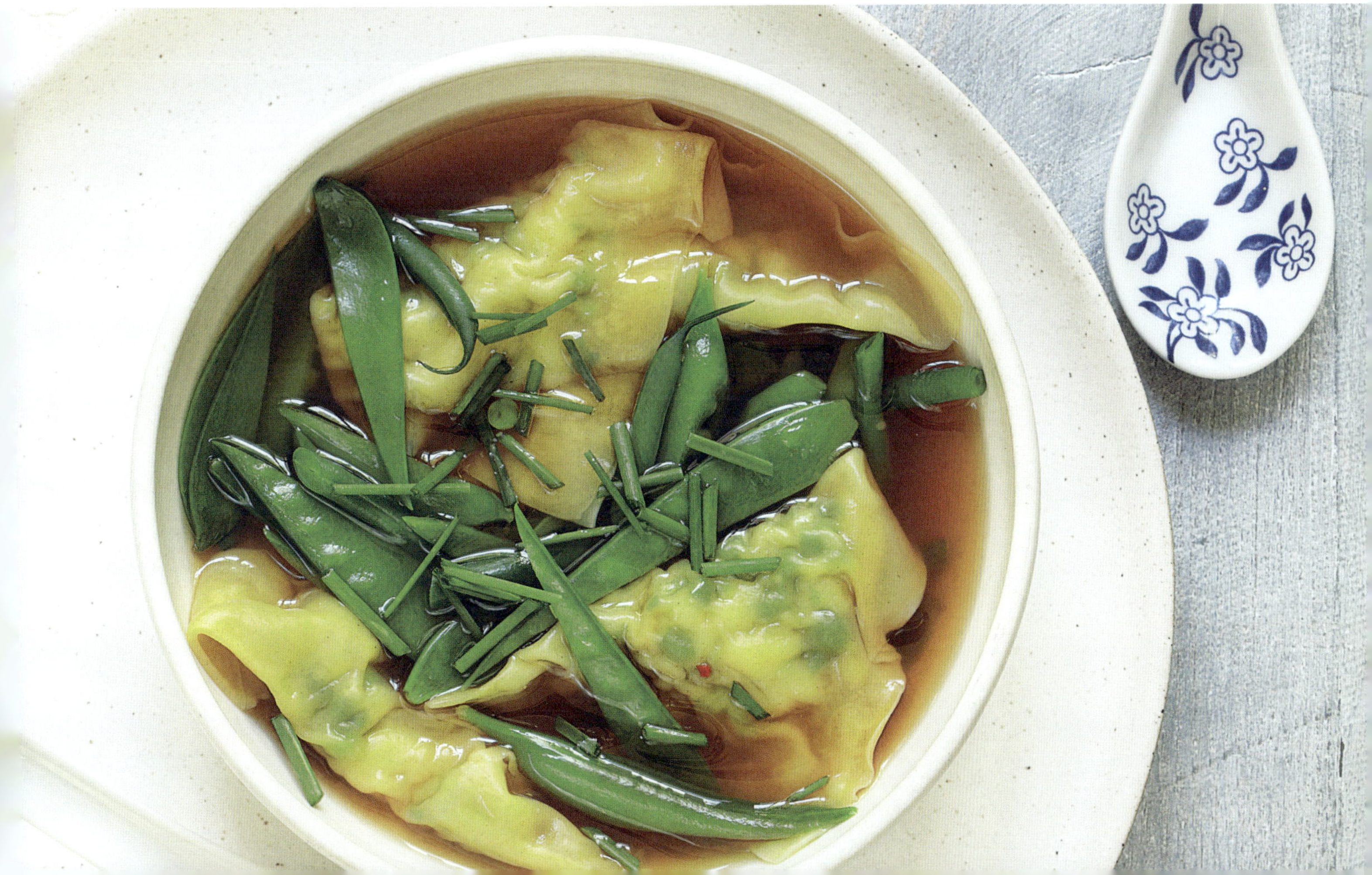

Ching He Huang's
STICKY HOISIN BROCCOLI AND PRAWNS WITH TOASTED ALMONDS

Prawns and sweet broccoli are tossed in a spicy orange and hoisin sauce, while toasted flaked almonds add a nutty bite. The trick is to char the broccoli in the wok to create smoky notes, as though it's been cooked on the barbecue. A satisfying dish perfect with added noodles (or rice), it also makes a great accompaniment to other sharing dishes.

Serves 2

150g (5½oz) wheat noodles (optional), to serve
1 teaspoon rapeseed oil
1 head of broccoli, broken into florets
handful of toasted almond flakes, to garnish
250g (9oz) cooked tiger prawns

For the sauce:
1 teaspoon freshly grated ginger
1 red chilli, deseeded and finely chopped
1 teaspoon golden syrup
zest and juice of ½ small orange
1 tablespoon hoisin sauce
1 tablespoon tamari or low-sodium light soy sauce
1 teaspoon toasted sesame oil
100ml (3½fl oz) cold vegetable stock
1 tablespoon cornflour

If you are adding wheat noodles, cook according to the packet instructions, and set aside.

Place all the sauce ingredients in a small jug and mix together to combine. Set aside.

Heat a wok over a high heat until smoking, then add the rapeseed oil. Once hot, add the broccoli florets and cook, stirring, for 1 minute, charring the edges slightly. Then add about 2 tablespoons water around the edges of the wok. This will create some steam to help cook the florets. Cook for another minute to bring the broccoli to an al dente texture.

Now pour in the sauce and stir, coating the broccoli florets well but taking care not to break them up. Bring the sauce to the boil and cook until glossy. Add the prawns and stir to warm through. If you are adding noodles, add them now and toss to warm through.

Finally, garnish with toasted almond flakes and serve immediately.

Nutritional information:
(including noodles and a handful almonds)
Energy 695 kcal/2907 kJ **Protein** 52g **Fat** 15g
Sat. Fat 1.8g **Carbohydrate** 97.3g **Fibre** 11.6g

WATERMELON GAZPACHO WITH FETA CREAM

For the gazpacho:
750g (26½oz) watermelon, *peeled and deseeded*
150ml (5fl oz) passata
2 very ripe tomatoes, *peeled and deseeded*
½ cucumber, *peeled, deseeded and diced*
2 celery sticks, *roughly chopped*
1 piece fresh ginger, *the size of a pound coin, grated*
1 red chilli, *chopped*
Juice of **1** lime
Handful of basil leaves
Handful of mint leaves
Salt and freshly ground black pepper

For the feta cream:
50g (2oz) feta cheese, *crumbled*
1 tablespoon crème fraîche
A few drops of lime juice

For the garnish:
Olive oil
Mint and basil leaves
Smoked paprika

This is a lovely variation on the traditional tomato gazpacho. The watermelon adds sweetness, which mellows the heat from the ginger and chilli, and makes it a wonderfully refreshing soup for a hot summer's day. Eat straightaway for maximum vitamin C!

Serves 6

Put all the ingredients for the gazpacho in a blender and blitz until smooth. If you want to make sure the soup is completely smooth, you can also put it through a sieve. Pour into chilled serving bowls.

For the feta cream, blitz together the feta, crème fraîche and lime juice. The consistency should be similar to that of cream cheese. Dollop dessertspoonfuls of it into the soup, drizzle over a little olive oil and sprinkle over a few mint and basil leaves and some smoked paprika.

TIP

- This soup can be frozen, but it won't taste quite as fresh on defrosting. In fact, I think it will actually taste better if you heat it! Remember that ginger and chilli will intensify on freezing, so use sparingly if you don't want the soup to taste too hot.

Energy 92 kcal/388 kJ **Protein** 2.5g **Fat** 3.8g
Sat. Fat 2.1g **Carbohydrate** 12.4g **Fibre** 0.9g

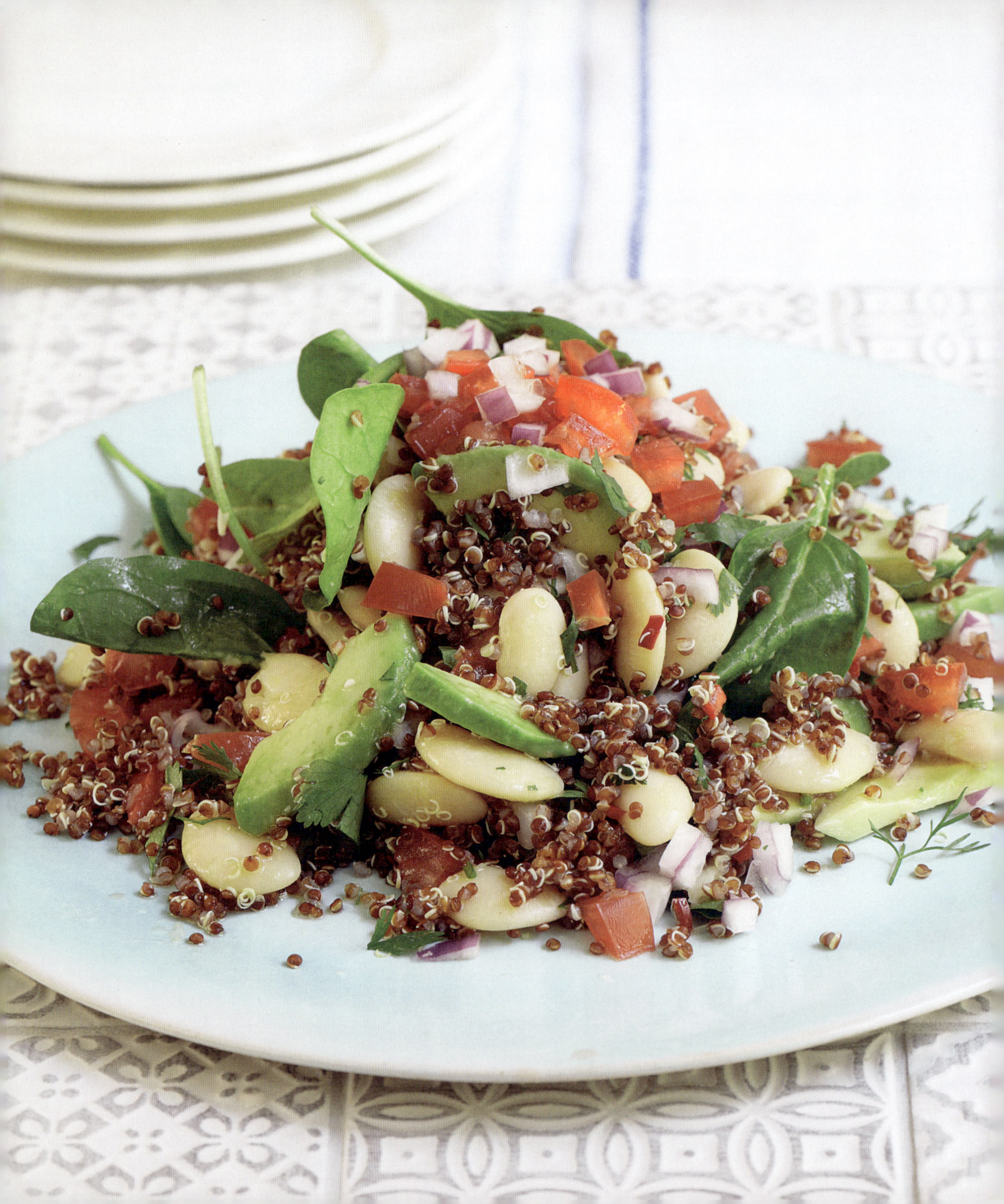

Martin Morales' QUINOA, AVOCADO, CHILLI AND HONEY SALAD

150g (5½oz) quinoa
400g (14oz) can butter beans, *drained and rinsed*
25g (¾oz) coriander leaves, *finely chopped*
1 chilli, *deseeded and finely chopped*
1 ripe avocado
½ red onion, *finely diced*
1 large tomato, *deseeded and finely diced*
Salt

For the dressing:
Juice of **2** limes
1 red chilli, *deseeded and finely chopped*
1 tablespoon extra virgin olive oil
1 teaspoon honey

Energy 286 kcal/1202 kJ
Protein 12.3g
Fat 10.2g
Sat. Fat 1.7g
Carbohydrate 38.7g
Fibre 8.0g

This is can either be a moulded or free-form salad. If you want to mould it, arrange avocado slices in the bottom of four 10cm round moulds on four plates, then add the quinoa mix, onion and tomato, pressing down as you go. Drizzle over the remaining dressing once you've taken the moulds off. This would be good with some baby salad leaves.

Serves 4

Wash the quinoa in cold water until it starts to run clear. Put in a saucepan, cover with cold water, add a pinch of salt and bring to the boil over a medium heat. Simmer for around 14 minutes until the quinoa is well cooked and has unfurled its tail. Drain, cool and set aside until needed.

In a bowl, mix all the dressing ingredients except the honey.

Add the butter beans, coriander and chilli to the quinoa and mix well. Add 3 tablespoons of the dressing, but don't soak the quinoa mixture too much.

To assemble the salad, cut the avocado into chunks, mix with the quinoa and butter beans, and sprinkle the dressing and the tomato/red onion garnish over the top, then drizzle the honey over each portion as a final touch.

Martin Morales (martinmorales.co.uk) is Chef and Founder of Ceviche and Andina, Peruvian restaurants in London. He is the award-winning author of *Ceviche: Peruvian Kitchen*. cevicheuk.com

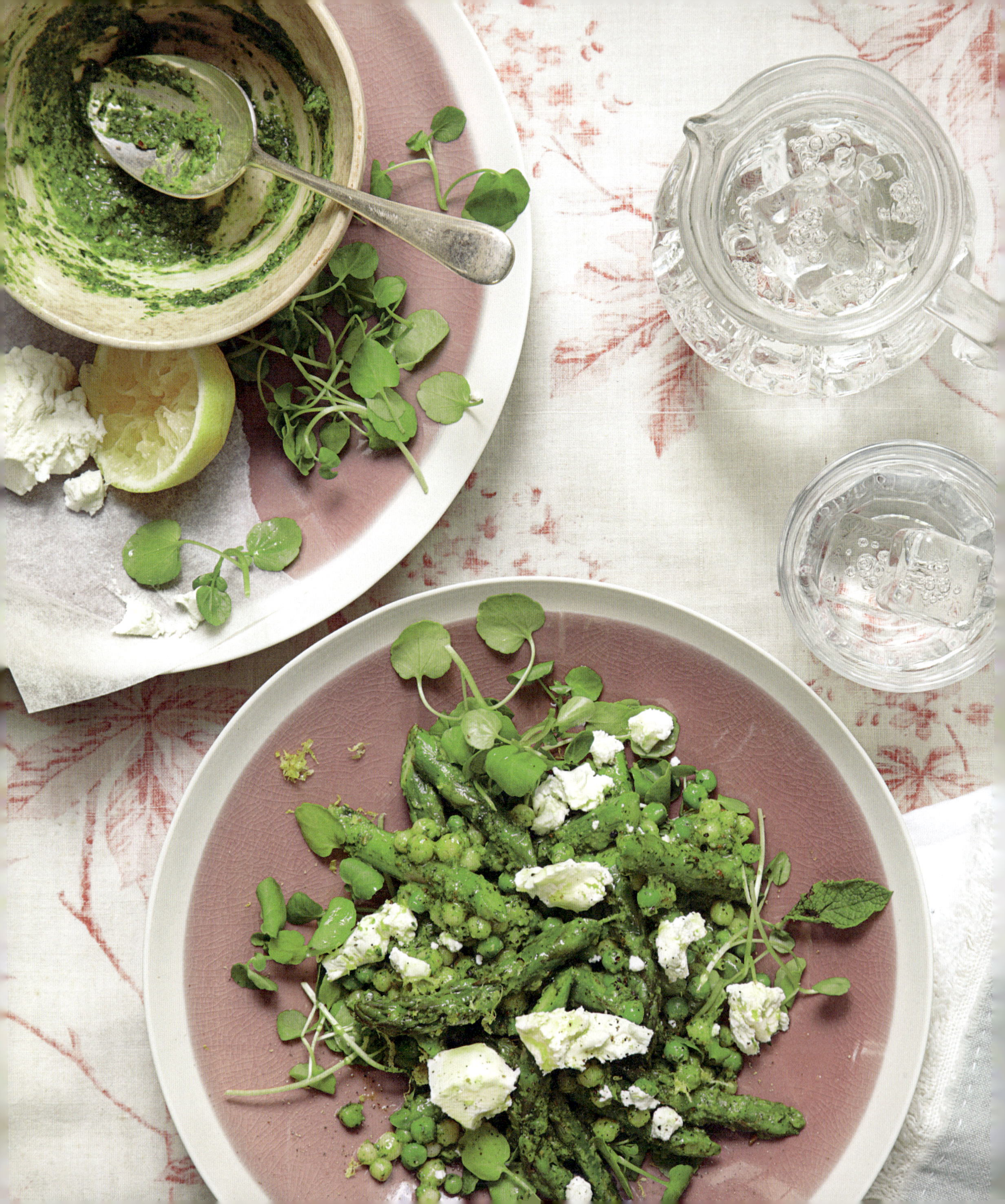

Lucas Hollweg's ASPARAGUS, PEA, GOAT'S CHEESE AND GIANT COUSCOUS SALAD

For the salad:
100g (3½oz) giant or Israeli couscous
250g (9oz) asparagus, *stalks trimmed*
6 handfuls of small peas (fresh or frozen)
Grated zest of ½ unwaxed lemon and **3 tablespoons** juice
5 tablespoons extra virgin olive oil
Handful of mint leaves
4 generous handfuls of watercress
125g (4½oz) fresh, rindless goat's cheese (or goat's curd)
¼ teaspoon fine salt, or to taste
Freshly ground black pepper

For the watercress pesto:
75g (2½oz) watercress, *stalks included*
Handful of mint leaves
25g (¾oz) pine nuts
40g (1½oz) pecorino cheese, *grated*
1 garlic clove, *crushed*
Finely grated zest of 1 unwaxed lemon and **1½ tablespoons** juice
5 tablespoons extra virgin olive oil

Energy 580 kcal/2402 kJ
Protein 19.0g
Fat 44.9g
Sat. Fat 10.2g
Carbohydrate 26.3g
Fibre 6.0g

This is the perfect summer salad – fresh, green and lively. You can substitute the couscous with spelt if you like – it will give the salad a nuttier flavour. Just bear in mind it will need cooking for longer. This recipe is high in vitamins and minerals but also a little higher in fat, but this is due to the generous portions of olive oil. The fat from the olive oil is mainly monounsaturated, which is good if you are trying to gain weight. If you are trying to watch your weight, then avoid using the last oil dressing. This salad will keep very well in the fridge for a few days and is a good one for the lunchbox, not least because it's best eaten at room temperature. Any leftover pesto will keep in the fridge or can be frozen.

Serves 4

Pour the couscous into a saucepan of salted boiling water and cook until the grains are soft (timings vary – follow the packet guidelines). Drain well and leave to cool. Wipe out the saucepan.

Meanwhile, make the watercress pesto. Whizz together all the ingredients in a food-processor with some salt and pepper, scraping down the sides if necessary. You want to end up with a brilliant green paste.

Put the saucepan back on the hob and bring some salted water to the boil. Cut each asparagus stalk into three and throw into the boiling water. After 4 minutes, add the peas and cook for a further 2–3 minutes, or until the vegetables are just done. Drain in a sieve and quickly refresh under the cold tap for 30 seconds to stop the cooking. Drain again, shaking off any water.

Put the pesto in a mixing bowl, along with 3 tablespoons lemon juice and 2 tablespoons of the olive oil. Add the drained couscous, mint, peas and asparagus and stir until everything is combined. Taste and season well – you'll need at least ¼ teaspoon fine salt – then toss in the watercress.

Divide the salad between plates or wide bowls. Add a couple of pinches of lemon zest to each one, plus a few blobs of the goat's cheese. Splash with the remaining olive oil and finish with a grind of black pepper before serving.

Ming's
SHIITAKE BROWN RICE PILAF

250g (9oz) brown rice
2 tablespoons extra virgin olive oil
3 garlic cloves, *finely chopped*
4 shallots (approx. **100g (3½oz)**) *finely chopped*
500ml (17fl oz) hot chicken stock
½ stick of cinnamon
120g (4½oz) shiitake mushrooms, *sliced*
Sprig of fresh or dried bay leaves
Kosher salt and freshly ground black pepper

Energy 251 kcal/1060 kJ
Protein 5.5g
Fat 5.3g
Sat. Fat 0.9g
Carbohydrate 48.1g
Fibre 1.6g

This pilaf would pair very nicely with Ching's choi sum stir-fry (see page 188), but it is equally good on its own. If you don't want to switch on the oven, you can simply simmer it very gently on the hob until all the liquid is absorbed. Brown rice has a greater concentration of B vitamins compared to white rice. A good source of fibre and being low in fat makes it an excellent source of starchy carbohydrate.

Serves 6 as a light meal or side dish

Rinse the rice and soak in fresh cold water for 1 hour. Drain in a colander until dry.

Preheat the oven to 160°C/gas mark 3/325°F.

Heat the oil in a large casserole or stockpot. Add the garlic and shallots and season well with salt and pepper. Sauté for about 30 seconds until the aroma and oils are released. Add the rice, sauté for a further 1–2 minutes, stirring, until the rice is golden brown. Add the stock, cinnamon stick, shiitake mushrooms and bay leaves, and bring to a simmer. Scrape down any grains of rice from the side of the pot to prevent them from burning. Taste the liquid and adjust the seasoning if necessary. Cover with a lid, place in the oven and cook for 20–25 minutes until all the liquid is absorbed.

Fluff up with a fork, remove the bay leaves and serve immediately.

TIP

- This makes quite a large quantity, but it's a very versatile side dish, so it's definitely worth freezing a few individual portions. Just make sure that you transfer it to the freezer as soon as the rice has cooled down.

Felicity Cloake's
SPINACH AND TOMATO DAL

250g (9oz) chana dal (yellow split peas can be substituted)
2 tablespoons vegetable or sunflower oil, *plus a splash more*
1 small onion, *finely sliced*
1 small chunk of fresh ginger, *grated*
2 garlic cloves, *crushed*
½ teaspoon turmeric
1 teaspoon garam masala
1 teaspoon brown mustard seeds
150g (5½oz) spinach, *washed and trimmed if necessary*
Handful of cherry tomatoes, *halved*
Small bunch of coriander, *to serve (optional)*

Energy 144 kcal/602 kJ
Protein 6.8g
Fat 7.4g
Sat. Fat 0.8g
Carbohydrate 14g
Fibre 1.6g

'Hot, comforting and wonderfully easy to make, for me, dal is the culinary equivalent of a warm duvet – I could eat it by the panful, and frequently do. This version uses chana dal, or split chickpeas, which are not only packed with fibre and protein, but also boast a remarkably low glycaemic index, so they'll keep you feeling fuller for longer. Chana dal is widely available in the Indian section of larger supermarkets, or at Asian grocers, but you could substitute yellow split peas if you can't find them. I've also added spinach, because just looking at it makes me feel healthier, tomatoes, and two immune-boosting spices – turmeric and mustard seeds. This is a very easy-going recipe; feel free to play around with the veg to suit your taste, or to add a few chilli flakes to the spices if you fancy something a bit punchier. I'm quite happy to eat it on its own, but flatbreads or brown rice would also work well.' *Felicity Cloake*

Serves 4 (small portions)

Rinse the chana dal under the cold tap until the water runs clear. Put in a large pan with 800ml (27fl oz) water and bring to the boil. Skim any scum from the top, then turn down the heat and simmer for 45–55 minutes until very tender. (Add more water if necessary.)

Meanwhile, heat the oil in a frying pan over a medium heat and add the onion. Cook until soft and golden brown, stirring often – this should take about 20 minutes.

Add the ginger and garlic, and cook for a couple of minutes, then set aside until the dal is ready. Once the dal is very soft, mash it roughly (if using the softer split peas, you may not need to do this), then leave it gently simmering and thickening on a medium-low heat. Add a splash more oil to the onion pan, bring it back to a sizzle, then add the spices. Cook for a couple of minutes, stirring, until aromatic.

Pour the spiced onion mixture into the dal, and add the spinach and tomatoes. Cover and leave to wilt for a couple of minutes, then stir it all together and season to taste. Garnish with fresh coriander to serve.

HOMEMADE POT NOODLES

1 small carrot, *peeled*
½ courgette
½ red pepper
1 spring onion
Handful of beansprouts
A few leaves of spinach
Some leftover cooked chicken *(optional)*
1 teaspoon finely chopped fresh ginger
1 garlic clove, *finely chopped*
A few coriander leaves
½ chicken stock cube or vegetable bouillon, or 1 sachet of miso paste
1 nest/strip of quick-cook egg noodles
Dash of soy or fish sauce
Squeeze of lime *(optional)*

Energy 326 kcal/1376 kJ
Protein 21.6g
Fat 6.6g
Sat. Fat 1.7g
Carbohydrate 47.8g
Fibre 6.4g

This is a very quick, easy lunch to make when you have lots of vegetables in the fridge, perhaps some you can spare from a stir-fry or something similar. Use the list here for guidance only – you can add any vegetables that need minimal cooking, or taste good eaten fairly crunchy, such as peas, cabbage and baby corn. You can also vary the flavours a lot – for example, instead of chicken stock and soy sauce, you could use a sachet of miso soup. You could even use cooked rice instead of noodles. This is a great source of vitamin B, iron and beta-carotene. The fresher the ingredients, the better the vitamin C content.

Serves 1

Shred the carrot, courgette, red pepper and spring onion, and layer them in a tall airtight box or preserving jar. Add the beansprouts, spinach and any other vegetables you might be using, along with the leftover chicken, if you have any. Sprinkle over the ginger, garlic, coriander and your choice of stock cube, then squash in the noodles. Seal well and leave until you are ready to eat it.

Boil a kettle and pour boiling water over your noodles until they are just covered. Give everything a quick stir or prod with a fork or chopsticks, then cover again and leave for a minimum of 5 minutes. Check to see if the noodles are soft enough and leave for a couple more minutes if necessary.

Season with soy or fish sauce to taste and add a squeeze of lime, if you like.

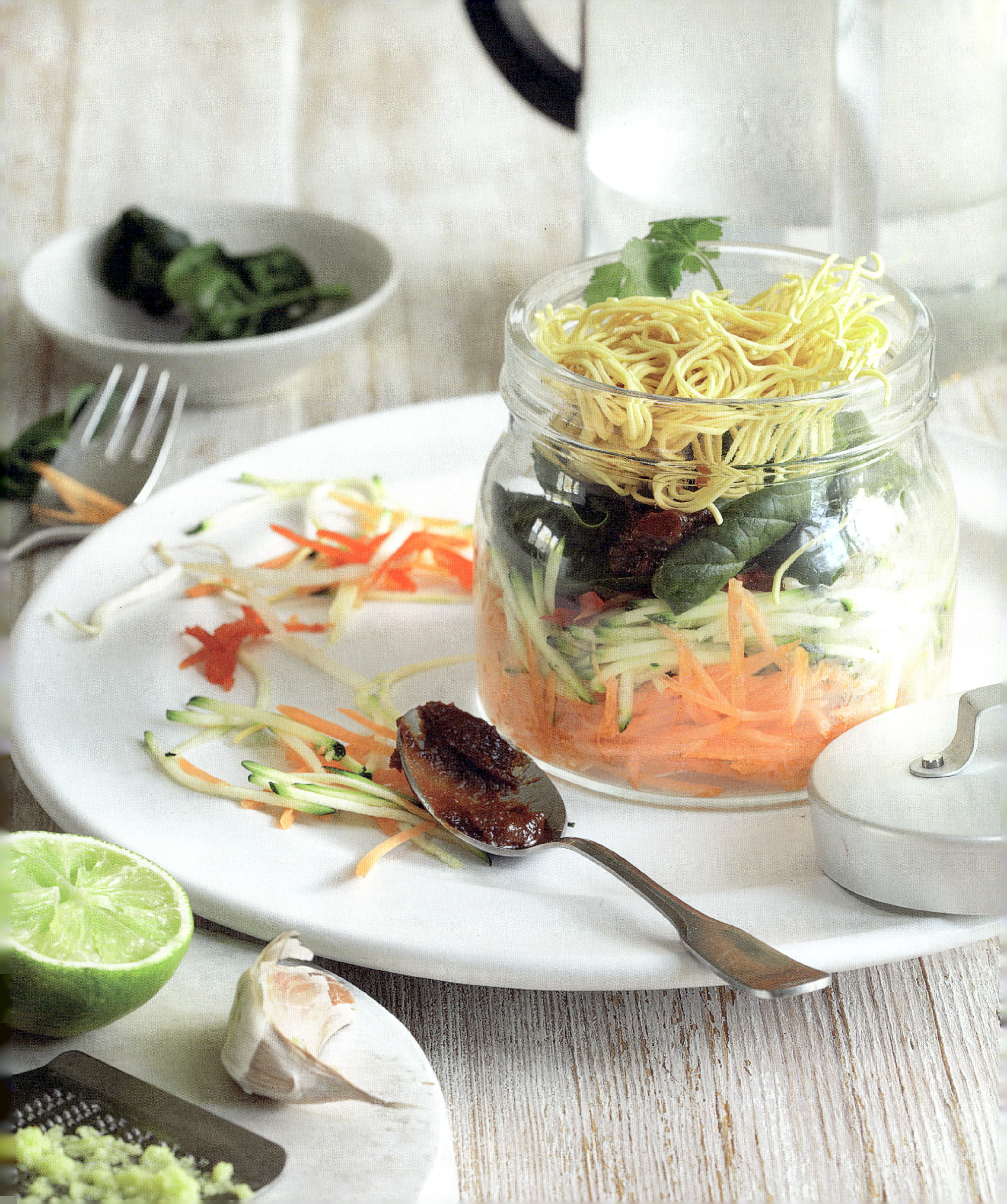

Gwyneth Paltrow's CHINESE CHICKEN SALAD

4 coin-sized pieces of fresh ginger, *crushed with the side of a knife*
2 garlic cloves, *crushed with the side of a knife*
6 spring onions, *2 bruised with the side of a knife and the other 4 finely sliced lengthways*
½ star anise
1 teaspoon five-spice powder
2 chicken breasts on the bone, *skin removed*
1 head of Little Gem lettuce (or **1** heart of cos), *core discarded, finely shredded*
1 head of green chicory, core discarded, *finely shredded*
1 head of red chicory, *core discarded, finely shredded (or just use another green one)*
Handful of mangetout, *thinly sliced lengthwise*
1 carrot, *peeled and cut into matchsticks*
3 tablespoons roughly chopped coriander
A little freshly minced red chilli *(optional)*
Big pinch of toasted black sesame seeds

Chinese Chicken Salad Dressing *(see right)*

'This recipe makes more than enough dressing, but whatever's left over is great on grilled fish or chicken, or on a bowl of brown rice. The preparation goes quickly if you prep the dressing and all your vegetables while the chicken steams. The steaming liquid can be strained and enjoyed as a light, wonderful broth.' *Gwyneth Paltrow*

Serves 2 generously

Bring a litre of water to the boil in a large wok or pot along with the ginger, the garlic, the two bruised spring onions, the star anise, and the Chinese five-spice powder. Turn the heat down and let the mixture simmer for 5 minutes. Set up a steamer (bamboo or whatever you have) above the fragrant broth and put the chicken breasts inside. Steam for about 45 minutes, then remove from the steamer. As soon as the chicken is cool enough to handle, shred the meat with your fingers.

Combine the shredded chicken with the 4 sliced spring onions, the Little Gem, chicory, mangetout, carrot, coriander, the chilli (if using), and the black sesame seeds, and stir to combine with as much of the dressing as you like.

CHINESE CHICKEN SALAD DRESSING

3 tablespoons hoisin sauce
5 tablespoons cold-pressed, untoasted sesame oil (or extra virgin olive oil)
1 tablespoon brown rice vinegar
60ml (2fl oz) water

Whisk everything together. Keeps well in a jar in the fridge for up to a week.

Energy 563 kcal/2376 kJ **Protein** 13.8g **Fat** 19.1g
Sat. Fat 9.8g **Carbohydrate** 91.1g **Fibre** 12.4g

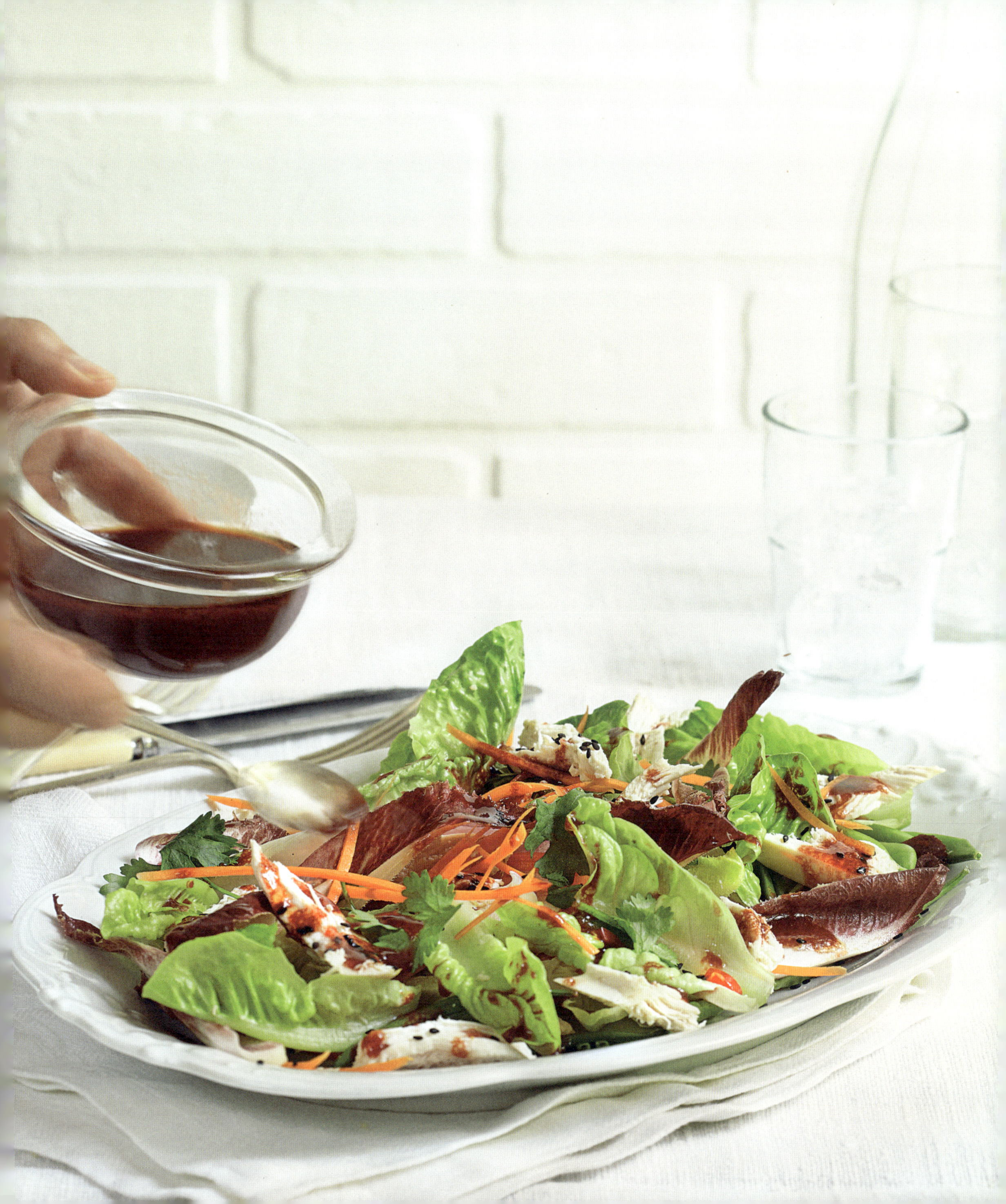

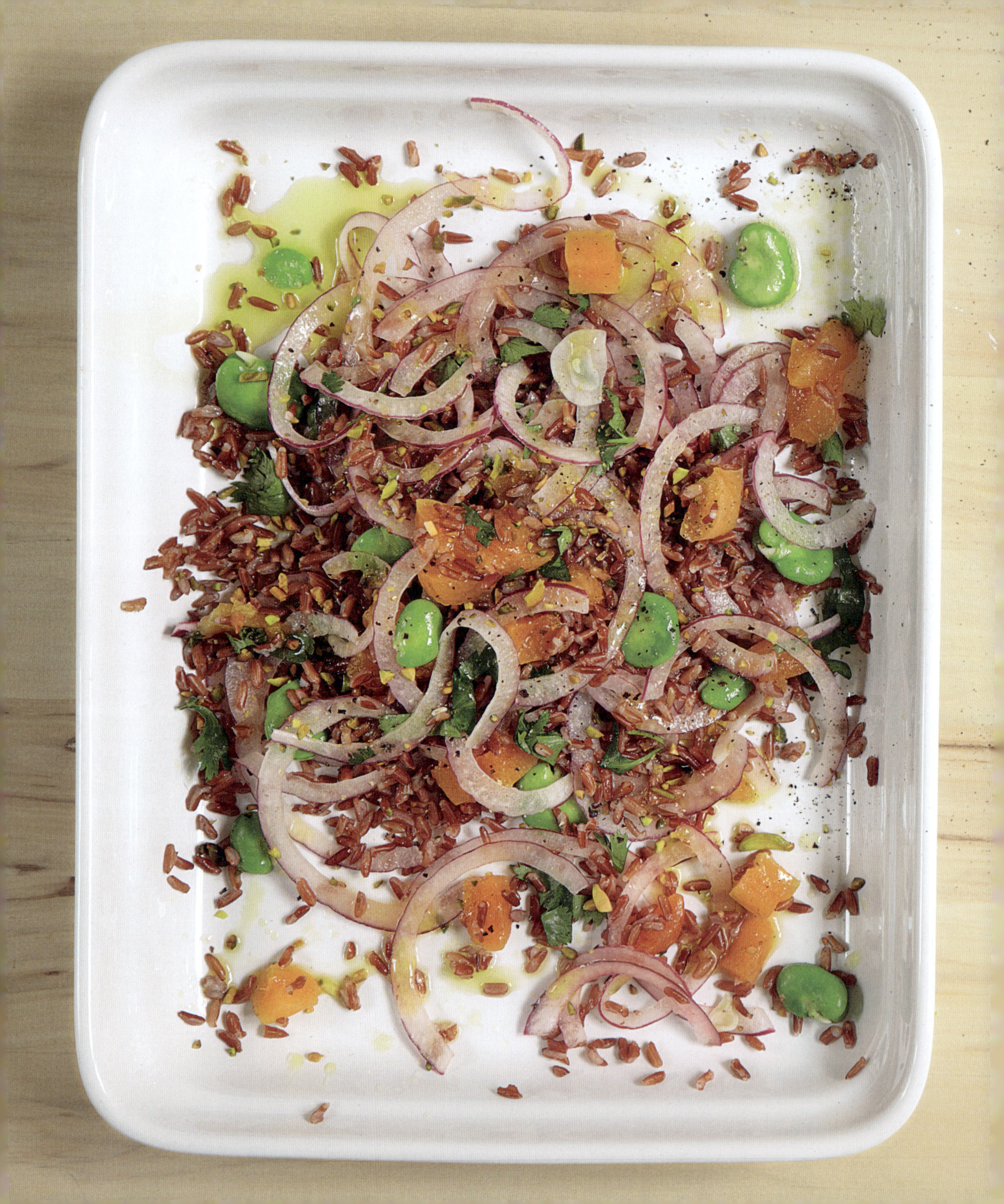

Henry Dimbleby's JACKSON POLLOCK SALAD

300g (10½oz) Camargue red rice
200g (7oz) podded broad beans
200g (7oz) red onions, *finely sliced*
200g (7oz) soft dried apricots, *chopped into raisin-sized pieces*
4 tablespoons olive oil
Juice of 1 lemon
100g (3½oz) unsalted pistachio nuts *(shelled weight)*
2 tablespoons chopped fresh coriander
Salt and freshly ground black pepper

Energy 295 kcal/1234 kJ
Protein 7.1g
Fat 10.4g
Sat. Fat 1.3g
Carbohydrate 43.8g
Fibre 5.6g

'A beautiful burst of colour to serve on a summer's day, on its own or alongside a barbecue.'

'Dimbleby Cancer Care offers practical and psychological support to people living with cancer through its Information and Support Services at Guy's and St Thomas' Hospital. Every donation makes a difference, visit www.dimblebycancercare.org to find out more.' *Henry Dimbleby*

Serves 8

Cook the rice in boiling salted water for 30 minutes, or until tender but still chewy. Drain well.

Bring a pan of salted water to the boil. Add the broad beans and cook for 1–2 minutes until tender, then drain in a colander and refresh under cold water. Skin the larger beans.

Put the rice in a large bowl and add the onions, broad beans, apricots, oil and lemon juice. Season well.

Just before serving, toast the pistachios for 2 minutes in a frying pan over a medium heat. Allow to cool, then crush with a rolling pin and mix into the salad. Stir in the coriander. Check the seasoning and serve.

TIP

- Camargue red rice is very easy to get hold of, but you could also use wild or brown rice, barley or spelt instead, if you like. In fact, this is an infinitely variable salad – you could swap the broad beans for runner or green beans or even peas, while parsley, mint or a strong-flavoured salad leaf such as rocket or mustard would be wonderful in place of the coriander.

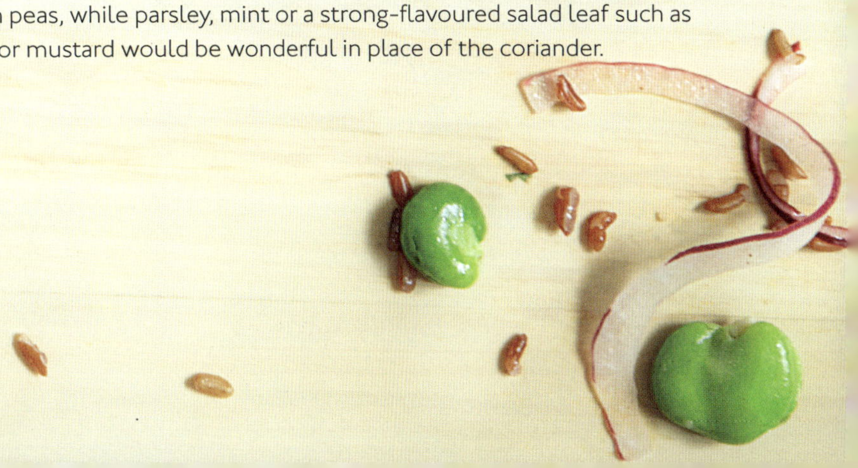

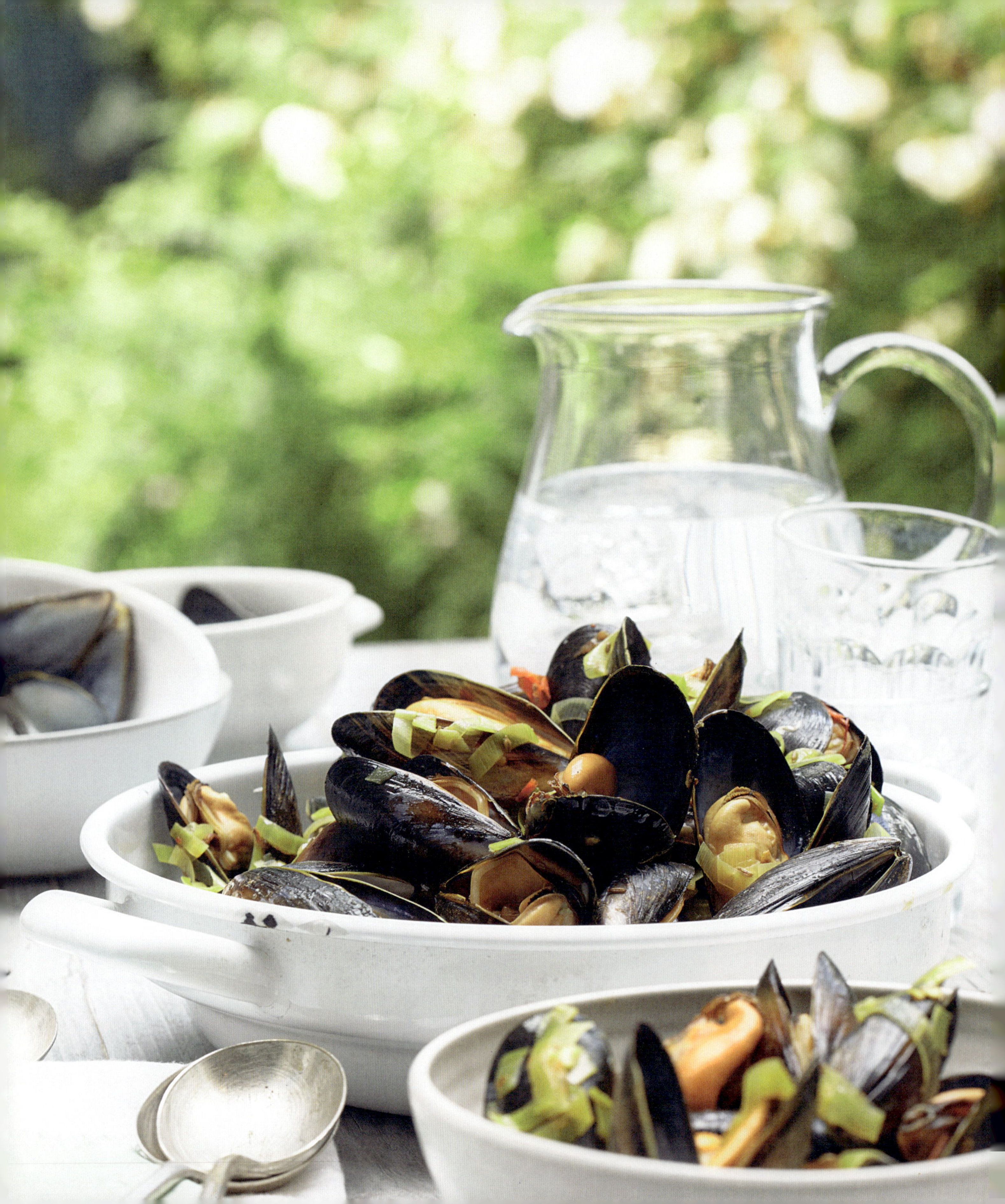

MUSSELS IN BROTH

1.5kg (50fl oz) mussels
1 tablespoon olive oil
Small knob of unsalted butter
2 leeks, *finely sliced into rounds*
2 garlic cloves, *finely chopped*
2 dried chillies, *crumbled* (or **½ teaspoon** chilli flakes)
1 teaspoon cumin seeds
1 teaspoon fennel seeds
Large pinch of saffron, *soaked in a little water*
Pinch of turmeric
1 teaspoon mild curry powder
2 very ripe tomatoes, *cored and chopped*
150ml (5fl oz) white wine
200ml (7fl oz) hot fish stock or water
1 tablespoon Pernod *(optional)*
Small bunch of coriander or parsley, *to serve*

Energy 215 kcal/910 kJ
Protein 19.4g
Fat 7.6g
Sat. Fat 1.8g
Carbohydrate 9.5g
Fibre 3.7g

Mussels are a great ingredient if you want a really easy, impressive dish, because they're very cheap, look amazing and are highly nutritious. The preparation is simple – just make sure you discard any that won't close before they are cooked, and any that don't open after they've been cooked. That way you can't go wrong. These mussels are served in a very slightly spicy, warming broth, reminiscent of the Mediterranean. This is a low-fat, high-protein dish with a whole range of micronutrients, including iron, selenium, iodine and vitamins E and B.

Serves 4

To prepare the mussels, wash them under plenty of cold water. Get rid of any that won't close when tapped. Pull out the beard and, if you have the energy, scrape off any barnacles. You could just give them all a quick scrub instead.

Heat the olive oil in a lidded saucepan or casserole large enough to hold all the mussels. Add the butter and, when it has melted, add the leeks. Cover and sweat for a few minutes over a low heat until the leeks have softened. Turn up the heat slightly. Add the garlic, chillies, cumin and fennel seeds and sauté for a couple of minutes. Pour in the saffron and its water, add a pinch of turmeric and the curry powder, then the tomatoes, wine and stock. Season with salt and pepper and bring to the boil. Simmer for 5 minutes.

Add the Pernod, if using, then throw in all the mussels. Cover and leave the mussels to steam for 3–4 minutes, giving the pan a good shake every so often. The mussels are done when they are open.

Serve in large shallow bowls with the broth poured over and sprinkled with the fresh herbs. Make sure you discard any mussels that haven't opened.

SMOKED MACKEREL, BEETROOT AND APPLE SALAD

This is a very good, multi-textured winter salad; it is excellent with salad greens, but you can also pile it on top of chicory leaves for an extra flavour hit of bitterness. It is very quick to assemble if you use vacuum-packed beetroot and canned lentils. If you happen to have some raw beetroot, however, it is well worth roasting it for this salad, as you can control how long you cook it – I prefer my beetroot slightly firmer than the vacuum-packed variety. An ideal light or packed lunch, this certainly does deliver on nutrients. The oily fish is a great source of omega-3 fatty acids, vitamin D and iron, and the lentils provide low GI carbohydrate.

Serves 4

400g (14oz) fairly small beetroot, *well scrubbed*, or **250g (9oz)** pack of cooked beetroot *(not pickled)*
1 tablespoon olive oil, *if roasting*
Salt, *if roasting*
1 thyme sprig, *if roasting*

For the dressing:
4 tablespoons oil *(preferably a nutty one, but olive oil is fine)*
2 tablespoons cider vinegar
1 tablespoon Dijon mustard
1 teaspoon honey
Salt and freshly ground black pepper

100g (3½oz) cooked Puy or green lentils
1 green apple, *cored, halved horizontally and thinly sliced*
1 small red onion, *finely sliced*
3 mackerel fillets, *skinned and torn into chunks*
1 tablespoon capers *(optional)*
Salad leaves – *watercress, rocket, spinach and chicory are all good*

Chopped dill or parsley, *to serve*

If you are roasting your beetroot rather than using the ready-cooked sort, preheat the oven to 200°C/gas mark 6/400°F, then put the unpeeled beetroot into a roasting tin. Drizzle over the oil and sprinkle with salt and thyme. Roast, uncovered, for 1 hour. Allow the beetroot to cool a little, then rub off the skins. Cut each beetroot into small wedges.

Make the dressing by whisking together all the ingredients. If you feel it is slightly thick, add a splash of water.

Put the lentils in a bowl, then add the beetroot, apple, onion, mackerel and capers, if using. Arrange the salad leaves on a large plate or bowl and pile the remaining ingredients on top. Drizzle over the dressing. Sprinkle over a little chopped dill or parsley.

Energy 487 kcal/2029 kJ **Protein** 27.6g **Fat** 34.0g
Sat. Fat 6.7g **Carbohydrate** 18.3g **Fibre** 5.0g

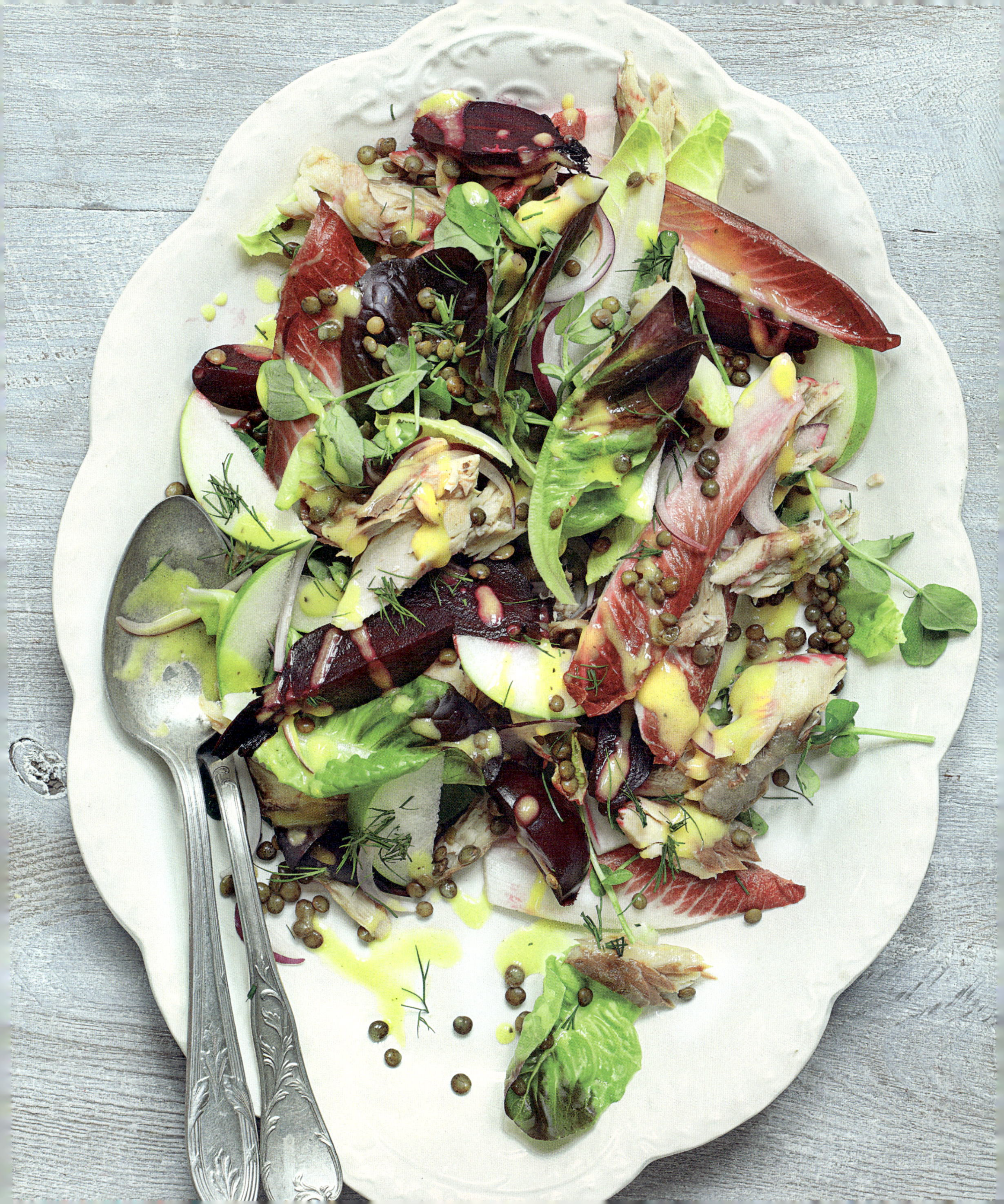

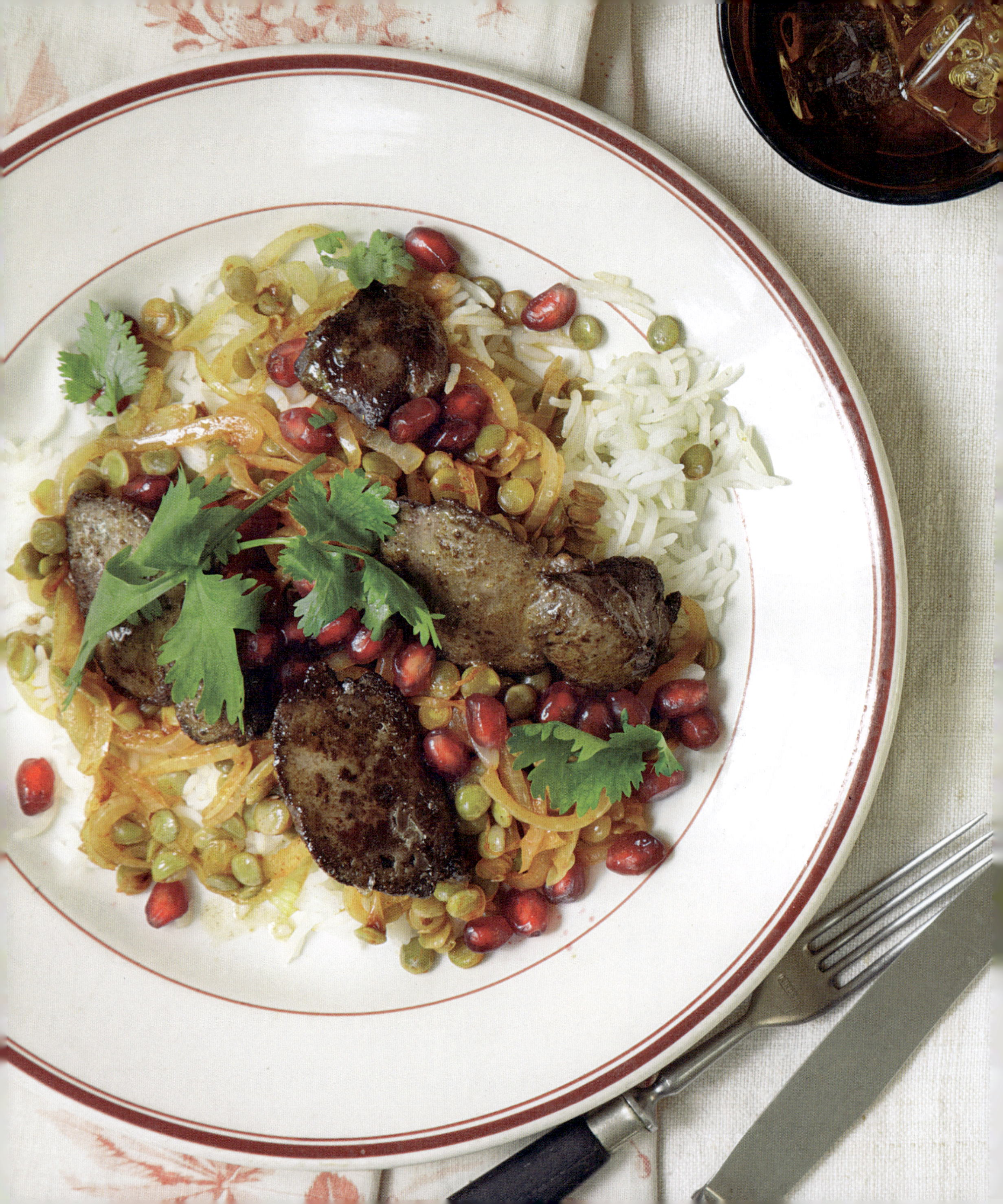

Thomasina Miers' WARM SPICED LENTILS AND RICE

with Chicken Liver and Pomegranate

120g (4½oz) green or brown lentils
250g (9oz) chicken livers
1 teaspoon ground cumin
40g (1½oz) unsalted butter
2 tablespoons vegetable oil
2 onions, *halved and finely sliced*
½–1 teaspoon cayenne pepper
2 teaspoons sweet smoked paprika
Juice of **1** lemon
Salt and freshly ground
black pepper

To serve:
225g (8oz) basmati rice, *cooked*
Seeds of **1** pomegranate
Small bunch of coriander,
roughly chopped
Pinch of sweet smoked paprika

Energy 452 kcal/1883 kJ
Protein 19.4g
Fat 16.3g
Sat. Fat 6.4g
Carbohydrate 57.3g
Fibre 3.1g

'There are few sights more splendid than this dish of sautéed chicken livers, sweet onions and steaming lentils and rice, topped with jewel-pink pomegranate seeds, paprika and green flecks of chopped coriander leaf. It is a homely, deeply restorative dish that takes very little time to make – luckily, as it seems to be a firm favourite in my house.' *Thomasina Miers*

Serves 4

Rinse the lentils in cold water and pour in a saucepan. Cover with at least 3cm (1¼in) of cold water, bring to the boil, then lower the heat and simmer until tender. (The cooking time will vary depending on what type of lentils you are using).

Meanwhile, sift through the livers with a sharp knife or pair of scissors, cutting out any bits of white gristle. Season them generously with salt and pepper and the ground cumin.

Heat a large frying pan over a high heat and, when the pan is smoking hot, add half the butter. Swirl the butter around the pan to melt it, then add half the livers and fry for about 30 seconds a side until they are brown and caramelised all over, then set aside. Repeat with the remaining livers.

Heat the same pan over a medium heat and add the oil and the rest of the butter. When the fat has melted, add the onions, cayenne and smoked paprika. Season with salt and pepper and cook for 15 minutes until the onions are sweet and soft.

Stir in the cooked lentils and lemon juice, and check the seasoning. Finally, add the chicken livers and about 100ml cold water and heat through for about 5 minutes.

Serve the lentils over piles of steaming hot rice, sprinkled with the pomegranate seeds, coriander and a dusting of the sweet smoked paprika.

SPICY BEEF SALAD

This salad makes a couple of steaks go a very long way as it will easily serve four people. You can use any salad ingredients you like here – treat this list as a suggestion only. Red meat has a reputation for being high in fat but by choosing lean meat this dish is low in total fat and saturated fat. Lean red meat is a good source of iron, zinc and B vitamins, and the addition of the salad makes this recipe high in beta-carotene and vitamin C.

Serves 4

2 sirloin steaks (**160g (5½oz)** each)

For the salad:
1 large heart of cos lettuce (or **3** Little Gems), *shredded*
½ courgette, *cut into fine strips*
1 large carrot, *cut into fine strips*
¼ red or white cabbage, *finely chopped*
1 red pepper, *very finely sliced*

For the dressing:
2 tablespoons soy sauce
1 tablespoon rice wine vinegar
1 teaspoon sugar
½ teaspoon grated fresh ginger
1 garlic clove, *crushed or grated*
Juice of **1** lime
1 chilli, *finely sliced*
1 teaspoon sesame oil

To serve:
4 spring onions, *shredded*
1 teaspoon sesame seeds

Heat a griddle pan until too hot to hold your hand over.

Arrange all the salad ingredients over a large serving platter.

Whisk together all the dressing ingredients.

Grill the steaks. It is entirely up to you how well done they are, but medium-rare to rare will work best with this dish, so cook for around 2 minutes on each side. Leave the steaks to rest for a few minutes, then slice into strips. Arrange these strips over the salad ingredients and add any meat juices to the dressing.

Pour over the dressing, then sprinkle over the spring onions and sesame seeds.

Energy 180 kcal/752 kJ
Protein 21.7g
Fat 5.8g
Sat. Fat 2.0g
Carbohydrate 10.5g
Fibre 3.9g

FRITTATA

2 red onions, *cut into wedges*
1 courgette, *cut into rounds*
1 red pepper, *sliced lengthways*
200g (7oz) butternut squash or sweet potato (peeled weight), *diced*
2 tablespoons olive oil
1 teaspoon dried herbs – *oregano or sage is good, as is a mixture*
6 free-range eggs, *beaten*
6 cherry tomatoes, *halved*
A few basil leaves, *torn*
Salt and freshly ground black pepper

Energy 256 kcal/1064 kJ
Protein 14.1g
Fat 16.2g
Sat. Fat 3.7g
Carbohydrate 14.3g
Fibre 4.1g

This makes a very large frittata, but that's no bad thing. It will serve four for a light meal, but, as it's so portable, it makes perfect lunchbox food. Refrigerate and cut wedges as necessary, or freeze and reheat by wrapping in foil and putting in a hot oven. There are suggestions for all seasons, but the vegetables can be chopped and changed at will. A finely diced slice of bacon or some cooked leftover meat (especially chicken) are also good.

Serves 4

Preheat the oven to 200°C/gas mark 6/400°F. Line a baking tray or roasting dish with greaseproof paper. Add the onions, courgette, pepper and butternut squash and pour over 1 tablespoon of the olive oil Turn everything over with your hands, then spread evenly over the baking tray. Sprinkle over the herbs and season with salt and pepper. Transfer to the oven and roast for 30 minutes.

Preheat the grill to its highest setting. Heat the remaining tablespoon of olive oil in a large, preferably non-stick, frying pan. Arrange the roast vegetables over the base of the pan, then pour over the eggs. Dot the cherry tomatoes around, then sprinkle over some torn basil. Cook over a medium heat until the base is set and the edges have turned a deep brown. Put under the grill (you may need to protect the frying pan handle) and cook until the eggs have set and the frittata has puffed up slightly.

Variations:

Fry 200g (7oz) mushrooms with a little onion and garlic, and add 300g (10½oz) sprouting broccoli, and a tablespoon or two of Parmesan. (Cherry tomatoes are optional, but always good as they provide welcome bursts of sweetness.)

Energy 323 kcal/1347 kJ **Protein** 20.7g **Fat** 19.5g
Sat. Fat 5.4g **Carbohydrate** 17.4g **Fibre** 8.5g

Shred 250–300g (9–10½oz) of chard, kale or cavalo nero. Blanch in boiling water for 2–3 minutes. Drain thoroughly. Roast the butternut squash or sweet potato and onions as above. Make up the frittata with a grating of lemon zest.

With kale: **Energy** 281 kcal/1170 kJ **Protein** 16.6g **Fat** 17.4g
Sat. Fat 3.9g **Carbohydrate** 15.4g **Fibre** 7.2g

Grill the tender stems and tips of a bunch of well-washed asparagus. Make the frittata with 100g (3½oz) each of broad beans and peas and lots of fresh herbs, especially mint and basil. Add some cubed feta cheese, if you like.

Energy 313 kcal/1300 kJ **Protein** 19.0g **Fat** 18.1g
Sat. Fat 4.6g **Carbohydrate** 19.7g **Fibre** 8.4g

MAIN MEALS

The overall balance of main meals for a healthy choice is plenty of vegetables and plant-based foods, such as pulses, potatoes, sweet potatoes, wholegrain rice, quinoa, pasta and noodles. Many recipes can be adapted to reduce the quantity of fat. Use cooking methods such as steaming, grilling and baking when possible. Stir fry or shallow fry rather than deep-fat fry. Use protein sources such as chicken, fish, eggs, pulses and nuts. If using red meat, then choose lean cuts rather than processed meat. Keep portions of meat small, and always serve with plenty of vegetables, salad and a starchy carbohydrate, such as potatoes, sweet potatoes, brown rice, pulses, couscous, pasta or noodles. Here are some ideas:

- Choose extra-lean red meat in traditional dishes, such as cottage pie, bolognaise and meat cobbler
- Add pulses to stews or casseroles to use less meat and more plant foods
- Stir fry pork, chicken, prawns or cashew nuts with vegetables and serve with brown rice or noodles
- Grill chicken skewers and serve with pitta bread and salad
- Roast chicken (remove the skin) and serve with oven-roasted vegetables
- Chicken, turkey, fish or vegetable curry – homemade to ensure a good balance of ingredients
- White fish such as seabass, plaice, cod, haddock, hake – bake in the oven or grill and flavour with lemon juice or herbs such as dill, and serve with a fresh salsa
- Oily fish such as salmon, trout, sardines or mackerel – see page 218 for a stuffing recipe for whole fish
- Stuffed vegetables such as aubergine, tomatoes or peppers
- Vegetable stews or tagines – serve with brown rice or couscous
- Roasted vegetables are a great accompaniment to roast meat, chicken and white fish – add to pasta or couscous and stir in feta cheese or soft goat's cheese

STUFFED AUBERGINES

This is a handy vegetarian dish to add to the repertoire, as it can be made ahead of time. Simply assemble to the point of adding the mozzarella and pop in the fridge until you are ready to cook it. Any leftovers are best served at room temperature. Serve with a green salad or a big bowl of herby tabbouleh. This dish has a good source of vitamins and minerals, including calcium, beta-carotene and vitamin E, with extra vitamin C from the green salad.

Serves 4

2 very large aubergines, *cut in half lengthways*
2 tablespoons olive oil, plus extra for drizzling
1 large onion, *finely chopped*
2 garlic cloves, *finely chopped*
1 teaspoon ground cumin
¼ teaspoon ground cinnamon
¼ teaspoon smoked paprika
¼ teaspoon cayenne or chilli powder
2 tablespoons *finely chopped* parsley stems
100ml (3½fl oz) red wine *(optional, you can use water, chicken stock or vegetable stock instead)*
400g (14oz) can chopped tomatoes
2 tablespoons capers, *rinsed and drained*
50g (2oz) green olives, *sliced*
2 tablespoons *finely chopped* parsley leaves
2 fresh mozzarella balls, *sliced*
Salt and freshly ground black pepper

Energy 300 kcal/1249 kJ
Protein 15.4g
Fat 20.7g
Sat. Fat 9.7g
Carbohydrate 9.9g
Fibre 6.8g

Preheat the oven to 180°C/gas mark 4/350°F. Line a roasting tin with baking parchment.

Using a sharp knife, cut out most of the flesh in the aubergines, leaving behind a thickness of around 1cm. Put the aubergine 'boats' in the roasting tin. Drizzle with olive oil. Dice the scooped-out flesh.

Heat the olive oil in a saucepan. Add the onion and cook for about 5 minutes, until soft and translucent. Add the garlic, spices and parsley stems, fry for a further minute or two, then add the diced aubergine. Stir so that the aubergine becomes well coated in all the spices, then add the wine. Allow to bubble up, then simmer until the wine has reduced by about half.

Add the tomatoes, season with salt and pepper, and simmer for 15–20 minutes until the sauce is well reduced. Add the capers and olives for the last 5 minutes, then stir in the chopped parsley.

Spoon the mixture into the aubergine skins and top with the mozzarella slices. Bake for about 20 minutes, until the mozzarella has melted and browned.

SUMMER VEGETABLE STIR-FRY

1 tablespoon olive oil
A few baby leeks (about **120g (4½oz)**), *cut into 4cm lengths*
Large bunch of Swiss or rainbow chard, *leaves and stems separated and shredded*
1 small fennel bulb, *halved and shredded widthways*
1 courgette or several small ones, *cut diagonally into slices*
A few asparagus tips
100g (3½oz) French beans
100g (3½oz) baby broad beans or peas
2 garlic cloves, *finely chopped*
Zest of 1 unwaxed lemon
A few cherry tomatoes
Salt and freshly ground black pepper

To serve:
Squeeze of lemon juice or a drizzle of balsamic/sherry vinegar
Selection of summer herbs – basil, bronze fennel, chervil, tarragon and/or mint
A few edible flowers if you have them – borage is particularly good, or any herb flowers will do
A few shavings of Parmesan cheese

This dish is perfect for summer. It's something I like to eat completely on its own, but to make it more substantial you could serve it with some grilled meat or, if you are undergoing treatment or if you do not eat meat, you could add mozzarella pearls or even a burrata right at the end; just don't let them melt completely – they will be lovely just slightly softened.

You can add as many or as few of the vegetables as you like, or swap them for others. For example, blanched runner beans would work well in place of the French beans. This recipe is packed with vitamins and minerals from the fresh vegetables: there is plenty of niacin, beta-carotene, vitamin E and folate. Adding cheese will add protein and calcium. Serve with wholegrain rice, noodles, quinoa or couscous for a starchy carbohydrate.

Serves 2

Heat the olive oil in a wok. Add the leeks, Swiss chard stems, the fennel, courgette, asparagus tips and French beans. Stir-fry over a high heat for about 3 minutes, then add the broad beans or peas, garlic and lemon zest. Season with salt and pepper and pour over 50ml (1½fl oz) cold water. After a couple of minutes, add the Swiss chard leaves and cherry tomatoes.

When the chard leaves have wilted and the cherry tomatoes have softened and burst a little, remove from the heat. Squeeze over a little lemon juice or drizzle over a sweet balsamic or sherry vinegar.

Serve with lots of summery herbs and flowers, if you have them, and perhaps a few shavings of Parmesan.

Energy 145 kcal/604 kJ **Protein** 8.8g **Fat** 7.4g
Sat. Fat 1.1g **Carbohydrate** 12.1g **Fibre** 10.1g

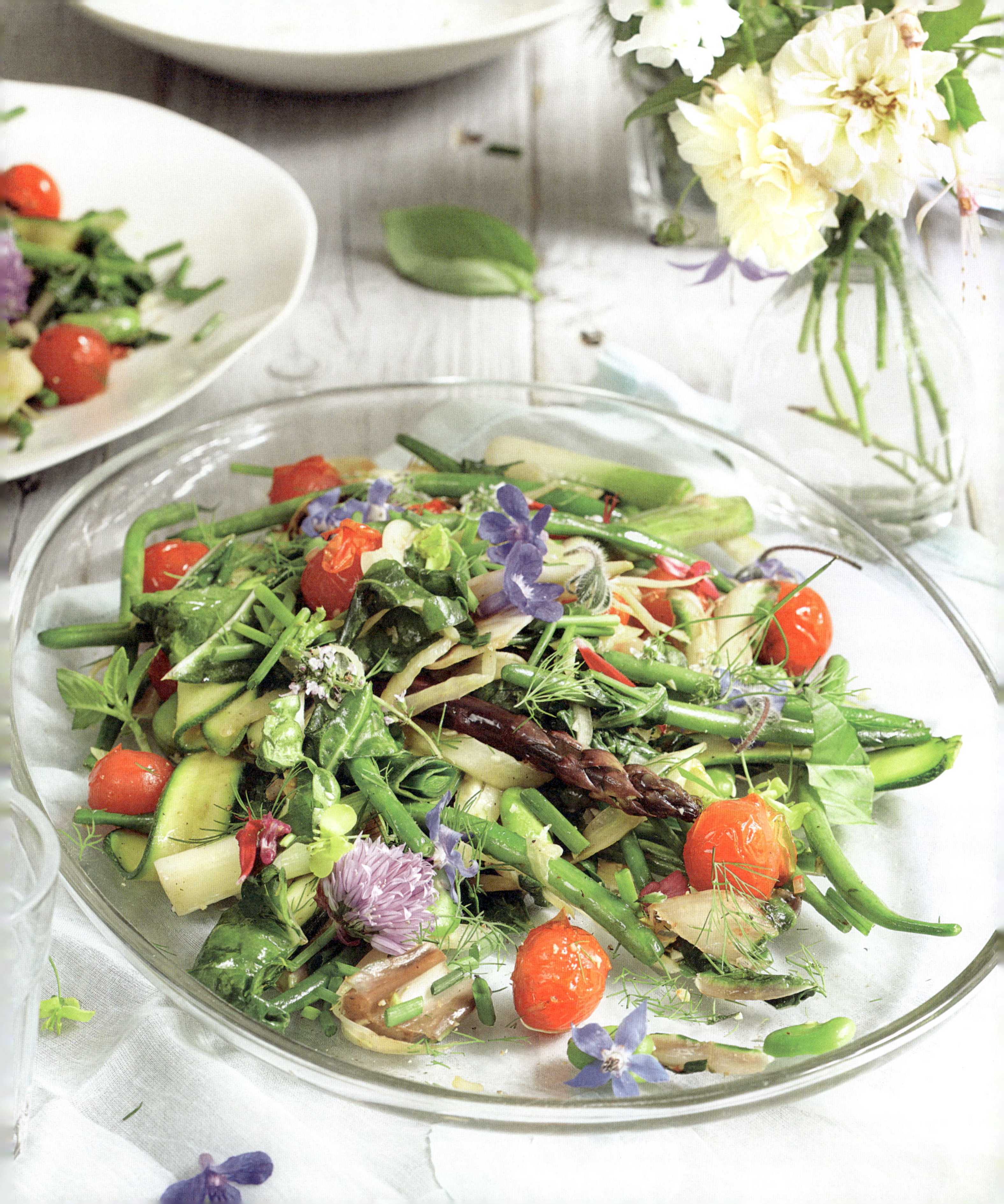

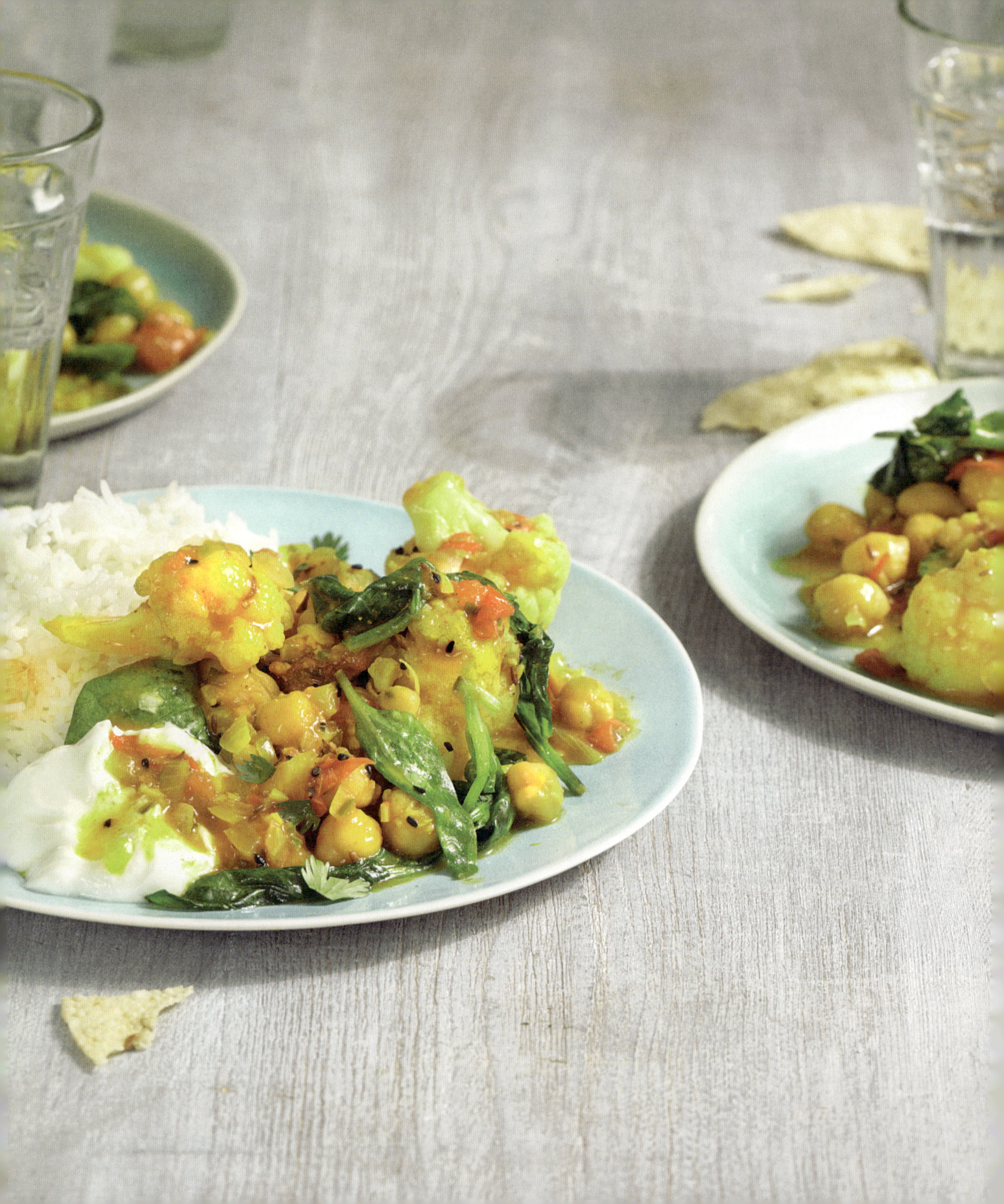

CAULIFLOWER, CHICKPEA AND SPINACH CURRY

1 cauliflower, *separated into small florets*
1 tablespoon vegetable oil
1 teaspoon cumin seeds
1 teaspoon nigella (black onion) seeds
1 onion, *finely chopped*
2 green chillies, *finely chopped*
1 piece fresh ginger, *grated*
2 garlic cloves, *finely chopped*
1 teaspoon ground coriander
½ teaspoon turmeric
½ teaspoon ground fenugreek
Pinch of ground cinnamon
150ml (5fl oz) hot vegetable stock or water
12 tomatoes, *finely chopped*
1 can chickpeas (about **240g (8½oz)** drained weight)
250g (8½oz) spinach leaves, *well washed*
Squeeze of lemon juice
Salt and freshly ground black pepper

To serve
Handful of coriander leaves
Greek yogurt

Energy 175 kcal/738 kJ
Protein 9.9g
Fat 6.4g
Sat. Fat 0.9g
Carbohydrate 21.7g
Fibre 8.4g

This is a very quick and simple curry, which is great on its own or served with some steamed rice. How hot it is depends on the type of chillies you use – if you do want it hotter, you can always add a little chilli powder along with the other spices. This curry has an excellent balance of nutrients, is low in fat, contains starchy carbohydrates with a low glycaemic index and has good amounts of vitamins and minerals, including folate and vitamin E. Serve with wholegrain rice for fibre and more B vitamins.

Serves 4

Bring a saucepan of water to the boil and add salt. Add the cauliflower florets and blanch for about 3 minutes until just al dente. Drain and refresh under cold water.

Heat the oil in a large saucepan. Add the cumin and nigella seeds, and fry for a minute, then add the onion, chillies and ginger. Cook for a few minutes until the onion has softened, then add the garlic and all the spices. Pour in the stock, add the tomatoes and season with salt and pepper. Simmer for 5 minutes, then add the cauliflower florets, chickpeas and spinach leaves. Don't worry about the spinach leaves crowding the saucepan, they will wilt down in no time.

When the spinach has wilted, taste for seasoning. Add more salt and pepper if necessary and then add a squeeze of lemon juice.

Serve with coriander sprinkled over and yogurt on the side.

TIP

- This dish is suitable for freezing – it can also be roughly blended with a little more liquid to make a curried vegetable soup.

Theo Randall's
SEA BASS IN A LEMON, BASIL AND VERMOUTH SAUCE

4 sea bass fillets or similar
8 thin slices of lemon
12 basil leaves
40g (1½oz) unsalted butter, *plus extra for greasing*
200ml (6¾fl oz) vermouth
Salt and freshly ground black pepper

Energy 280 kcal/1167 kJ
Protein 29.2g
Fat 12g
Sat. Fat 5.8g
Carbohydrate 1.7g
Fibre 0g

This dish could not be easier or quicker to make, but if you want to prepare ahead, you can make up the parcels, without the vermouth, and keep them in the fridge until you want to cook them. Then simply add the vermouth and bake. Serve with steamed new potatoes and greens.

Serves 4

Preheat the oven to 190°C/gas mark 5/375°F.

Cut four large squares of foil and butter them on one side. Place a fillet of fish on each buttered square, skin-side down. Top each fillet with two slices of lemon, three basil leaves, 10g (⅓oz) of butter and some seasoning. Fold the sides of the foil up, then pour 50ml (1¾fl oz) vermouth over each fillet. Crimp the edges of the foil together to create sealed parcels. Bake in the oven for 15 minutes.

Remove the fish parcels from the oven and keep warm. Strain the sauce into a saucepan and boil until reduced by half. Serve poured over the fish fillets.

BASIL AND LIME-CRUSTED SALMON

with Cherry Tomatoes and Courgette 'Spaghetti'

You can serve this with regular spaghetti if you wish, but the courgette version is very simple to make. There are devices that make perfect strands of vegetable spaghetti, but you don't need one. Simply use a cheap julienne slice or even a vegetable peeler for slices that you can cut to the width of tagliatelle.

Serves 4

For the salmon:
4 salmon fillets
4 tablespoons breadcrumbs
3 tablespoons pine nuts, *toasted and lightly ground (optional)*
Handful of basil leaves, *finely chopped*
Handful of parsley leaves
A few sprigs of tarragon, leaves only *(optional)*
1 teaspoon capers, *well rinsed*
1 garlic clove
Zest and juice of 1 unwaxed lime
1 tablespoon olive oil
20 cherry tomatoes on the vine
Salt and freshly ground black pepper

For the courgette spaghetti:
1 tablespoon olive oil
2 large courgettes, *cut into long, thin, ribbons*

Energy 331 kcal/1380 kJ
Protein 24.2g
Fat 19.4g
Sat. Fat 3.1g
Carbohydrate 15.8g
Fibre 2.4g

Preheat the oven to 200°C/gas mark 6/400°F. Line a baking tray with baking parchment and space the salmon fillets onto it, skin-side down.

Put the breadcrumbs, pine nuts, herbs, capers, garlic and lime zest into a food-processor and blitz until well combined. Season with salt and pepper, then pour in the lime juice. Mix to combine – if you squeeze it lightly, the mixture should clump together. Divide the mixture between the salmon and press it down firmly. Press a thin layer of this mixture over the salmon. Drizzle the olive oil over the crust.

Roast the salmon in the oven for 10–12 minutes until the crust is a golden brown and the salmon is just cooked through. Add the cherry tomatoes to the tray for the last 5 minutes of the cooking time.

Meanwhile make the courgette spaghetti. Heat the olive oil in a large frying pan or wok. Throw in the courgette and fry very quickly for 1–2 minutes, until it starts to brown very slightly around the edges and softens. You mustn't over cook this as it will go soggy very quickly. Remove from the heat and season with salt and pepper.

To serve, divide the courgette ribbons between four plates and top with the salmon and cherry tomatoes. Garnish with more fresh herbs, if you like.

Allegra McEvedy's STUFFED TROUT

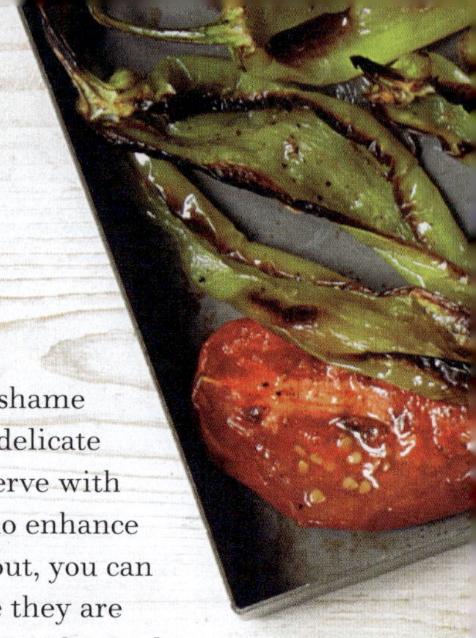

For the trout:
90g (3oz) basmati rice, *well rinsed*
2 spring onions, *sliced into 1cm rounds*
Large handful of parsley, *roughly chopped*
Small handful of dill, *chopped*
Large pinch of allspice
½ teaspoon sumac
35g (1oz) flaked almonds
20g (¾oz) currants
Zest of **1** unwaxed lemon
30g (1oz) unsalted butter
4 trout (each approx. 250g (9oz)), *gutted and scaled*
150ml (5fl oz) white wine
3 tablespoons extra virgin olive oil
Salt and freshly ground black pepper

For the roast vegetables:
4 long, green peppers, *halved*
1 red onion, *cut into thick rings*
Olive oil, *for drizzling*
4 tomatoes, *halved*

To serve:
Cos lettuce leaves
Lemon wedges

Energy 678 kcal/2838 kJ
Protein 55.0g
Fat 35.0g
Sat. Fat 8.7g
Carbohydrate 31.1g
Fibre 4.7g

We seem to eat much less trout these days, which is a shame as it is much cheaper than salmon, has a wonderfully delicate flavour and is just as good for you. You don't need to serve with the peppers and onion if you don't want to, but they do enhance the Turkish attributes of the dish. If you buy fresh trout, you can stuff a batch of these and freeze them. Just make sure they are thoroughly defrosted before you roast them. This dish can be made lower in fat by careful use of the butter and olive oil. Most of the fat comes from the olive oil, nuts and trout, so is a good source of monounsaturated and polyunsaturated fats. The dish also provides an excellent source of potassium, vitamins D and E in addition to other nutrients such as zinc and iron.

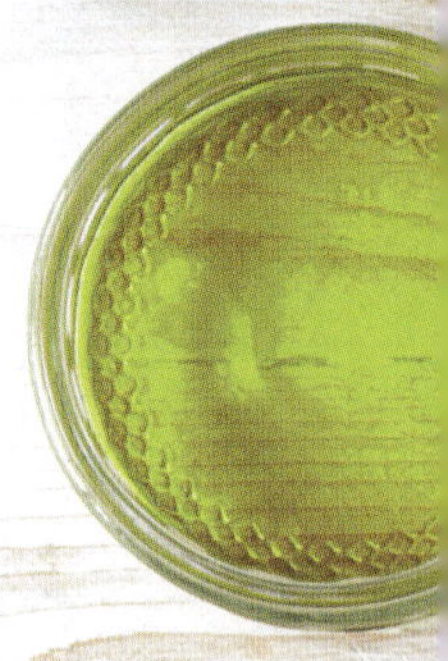

Serves 4

Preheat the oven to 180°C/gas mark 4/350°F.

Cook the rice according to the packet instructions.

Meanwhile, put the spring onions, herbs, spices, almonds, currants and lemon zest in a bowl. Add the drained rice while it is still hot and stir in the butter so it melts. Season with salt and pepper.

Season the inside of the trout, add the rice stuffing and secure with cocktail sticks. Put the trout on a baking tray – one should be able to hold them all. Mix 100ml (3½fl oz) cold water with the wine and season. Pour this over the fish and drizzle over the oil. Bake in the oven for 20 minutes and serve with the juices and the accompaniments.

To grill the vegetables, set your grill to its highest setting. Line a tray with greaseproof paper and arrange the peppers and onion rings on it. Drizzle with some olive oil and season with salt and pepper. Grill for about 5 minutes, then turn over and grill for a further 2 minutes. Add the cut tomatoes and grill those, along with the peppers and onions, for another 3 minutes.

Arrange a few lettuce leaves on four plates, top with the trout and vegetables and serve with lemon wedges for squeezing.

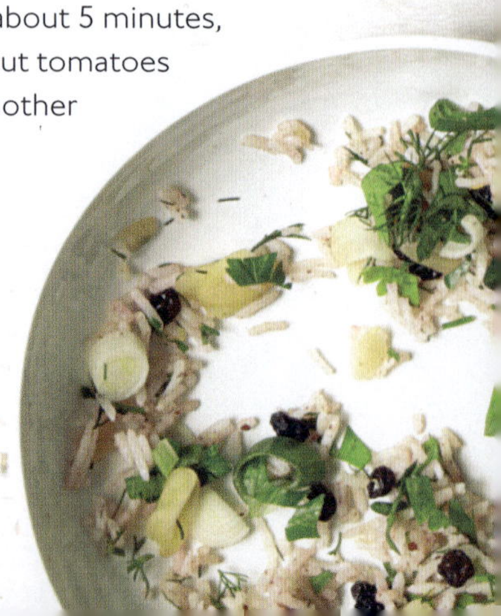

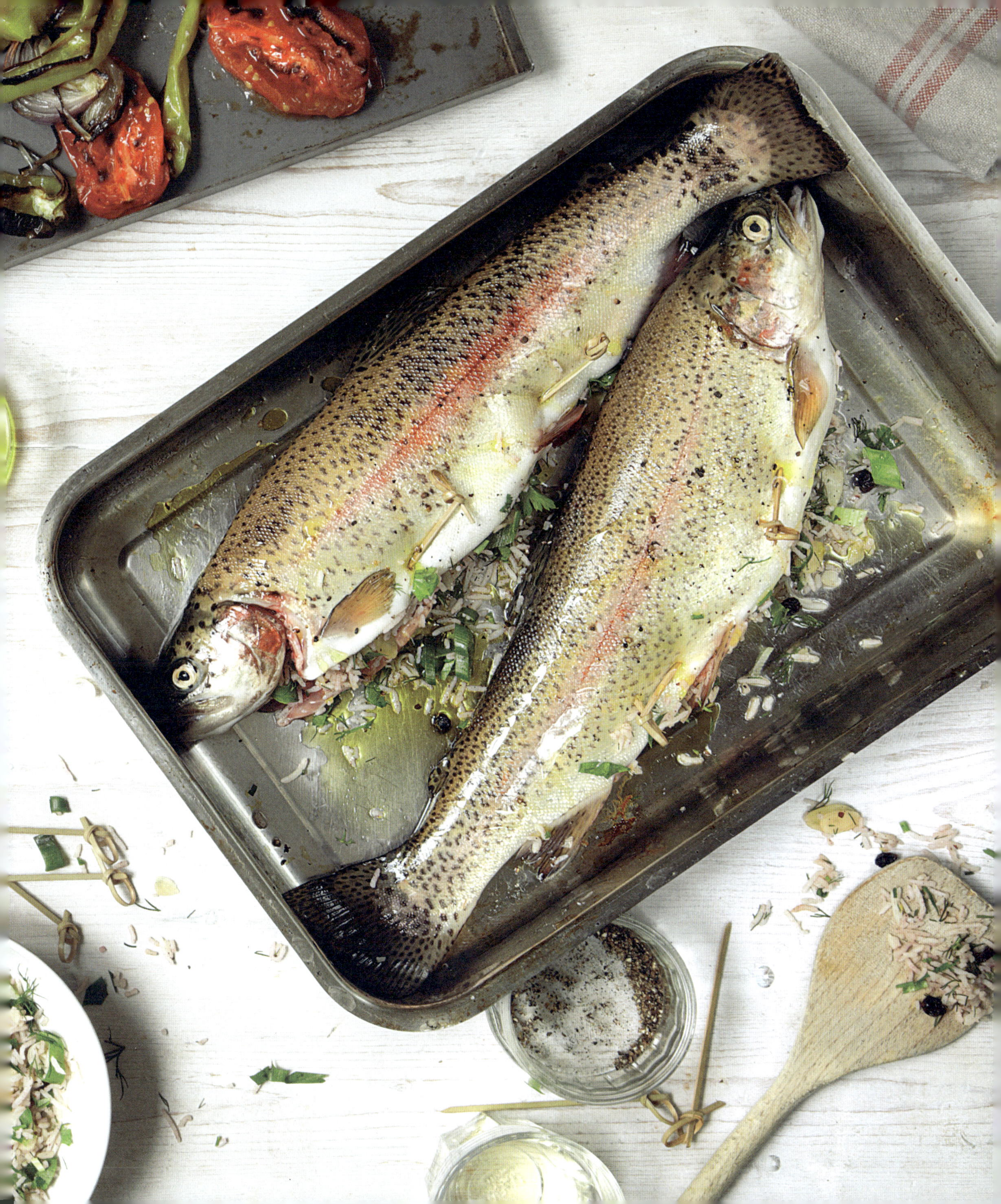

Sam & Sam Clark's BREAM

with Chickpeas, Currants, Turmeric and Dill

4 bream fillets
Juice and zest of **1** unwaxed orange
Juice and zest of **2** unwaxed limes
1 teaspoon ground cumin
1 teaspoon turmeric
½ teaspoon ground cinnamon
200g (7oz) Swiss chard, leaves only, *finely shredded*
Small bunch of dill, *finely chopped*
Bunch of spring onions, *sliced into thin rounds*
A few wild garlic leaves, *finely chopped* (optional)
50g (2oz) currants
120g (4½oz) (drained weight) canned chickpeas
Small knob of unsalted butter
200ml (7fl oz) fish or vegetable stock
Salt and freshly ground black pepper

Energy 241 kcal/1018 kJ
Protein 30.4g
Fat 7.0g
Sat. Fat 0.8g
Carbohydrate 16.0g
Fibre 2.2g

This recipe calls for wild garlic, which is only available in the spring. However, you can instead add ½ garlic clove or some garlic chives instead for a similar flavour. If you have a small amount leftover it will be very good with rice or any other grain such as couscous. This is low in fat and saturated fat but still packed with vitamins and minerals, including iron, B vitamins and beta-carotene.

Serves 4

Cut the bream into thin slices and put in a bowl with the citrus juices and zests, the cumin, turmeric and cinnamon. Season with salt and pepper and leave to marinate for 15 minutes.

Put a large saucepan over a high heat. Pour in the fish and all the marinade ingredients, followed by all the remaining ingredients. Cover and cook for 2–3 minutes until the fish has cooked through and the chard has wilted. Check for seasoning and serve immediately.

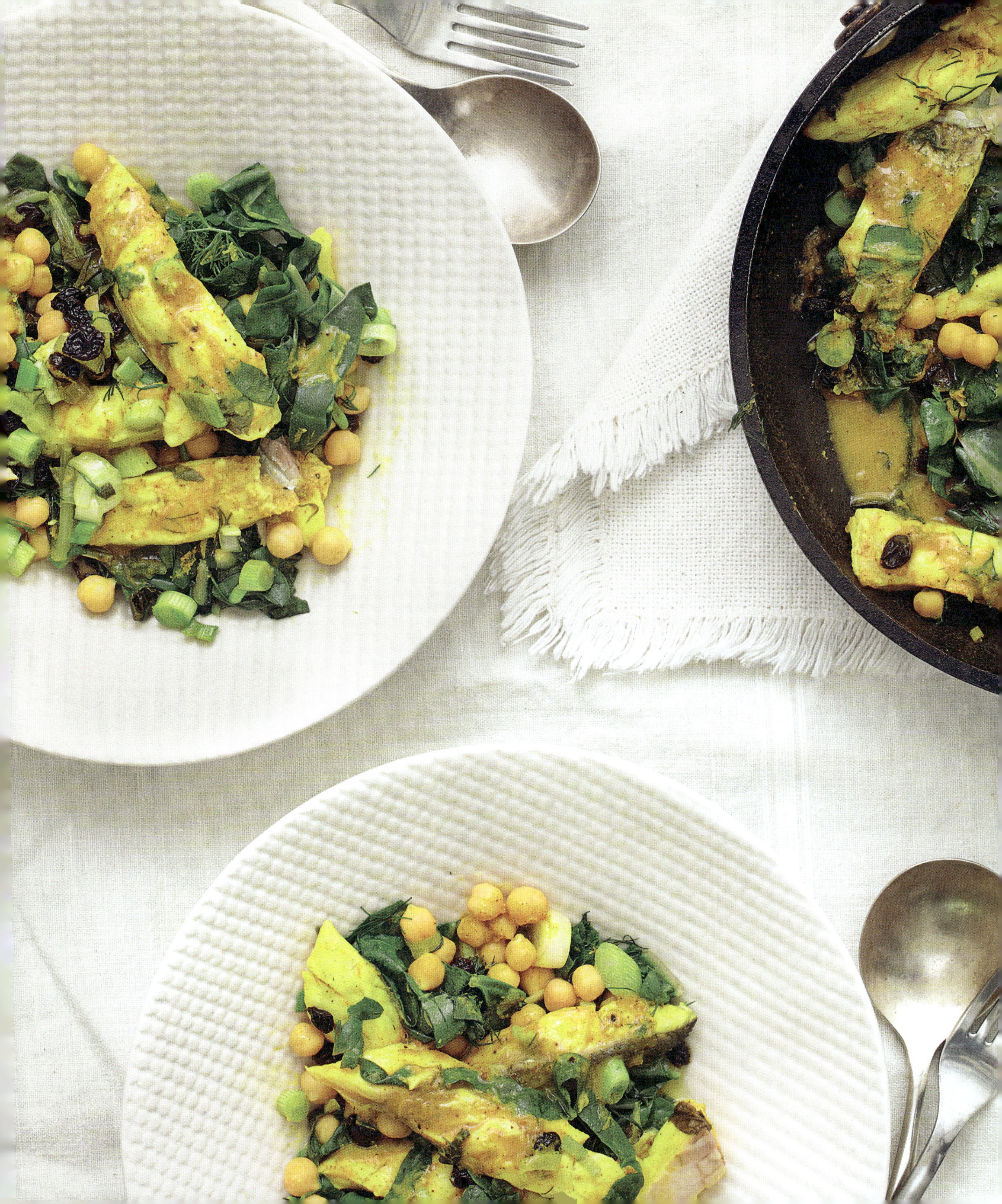

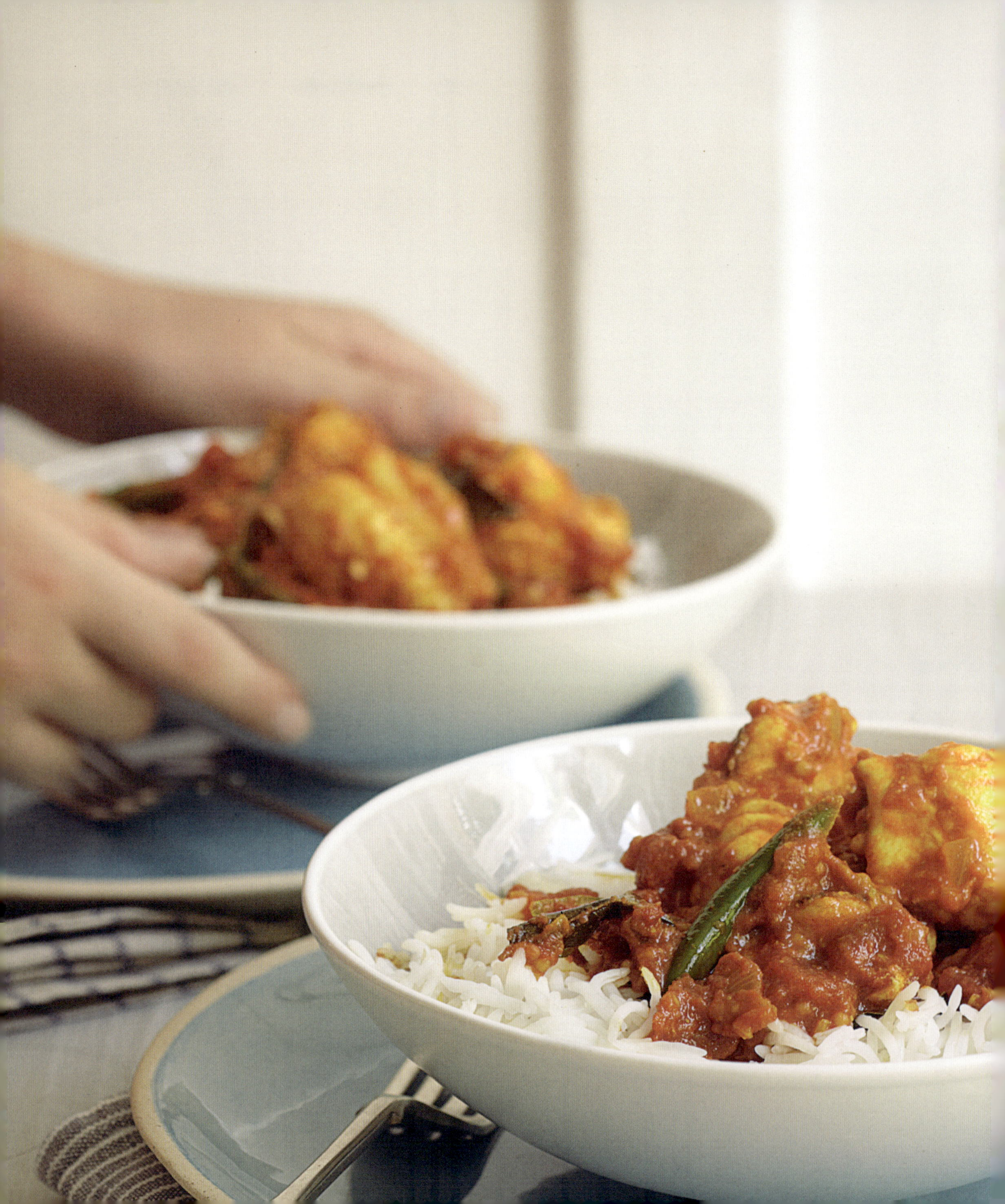

Rick Stein's MADRAS FISH CURRY OF SNAPPER, TOMATO AND TAMARIND

2 tablespoons vegetable oil
1 tablespoon yellow mustard seeds
1 large onion, *finely chopped*
3 garlic cloves, *finely crushed*
30 fresh curry leaves
2 teaspoons Kashmiri chilli powder or **½ teaspoon** hot chilli powder
2 teaspoons ground coriander
2 teaspoons turmeric
400g (14oz) can chopped tomatoes
100ml (3½oz) tamarind water (see right)
2 green chillies, *each sliced lengthways into 6 pieces, with seeds*
1 teaspoon salt
700g (25oz) snapper fillets, *cut into 5cm chunks*

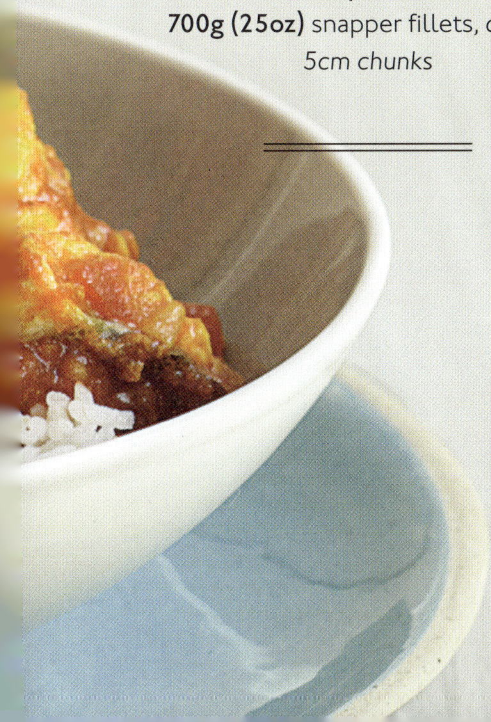

Kashmiri chillies are quite mild and are used for their deep red colour – if you can't find the powdered form, substitute it for around ½ teaspoon of regular chilli powder, which will give you a similar strength of heat. This recipe is low in fat but high in flavour. Choose wholegrain rice for extra fibre and B vitamins.

Serves 6

Heat the oil in a heavy-based saucepan over a medium heat. When hot, add the mustard seeds and fry for 30 seconds, then stir in the onion and garlic, and fry gently for about 10 minutes until softened and lightly golden. Add the curry leaves, chilli powder, coriander and turmeric, and fry for 2 minutes, then stir in the tomatoes, tamarind water, green chillies and salt. Simmer for about 10 minutes until rich and reduced. Add the fish, cook for a further 5 minutes or until just cooked through, and serve with plain rice.

Tamarind Water

You can buy jars of tamarind in liquid, just be careful it's not in concentrated form as it will be too strong. You can also prepare a liquid by steeping tamarinds (usually available in a block, a bit like dates) or tamarind concentrate with water. If using tamarinds, for 100ml (3.5fl oz) liquid, put 60g (2oz) of tamarinds in a bowl with 120ml (4fl oz) freshly boiled water. Leave to steep for about 15 minutes, then work everything together with your fingers, until the tamarinds have broken down. Push through a sieve, leaving behind the seeds and fibrous strands.

TIP

- You can freeze this dish as it is, as long as you are careful when you reheat it, because the fish will break up if you fiddle with it too much. Even better would be to just freeze some of the sauce – that way you can just defrost it and add some fresh fish. The sauce is also versatile enough to work with chicken or grilled vegetables.

Energy 196 kcal/828 kJ **Protein** 25.8g **Fat** 6.3g
Sat. Fat 0.9g **Carbohydrate** 12.2g **Fibre** 1.6g

Anjum Anand's BURMESE CHICKEN AND COCONUT CURRY

2 tablespoons vegetable oil
2 onions, *sliced*
30g (1oz) fresh ginger, *peeled weight, coarsely chopped*
7 large garlic cloves
2 rounded tablespoons gram (chickpea) flour
¾ teaspoon turmeric
1 tablespoon ground coriander
2 teaspoons ground cumin
2 teaspoons garam masala
250ml (8½fl oz) hot chicken stock
400ml (14fl oz) can coconut milk
500g (18oz) skinless, boneless chicken thighs, *each cut into 3 pieces*
1 large tomato, *finely chopped*
60g (2oz) creamed coconut
2 tablespoons lemon juice, *or to taste*
Salt

For the accompaniments:
Shop-bought crispy fried shallots
2 spring onions, *sliced*
3 hard-boiled eggs, *quartered*
2 long red chillies, *finely sliced*
Handful of roasted peanuts
Egg noodles (about **2** x **400g (14oz)** packets), *cooked according to the packet instructions*
Handful of chopped coriander leaves
Lime wedges

'I have never been to Burma, but this particular dish has well and truly made it to India and has become dinner party fare. I love it. It is impressive, but requires little more effort than making a curry and buying accompaniments.' *Anjum Anand*

Serves 4

Heat the oil in a large non-stick saucepan. Add the onions and cook until golden brown at the edges. Meanwhile, blend together the ginger and garlic with a small splash of water to help it become smooth (I use a hand-held blender). Add to the onions and cook until the water has dried off and the garlic has had a minute to cook; add a little water if it starts to stick. Spoon in the gram flour and stir for a minute before adding a good splash of water and the powdered spices. Cook for 3–4 minutes.

Add the chicken stock and coconut milk, bring to the boil, then lower the heat and simmer for 5 minutes. Add the chicken, tomato and creamed coconut, and bring back to the boil, then lower the heat and cook gently for a further 7–8 minutes, or until cooked through. Stir in the lemon juice, taste and adjust the salt and lemon juice accordingly.

Meanwhile, prepare as many of the accompaniments as you like or can be bothered to make, and offer them at the table in small bowls and dishes. These are what make this dish memorable, so the more the merrier!

TIP

- This will freeze well if you treat it gently when reheating.

Nutritional information for the basic curry recipe:
Energy 442 kcal/1853 kJ **Protein** 38.3g **Fat** 23.5g
Sat. Fat 8.5g **Carbohydrate** 21.8g **Fibre** 3.6g

YOGURT-MARINATED CHICKEN

8 chicken pieces, *on the bone, skinned*

For the marinade:
200ml (7fl oz) yogurt
Juice of **1** lemon
Juice of **1** lime
1 small onion, *finely chopped or grated*
2 garlic cloves, *crushed*
1 teaspoon ground cumin
1 teaspoon allspice
½ teaspoon turmeric
1 tablespoon chipotle paste

Lime wedges, *to serve*

Energy 187 kcal/785 kJ
Protein 24.0g
Fat 8.8g
Sat. Fat 2.7g
Carbohydrate 3.9g
Fibre 0.3g

Oven baking suits larger pieces of chicken much more than grilling or barbecuing, but if you would rather use either of these methods, buy chunks of filleted chicken instead. Serve with a big bowl of brown rice or quinoa with lots of coriander, mint and lime zest stirred through it. It would also be great with a watercress and orange salad or used in a packed lunch. Low in fat and saturated fat, this makes a great accompaniment to salad or cooked vegetables.

Serves 6

Mix all the marinade ingredients together. Make cuts into the chicken at regular intervals. Cover the chicken pieces in the marinade and massage in. Leave to marinate in the fridge for a few hours or overnight.

When you are ready to cook the chicken, preheat the oven to its highest setting. Line a baking tray with foil or greaseproof paper. Remove the chicken from the marinade, scraping off any excess as you go and place on the lined baking tray. Put in the oven and reduce the heat to 200°C/gas mark 6/400°F. Bake for 20–25 minutes until the juices run clear (test by piercing the thickest part of the leg) and the flesh has started to blacken in places. Serve with lime wedges.

TIP

- The chicken can be frozen raw in its marinade or cooked. It will also keep well in the fridge for a few days. Cut it up small and stir into some yogurt or mayonnaise for a tasty sandwich filling.

POT-ROAST CHICKEN

1 tablespoon olive oil
1 onion, *sliced*
1 leek, *cut into chunks*
1 large carrot, *peeled and cut into chunks*
2 celery sticks, *cut into chunks*
150ml (5fl oz) white wine
150ml (5fl oz) hot chicken stock
1 head of garlic, *broken into cloves, unpeeled*
2 thyme sprigs
2 large tarragon sprigs
1 chicken (approx. **1.2–1.5kg (44–52oz)**)
Wedge of lemon
Large knob of unsalted butter
Salt and freshly ground black pepper

Energy 452 kcal/1878 kJ
Protein 35.0g
Fat 27.1g
Sat. Fat 7.4g
Carbohydrate 11.5g
Fibre 3.7g

This way of roasting a chicken ensures succulent meat, sweet, melting vegetables and a beautifully creamy gravy. Any leftover gravy can be used in all kinds of things, but is particularly good added to stock for risotto, or made into a quick pasta sauce with some leftover chicken, some diced bacon and a cupful of peas. This is an easy way of combining chicken and vegetables to give a good balance of vitamins, including beta-carotene and vitamin A.

Serves 4

Preheat the oven to 200°C/gas mark 6/400°F.

Heat the oil in a lidded casserole large enough to hold the chicken. Add the vegetables and sauté over a medium heat until starting to soften and colour around the edges. Add the wine, allow to bubble away for a couple of minutes to reduce, then pour in the stock. Add the garlic cloves and half the herbs.

Season the chicken with salt and pepper, inside and out. Stuff the remaining herbs and the lemon in the cavity. Spread the butter over the chicken breasts, then put the chicken on top of the vegetables, pushing them to the sides as much as possible.

Put the lid on the casserole and transfer to the oven. Cook for about 45 minutes, then remove the lid and allow the chicken to brown and crisp up for a further 20 minutes.

Test that the chicken is cooked by piercing the thickest part of the leg and checking that the juices run clear. Remove the chicken and the vegetables to a serving platter and keep warm by covering with foil.

Take all the garlic cloves and squeeze the flesh out back into the casserole. Simmer the remaining liquid until it has reduced down and thickened – it should look quite creamy, thanks to the garlic. Sieve the gravy into a gravy boat, pushing through as much garlic as you can. Serve immediately with some new potatoes.

TIP

- Keep leftover chicken or gravy in the fridge for a few days, or you can also freeze. The gravy is best frozen in small pots or ice-cube trays as just one cube will enrich anything you add it to.

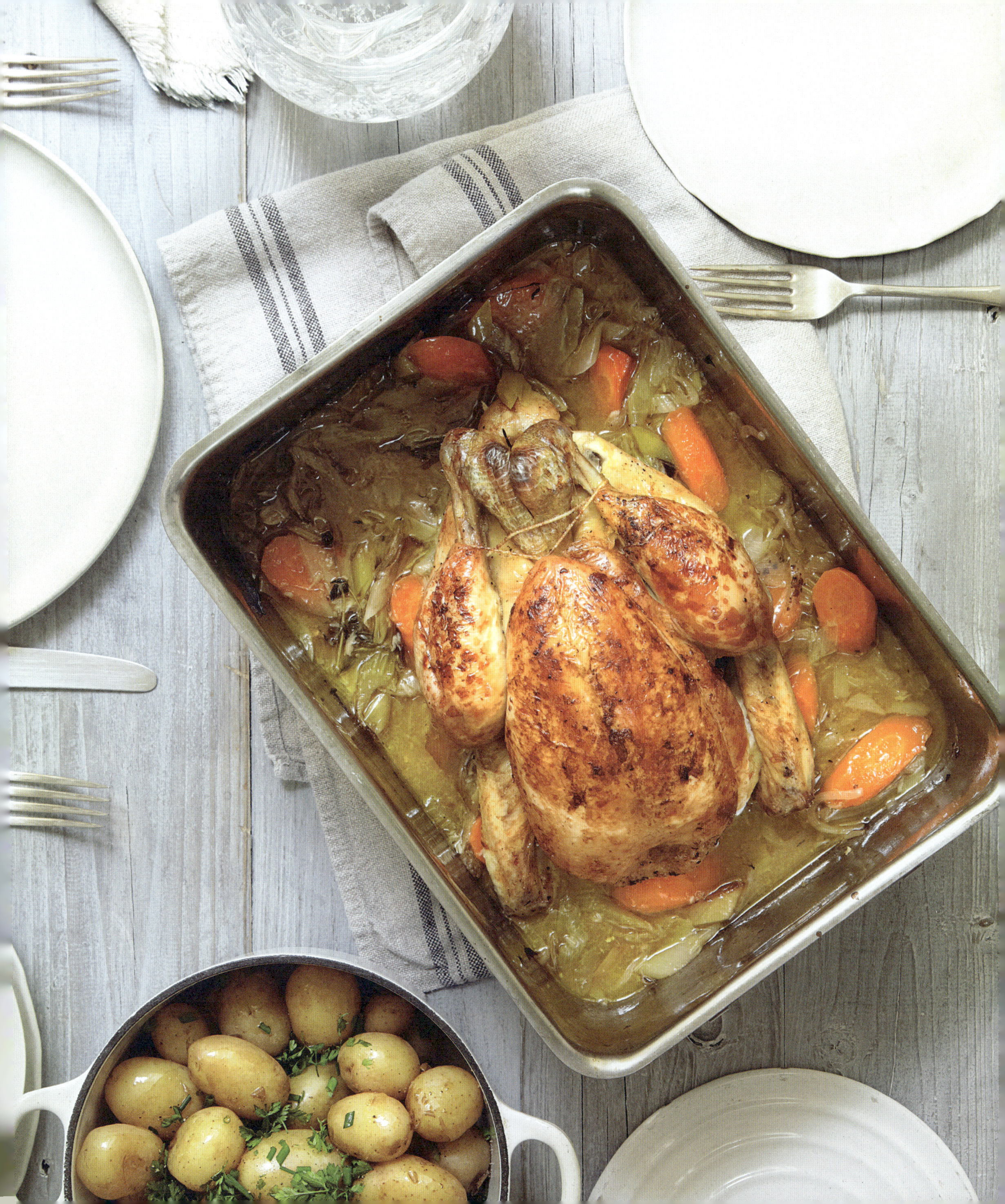

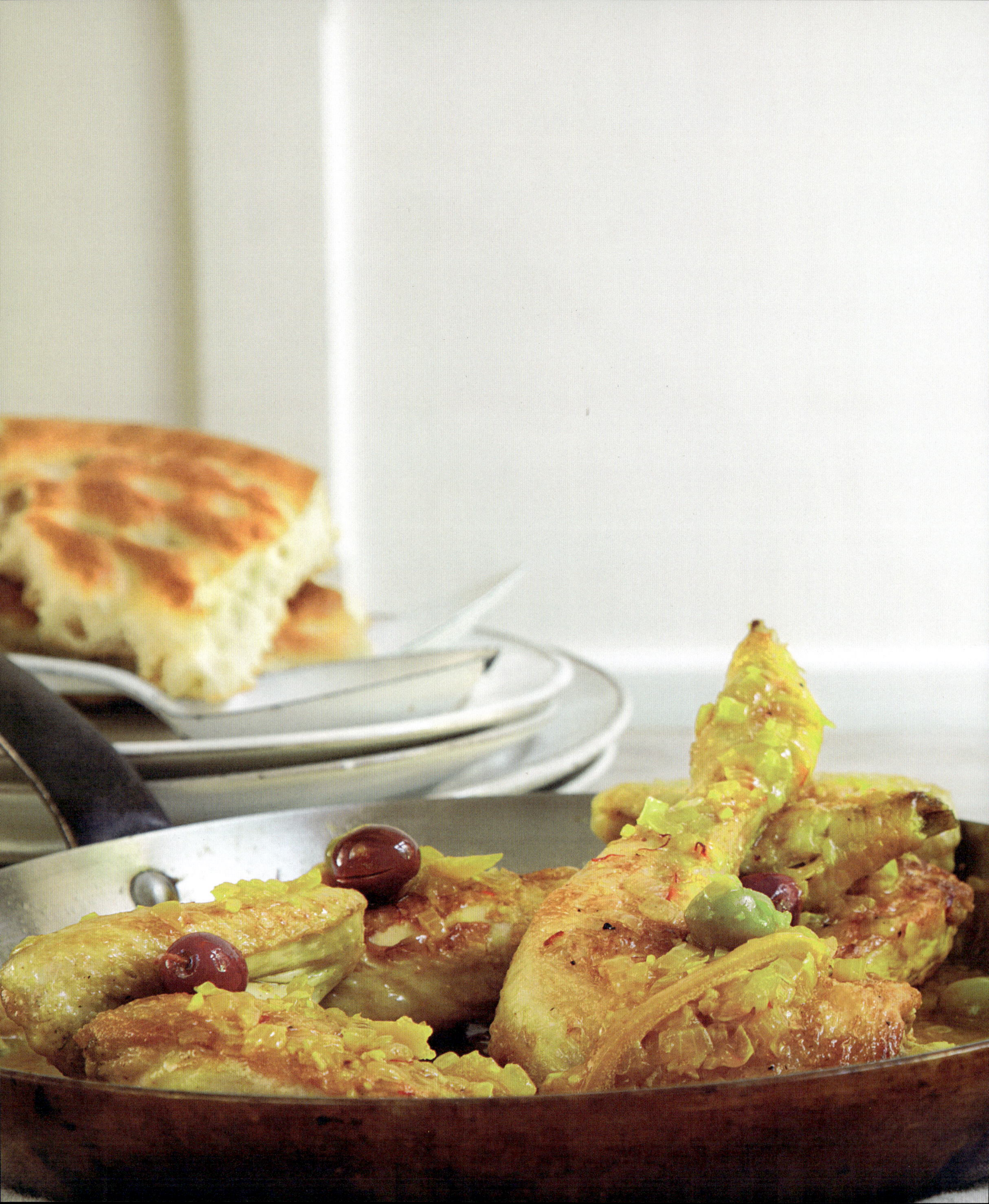

Claudia Roden's
TAGINE OF CHICKEN
with Preserved Lemons and Green Olives

3 tablespoons extra virgin olive oil
2 onions, *grated or very finely chopped*
2–3 garlic cloves, *crushed*
¼ teaspoon crushed saffron threads or good-quality saffron powder
¼–½ teaspoon ground ginger
1 chicken, *jointed and skinned* or **4** chicken quarters, *skinned*
Juice of ½ lemon
2 tablespoons chopped coriander
2 tablespoons chopped flat-leaf parsley
Peel of **1** large or **2** small preserved lemons, *cut into quarters or strips*
12–16 green or violet olives
Salt and freshly ground black pepper

'This is the best-known Moroccan chicken dish. It was the only one, apart from appetizers, served during an evening of Arab poetry and story-telling, accompanied by musicians, that I attended in a Paris restaurant. The olives do not have to be stoned. If you find them too salty, soak them in two changes of water for up to an hour.' *Claudia Roden*

Serves 4

Select a wide casserole or heavy-bottomed pan that can hold all the chicken pieces in one layer. Pour in the oil and heat before adding the onions. Sauté, stirring over a low heat, until they soften, then stir in the garlic, saffron and ginger.

Put in the chicken pieces, season with salt and pepper, and pour in about 300ml cold water. Simmer, covered, turning the pieces over a few times and adding a little more water if it becomes too dry. If using breasts, lift them out after about 20 minutes and put them to one side. Continue to cook the remaining pieces for a further 25 minutes or so before returning the breasts to the pan.

Stir the lemon juice, the chopped coriander and parsley, the preserved lemon peel and the olives into the sauce. Simmer, uncovered, for 5–10 minutes, until the reduced sauce is thick and unctuous. If there is too much liquid, lift out the chicken pieces and keep them to one side while you reduce the sauce further, then return the chicken to the pan and heat through.

Present the chicken on a serving dish with the olives and lemon peel on top of the meat.

TIP

- This dish will freeze well, with or without the herbs, but add more after reheating to freshen up the dish.

Energy 388 kcal/1417 kJ **Protein** 46.5g **Fat** 13.9g
Sat. Fat 2.6g **Carbohydrate** 7.3g **Fibre** 2.6g

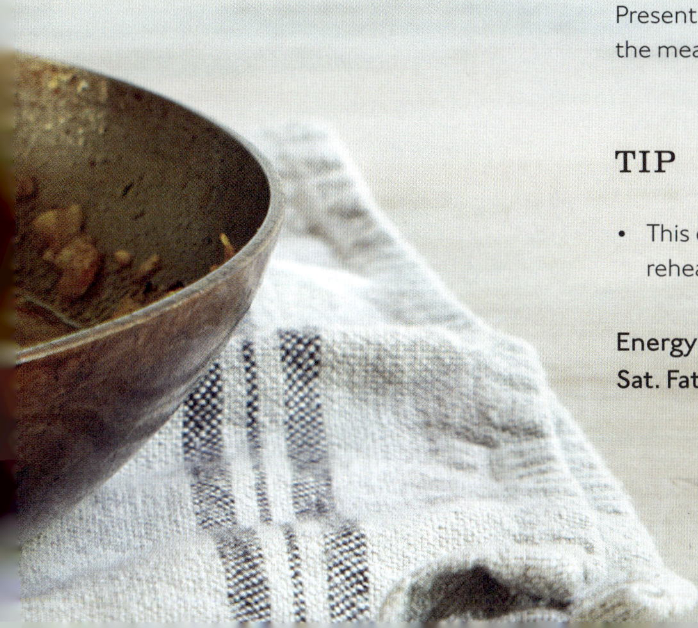

SHEPHERD'S PIE

This is a shepherd's pie with a difference. Replacing some of the lamb with cooked lentils reduces the fat content but makes a beautifully creamy ragu, while the sweet potatoes and lentils have a lower glycaemic index value than potatoes, so carbohydrate is absorbed into your bloodstream more slowly. This is a healthier version of a traditional recipe, still with the iron and B vitamins you would expect but also packed with beta-carotene. Serve with a leafy green vegetable, such as cabbage or spinach.

Serves 8

4 teaspoons olive oil
400g (14oz) lamb mince
1 onion, *finely chopped*
1 carrot, *finely chopped*
2 celery sticks, *finely chopped*
2 garlic cloves, *finely chopped*
¼ teaspoon ground cinnamon
1 teaspoon dried oregano
½ teaspoon fresh rosemary, *very finely chopped*
2 teaspoons tomato purée
2 teaspoons tomato ketchup
1 teaspoon Worcestershire sauce
250ml (8½fl oz) red wine or stock
250ml (8½fl oz) hot lamb or chicken stock
300g (10½oz) cooked brown lentils
Salt and freshly ground black pepper

For the mash:
2–3 sweet potatoes (approx. **1kg (35oz)**)
2 tablespoons crème fraîche
A little unsalted butter

Energy 319 kcal/1344 kJ
Protein 15.3g
Fat 10.9g
Sat. Fat 4.7g
Carbohydrate 37.3g
Fibre 7.1g

To make the ragu, heat 1 teaspoon of the olive oil in a large frying pan. Add the lamb and brown it thoroughly, searing it rather than letting it stew.

Heat the remaining 3 teaspoons of oil in a large casserole or saucepan. Add all the vegetables and cook for several minutes until beginning to soften. Add the garlic, cooked lamb, cinnamon and herbs, and cook for a couple more minutes. Add the tomato purée, ketchup and Worcestershire sauce. Pour over the wine and bring to the boil until the wine has reduced by about half. Add the stock and the lentils. Season with salt and pepper. Cover and simmer gently for about 45 minutes, checking regularly to make sure it doesn't require more liquid.

Meanwhile, make the mash. Preheat the oven to 200°C/gas mark 6/400°F.

Put the unpeeled sweet potatoes on a baking tray. Bake for 35–40 minutes until soft. Remove from the oven. As soon as they are cool enough to handle, break them open and scoop out the flesh into a bowl. Add the crème fraîche, season with salt and pepper and mash thoroughly.

To assemble, put the ragu into an ovenproof serving dish. Spoon the sweet potato mash on top, spreading it out with a palette knife and making sure that none of the ragu has bled through, then fluff up slightly with a fork for a rougher finish. Dot with a few small knobs of butter. Bake for about 25 minutes.

TIP

- You can freeze the ragu or the whole assembled pie very successfully, so if you would sooner make lots of individual portions, perhaps invest in some foil containers you can put straight from the freezer into the oven.

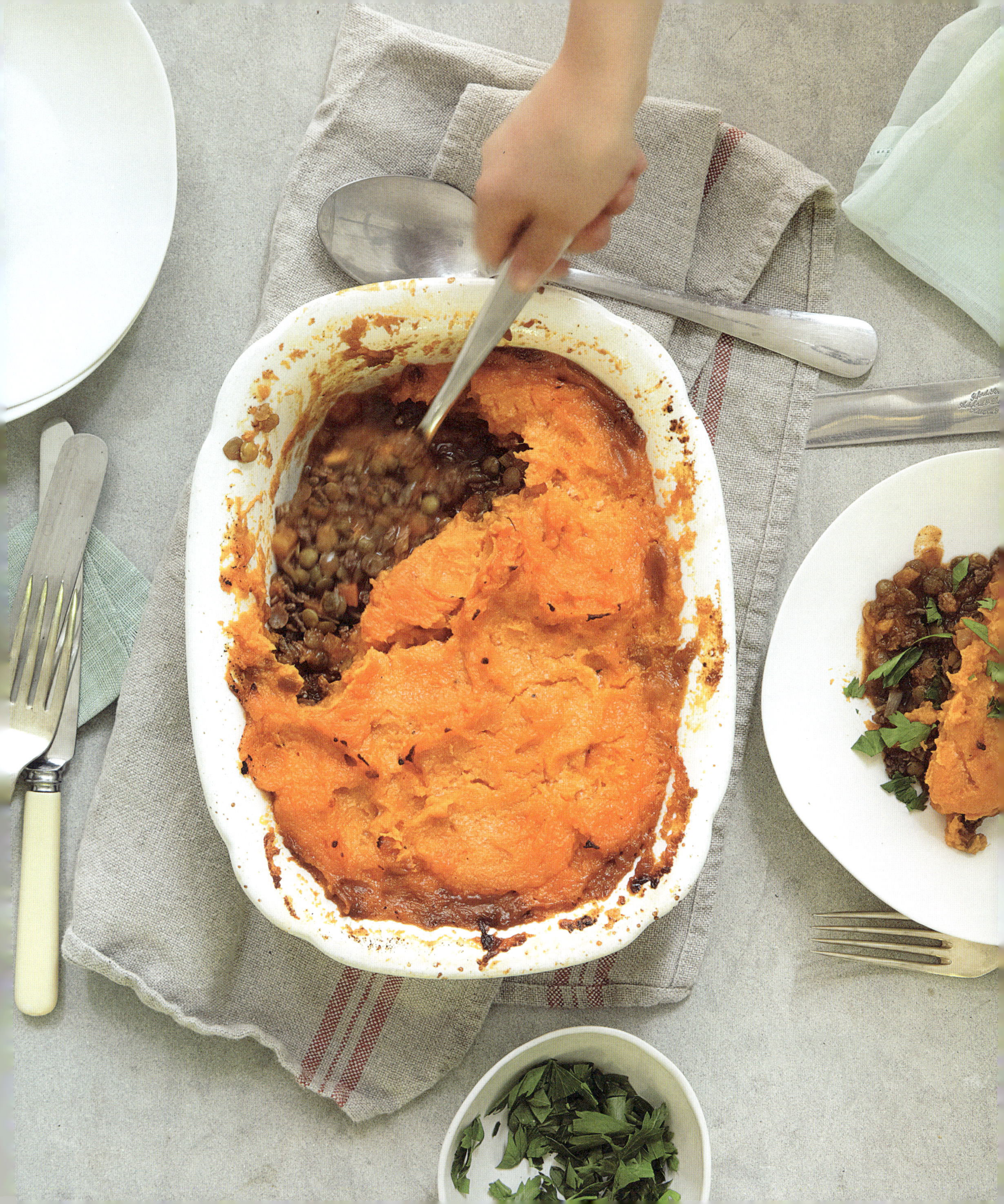

DESSERTS and BAKING

Fruit is an obvious choice for a healthy dessert. Choose fruits in season for the best flavour and make the most of the variety of fruits that are available, such as peaches, nectarines, apricots, mangos, berries, including strawberries, raspberries and blueberries, and currants, such as blackcurrants and redcurrants. If you want to add a topping, choose low-fat yogurt, fromage frais, low-fat Greek yogurt or sorbet. Alternatively, make fruit coulis and stir into yogurt or fromage frais.

In the winter, bake, stew or poach fruit such as apples, pears or plums. Add seasonal berries, such as blackberries, for extra colour and flavour. Use fruit that has been frozen during the summer months for stewing and in compôtes.

Dried fruit is a good choice in the winter months. Simmer with water and fruit juice, such as orange juice, until the fruit has absorbed some of the liquid and is soft. Add cinnamon, mixed spice and orange and lemon zest for extra flavour.

Other desserts are usually higher in fat and sugar, so have them occasionally. It is the overall balance of your intake over the weeks and months that is important, so, if your diet has a good balance for most of the time, then you can afford to treat yourself occasionally.

BLACKBERRY AND APPLE SORBET

The flavours of this sorbet are beautifully fresh on their own, but adding a tablespoonful of alcohol, sloe gin or a blackberry eau de vie or liqueur would be lovely. This is a delicious way to eat fresh, seasonal fruits providing a range of vitamins and minerals.

125g (4½oz) caster sugar
Juice of **2** limes
2 large Granny Smith apples, *peeled, cored and sliced*
300g (10½oz) blackberries, *fresh or frozen*
Handful of mint leaves
1 tablespoon sloe gin or blackberry liqueur *(optional)*

Energy 88 kcal/375 kJ
Protein 0.5g
Fat 0.1g
Sat. Fat 0g
Carbohydrate 22.7g
Fibre 2.4g

Serves 8

Put the caster sugar in a saucepan and add 200ml (7fl oz) freshly boiled water and the lime juice. Simmer over a very low heat until the sugar has dissolved. Drop the apples straight into the sugar syrup to stop them browning. Poach until very soft. Add the blackberries and simmer for 2–3 minutes. Add the mint leaves, then remove from the heat and allow to cool. Blitz the mixture and pass through a sieve until smooth. Add the alcohol, if using.

Churn in an ice-cream maker until thick and aerated, or pour straight into a freezerproof container and whisk regularly during the freezing process.

VANILLA POACHED PEARS WITH CHOCOLATE SAUCE

6 firm pears

For the poaching liquor:
500ml (17fl oz) apple juice (cloudy or clear)
1 vanilla pod, *split lengthways*
1 teaspoon black peppercorns, *lightly crushed*

For the chocolate sauce:
150g (5½oz) dark chocolate
½ teaspoon vanilla extract

Nutritional Information for 1 pear:
Energy 51 kcal/215 kJ
Protein 0.5g
Fat 0g
Sat. Fat 0g
Carbohydrate 11g
Fibre 2.1g

Nutritional Information for 1 tablespoon chocolate sauce:
Energy 51 kcal/215 kJ
Protein 0.5g
Fat 2.8g
Sat. Fat 1.7g
Carbohydrate 6g
Fibre 0g

This dessert can look very elegant: whole pears swathed in sauce, but you can also simplify things by just halving the pears and scooping out the cores. If you do this, you can also make quite a large batch – they will keep in the fridge for at least a week.

Serves 6

For the poaching liquor, put all the poaching ingredients, along with 200ml (7fl oz) cold water, into a saucepan large enough to hold all the pears. Heat gently.

Prepare the pears by peeling them. To make the dessert look very elegant, you can core them while leaving the stem intact. Simply use a very small, sharp knife to cut out the core, starting at the base of the pear and working your way up. Otherwise, cut them in half and remove the core.

Add the pears to the poaching liquor as you prepare them so they don't discolour. Make sure they are completely submerged. If they aren't, add a little more water. To stop the pears from floating, you can also cover them with an upturned plate that fits inside the pan. Simmer the pears for 20–30 minutes – how long they take will depend entirely on how ripe they are.

To make the sauce, break the chocolate into a small saucepan and add the vanilla extract and 75ml (2½fl oz) cold water. Melt everything together over a very low heat, stirring constantly, until you have a rich, glossy sauce.

Remove the pears from the poaching liquor and allow to cool. Serve with the sauce.

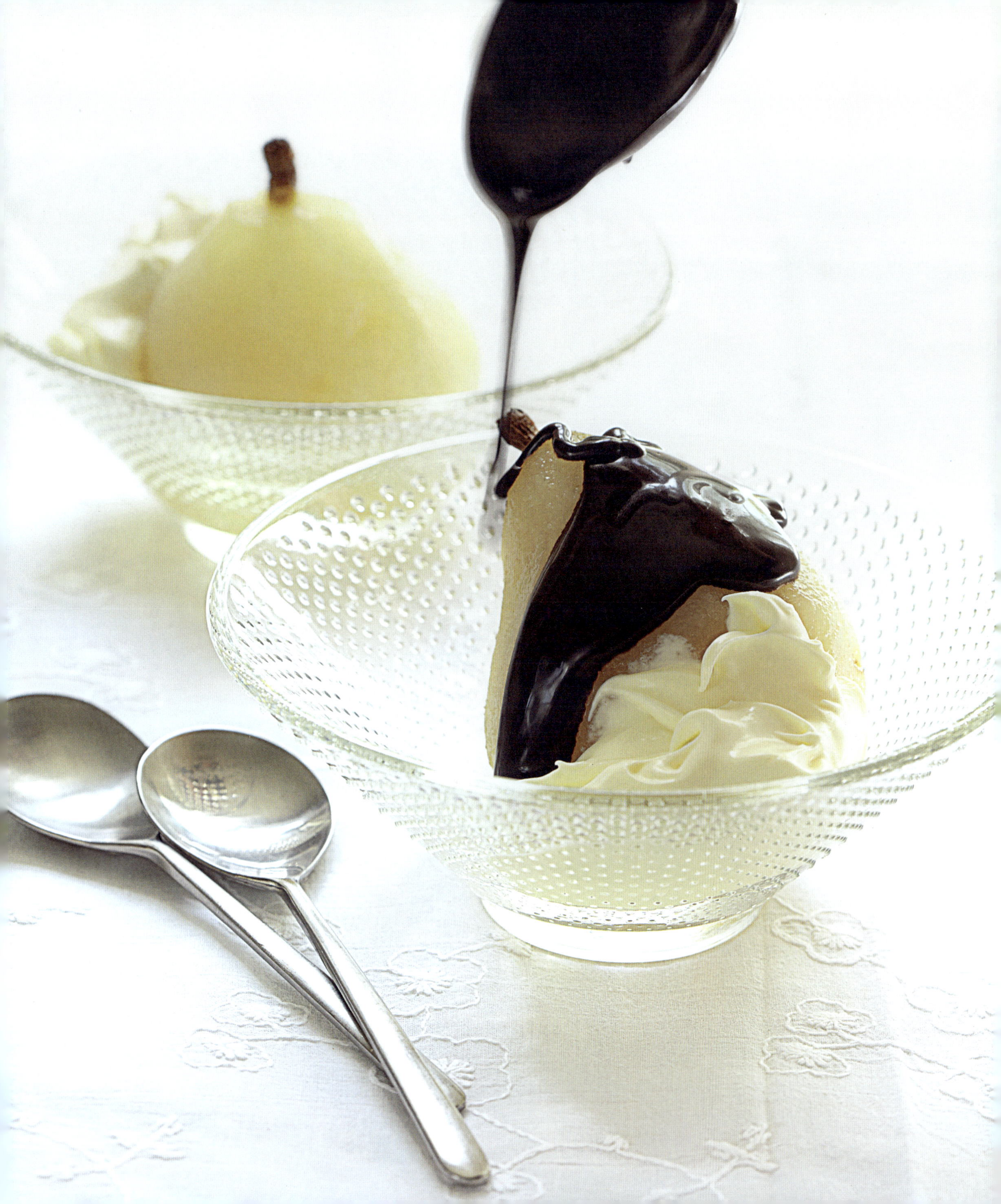

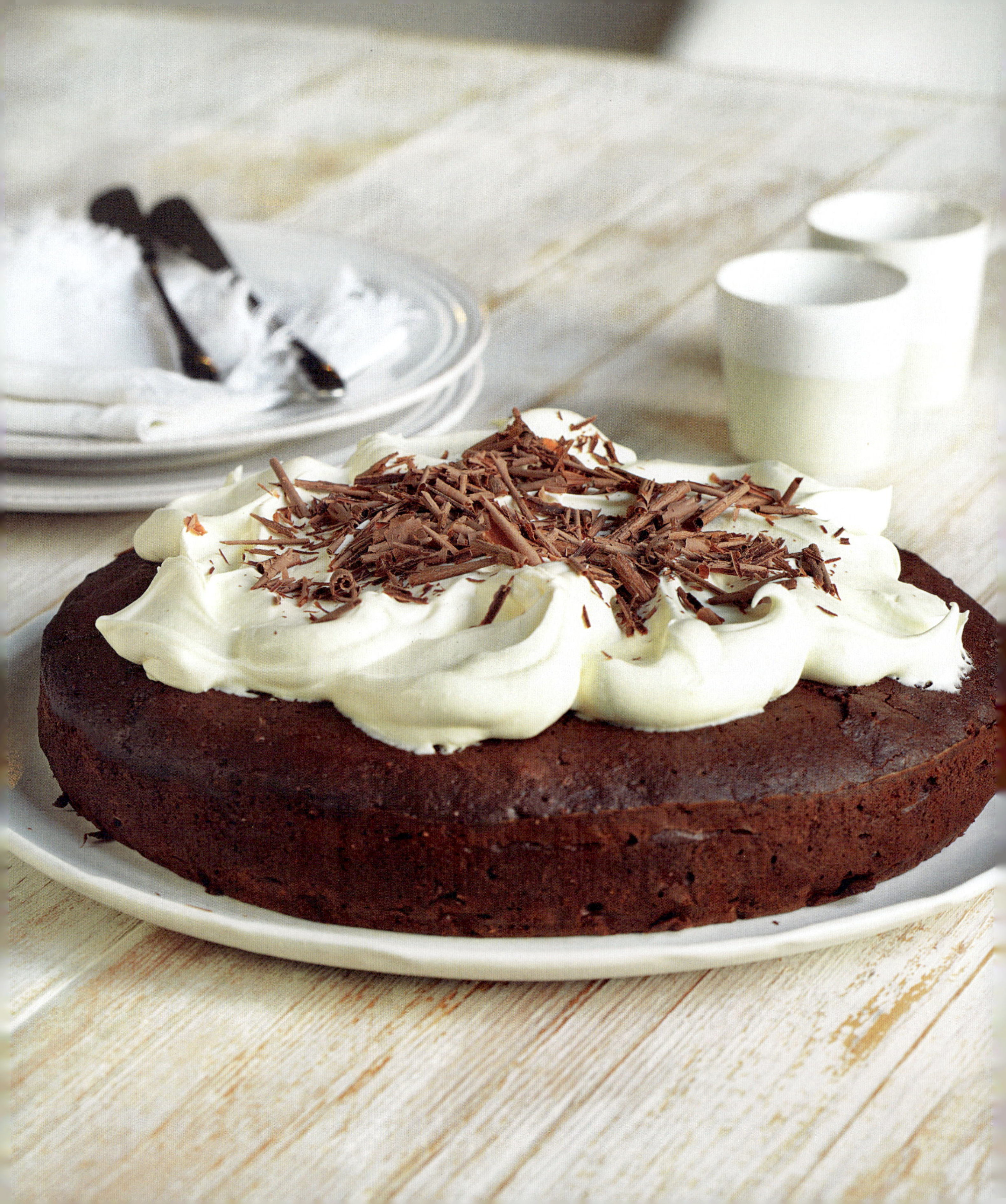

CHOCOLATE AND BEETROOT CAKE

225g (8oz) self-raising flour
50g (2oz) cocoa powder
100g (3½oz) dark chocolate
125g (4½oz) unsalted butter, *softened, diced*
200g (7oz) soft, light brown sugar
50g (2oz) runny honey
3 free-range eggs
200g (7oz) cooked beetroot, *puréed*
2 teaspoons espresso powder dissolved in **2 tablespoons** hot water *(optional)*

For the topping
200ml (7fl oz) double cream
100ml (3½fl oz)thick crème fraîche
1 tablespoon runny honey
Dark chocolate

Energy 422 kcal/1763 kJ
Protein 5.7g
Fat 26.2g
Sat. Fat 15.8g
Carbohydrate 44.2g
Fibre 2.2g

Nutritional information for 1 slice with no filling:
Energy 298 kcal/1251 kJ
Protein 5.2g
Fat 13.7g
Sat. Fat 7.9g
Carbohydrate 41.7g

This is a cake for a special occasion, with its delicious moist consistency. This recipe cuts the usual amount of sugar by using beetroot in the ingredients. The result is a cake that is very moist, with a dark, rich chocolate flavour. Consequently, it makes a good dessert. If you wish to reduce the fat content, then do not decorate it, just serve slightly warm with low-fat crème fraîche or natural yogurt on the side. This way it will keep better, too. The addition of a vegetable to this traditional recipe increases the vitamin content and provides some dietary fibre.

Makes 1 × 23cm (9in) cake/ 12 slices

Line a loose-based 23cm (9in) round cake tin with baking parchment. Preheat the oven to 180°C/gas mark 4/350°F.

Sift the flour and cocoa powder into a small bowl. Break the chocolate into a heatproof bowl and melt over a simmering pan of water.

Cream together the butter and sugar until light and fluffy. Add the honey, then start adding the eggs with alternate tablespoons of flour and cocoa, mixing well in between, then add in the remaining flour and cocoa.

Pour in the melted chocolate, the beetroot and the espresso, if using. Make sure everything is evenly incorporated, then pour the batter into the prepared cake tin.

Bake for 40–50 minutes. If after 30 minutes you feel the top of the cake is in danger of burning, cover the tin with a sheet of foil. The cake will be done when the top is springy in the middle and it has shrunk away from the sides slightly. Leave the cake to cool in the tin for 10 minutes, then turn out onto a cooling rack.

For the filling, if using, lightly whip the cream until it is almost at the soft peak stage, then add the crème fraiche and honey. Continue to whisk until it is stiff enough to hold its shape. Pile onto the top of the cake and swirl around with a spatula to cover. Grate or shave chocolate to sprinkle on top.

TIP

- This cake can be frozen – either whole or portioned out and individually wrapped. Once defrosted, it is particularly good served warm.

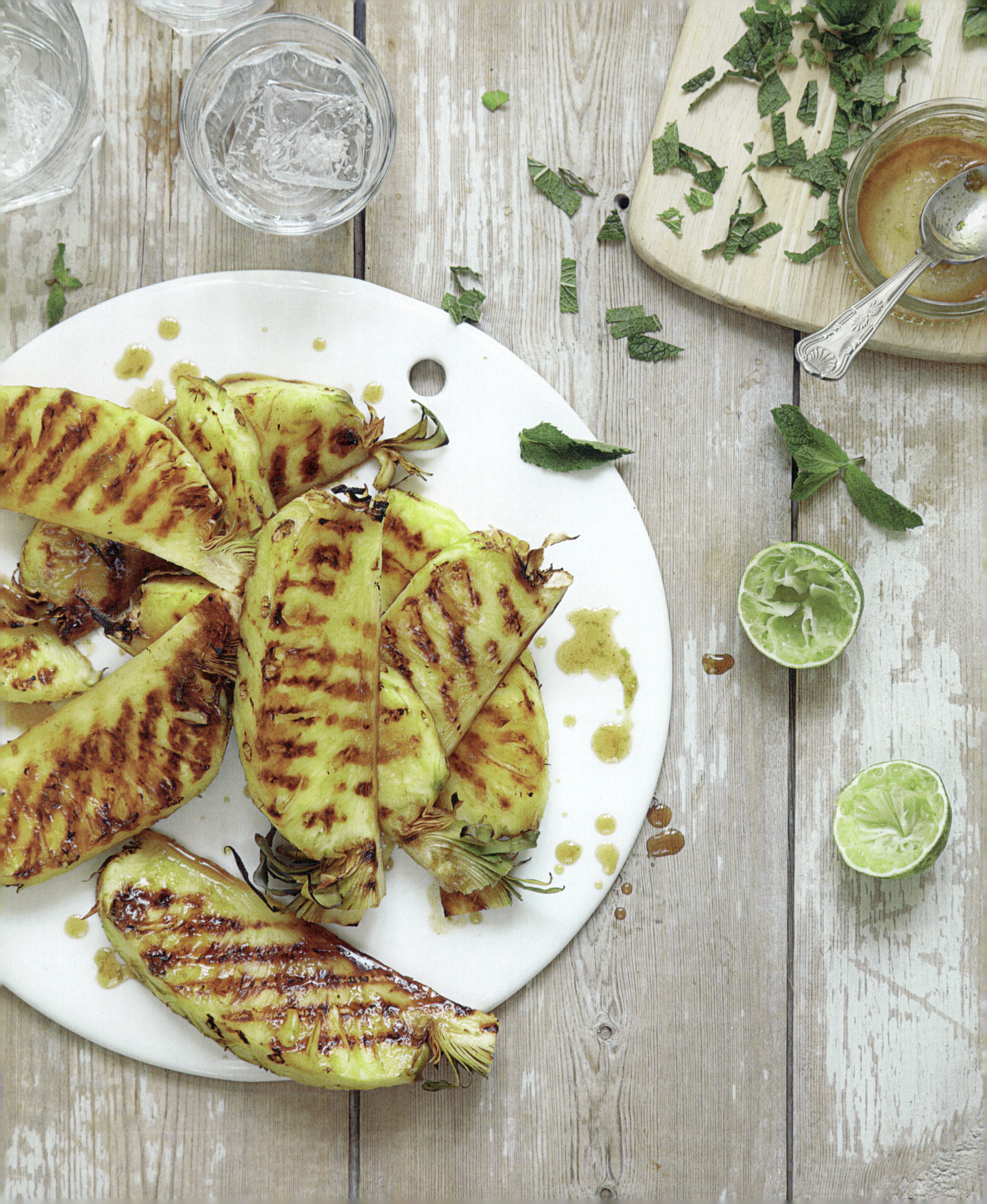

GRILLED PINEAPPLE

with Ginger, Mint and Chilli

2 tablespoons runny honey
2 tablespoons rum *(optional)*
Zest and juice of 1 unwaxed lime
½ **teaspoon** ground ginger
1 mild red chilli, *deseeded and finely chopped*
1 large ripe pineapple, *peeled, cored and cut into long wedges*

A few mint leaves, *to serve*

Energy 86 kcal/369 kJ
Protein 0.7g
Fat 0.3g
Sat. Fat 0g
Carbohydrate 21.6g
Fibre 2.4g

This is fantastically easy, very tasty and healthy. It's best eaten on its own – or perhaps with some coconut ice cream on the side. This is also a great dish for the barbecue. If you are cooking indoors and don't have a griddle pan, you can pop the pineapple under a hot grill instead.

Serves 6

Mix together the honey, rum (if using), lime juice and zest, ground ginger and chilli. Add the pineapple and make sure it is completely covered with the marinade. Leave for stand for at least 1 hour.

Heat a large griddle pan. Drain the pineapple, reserving the marinade, and griddle for about 2–3 minutes on each side. Serve with the reserved marinade spooned over and a sprinkling of torn mint leaves.

BAKED APPLES WITH TOASTED OATS AND HONEY

4 large Bramley apples, *cored*
2 tablespoons runny honey or maple syrup
50g (2oz) porridge oats
25g (1oz) raisins
Pinch of ground cinnamon
A few knobs of unsalted butter, *plus extra for greasing*
2 teaspoons soft, light brown sugar

Energy 211 kcal/890 kJ
Protein 2.4g
Fat 4.4g
Sat. Fat 2.0g
Carbohydrate 43.2g
Fibre 5.0g

This dessert would also be a good dish to eat at breakfast time as, thanks to the oats, it will set you up with plenty of slow-release energy. The raisins give sweetness so you can reduce the amount of honey, maple syrup or brown sugar if you prefer this less sweet. Serve with dollops of natural yogurt. An excellent low-fat dessert with soluble dietary fibre.

Serves 4

Preheat the oven to 180°C/gas mark 4/350°F. Grease a baking or roasting dish with butter. Set the apples upright in the dish.

Heat the honey with 2 tablespoons water until very runny, then stir in the porridge oats, raisins and cinnamon. Stuff this mixture into the apple cores. Top the apples with a small knob of butter and sprinkle with the sugar. Bake in the oven for 35–40 minutes. Serve with any escaped juices spooned over.

SNACKS & DRINKS

Finding healthier snacks can be challenging. Dried fruit, nuts and seeds are great if you want something that travels well and will keep without perishing. Avoid salted varieties if possible and remember that they can be high in energy – great if you want to gain weight but not so good if you are trying to lose weight! See the recipe for fruit leather on page 248 to see how to use seasonal fruits for a delicious snack.

High in dietary fibre and low in fat, popcorn is filling and does not need to be weighed down with sugar, fat and salt to be delicious. A great flavour for popcorn is seaweed – take nori sheets and blitz them with a teaspoon of dried miso and 1 teaspoon of lemon zest. You can add a splash of soy sauce or tamari just before serving.

Kale chips are a healthy, low-calorie alternative to the potato or corn version and really hit the spot when you fancy a savoury snack. They will keep quite well in an airtight container, but you can always pop them back in the oven for a minute if you want to recrisp them. This savoury snack is bursting with beta-carotene and potassium. Tear the kale leaves into large bite-sized pieces, drizzle with olive oil and season well. If you want to add any liquid flavouring and/or citrus zest to the kale, add them now. Mix thoroughly. Spread the kale over baking parchment lined baking trays. Bake in the oven for 10–15 minutes at 180°C. The crisps are ready when they start to turn a light golden brown in patches and around the edges only. Remove from the oven and allow to cool. Put in a large bowl and add any dry seasonings you like. (Try mixing dried herbs and spices with salt, making an approximation of salt and vinegar crisps by using a combination of lemon juice or cider vinegar with salt, or different kinds of ground chilli – everything from cayenne to chipotle. You can add garam masala, Chinese five-spice, ras el hanout…the possibilities are endless.)

Rice cakes, wholemeal crackers, oatcakes and crispbreads are ideal to eat with low-fat toppings if you need something a little more substantial.

If you are looking for something sweet, then perhaps sneak a chocolate drop from the during treatment section (see page 147) to satisfy cravings.

Katie and Giancarlo Caldesi's ZHUG

60g (2oz) fresh coriander leaves
40g (1½oz) parsley leaves
2 green chillies (or red chillies, for a red zhug)
3 garlic cloves, *peeled*
2 tablespoons lemon juice
5 tablespoons extra virgin olive oil
1 teaspoon coriander seeds
½ teaspoon cumin seeds
½ teaspoon cardamom pods
4 cloves
½ teaspoon salt

Nutritional value for $^1/_{16}$th of the recipe (16g)
Energy 34 kcal/141 kJ
Protein 0.4g
Fat 3.6g
Sat. Fat 0.5g
Carbohydrate 0.4g
Fibre 0.2g

'This originates from the Yemen and is a spicy, Middle Eastern version of pesto. We love Middle Eastern cooking and so use it quite frequently with couscous, harissa and North African merguez sausages, or over halved boiled eggs and roasted vegetables. It is really versatile and you can alter the strength of the heat by adding or subtracting chillies as you like.'
Katie and Giancarlo Caldesi

This is used only in small amounts but the fresh ingredients provide a little iron, beta-carotene and vitamin E.

Put the herbs, chillies, garlic cloves, lemon juice and olive oil in a food-processor and blitz to a paste. Grind the spices and salt to a powder in a pestle and mortar or a spice grinder, discarding the cardamom husks once they have released their seeds. Add the spices to the food-processor and blitz again – it doesn't have to be completely smooth.

You can use it straight away, or spoon it into a sterilized jam jar and top up with olive oil. Store in the fridge for up to a week or freeze cubes of it in an ice-cube tray for up to 3 months.

A MEDITERRANEAN SELECTION OF BRUSCHETTE

Each topping is enough for four small bruschette

You can put pretty much anything on toasted sourdough, but these suggestions all taste very fresh, and are very quick and easy to make, despite the number of ingredients. They can also all be prepared in advance and kept in the fridge until you need them. Nutritional information overleaf.

For the bruschette:
4 slices of good sourdough or other firm wholemeal bread
1 garlic clove, *halved lengthways*
Extra virgin olive oil

To make the bruschette, toast the slices of bread. Rub one side of each slice with the garlic, then drizzle with a little olive oil.

For the broad bean, mint and ricotta topping:
100g (3½oz) broad beans, *cooked, skinned*
75g (2½oz) peas, *cooked*
Zest of ½ unwaxed lime
A few mint leaves, *torn*
2 tablespoons olive oil
Squeeze of lime
4 tablespoons fresh ricotta cheese

To make the broad bean, mint and ricotta topping, put the cooked beans and peas in a bowl. Add the lime zest, mint leaves and olive oil and a little squeeze of lime juice. Mix together. Spread a tablespoon of ricotta over each slice of toast and top with the bean and pea mixture. Drizzle with a little more olive oil and serve immediately.

For the courgette, mushroom and shrimp topping:
1 tablespoon olive oil
1 small courgette, *finely sliced into rounds*
150g (5½oz) mushrooms, *finely sliced*
1 garlic clove, *finely chopped*
100g (3½oz) brown shrimp
Zest of ½ unwaxed lemon
Handful of basil
Fine grating of nutmeg
Shaved Parmesan cheese *(optional)*
Salt and freshly ground black pepper

To make the courgette, mushroom and shrimp topping, heat the olive oil in a large frying pan. Add the courgette and mushroom slices, and sauté over quite a gentle heat until both are soft. The mushrooms will give out quite a lot of water, so cook until most of this has evaporated. Don't worry about the courgettes collapsing – the point here is for them to be soft and creamy, rather than brown and firm. Add the garlic and cook for a further couple of minutes, then stir in the shrimp, lemon zest and basil. Grate in a little nutmeg and season with salt and pepper. Pile onto the prepared bruschetta and add a few shavings of Parmesan, if you like.

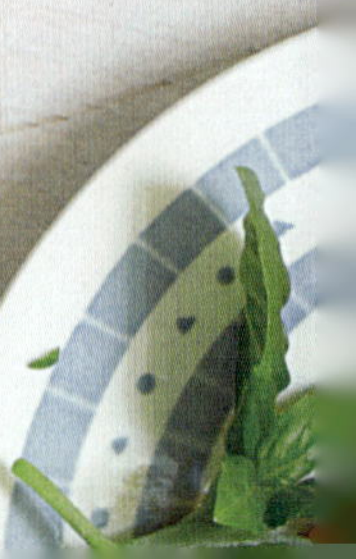

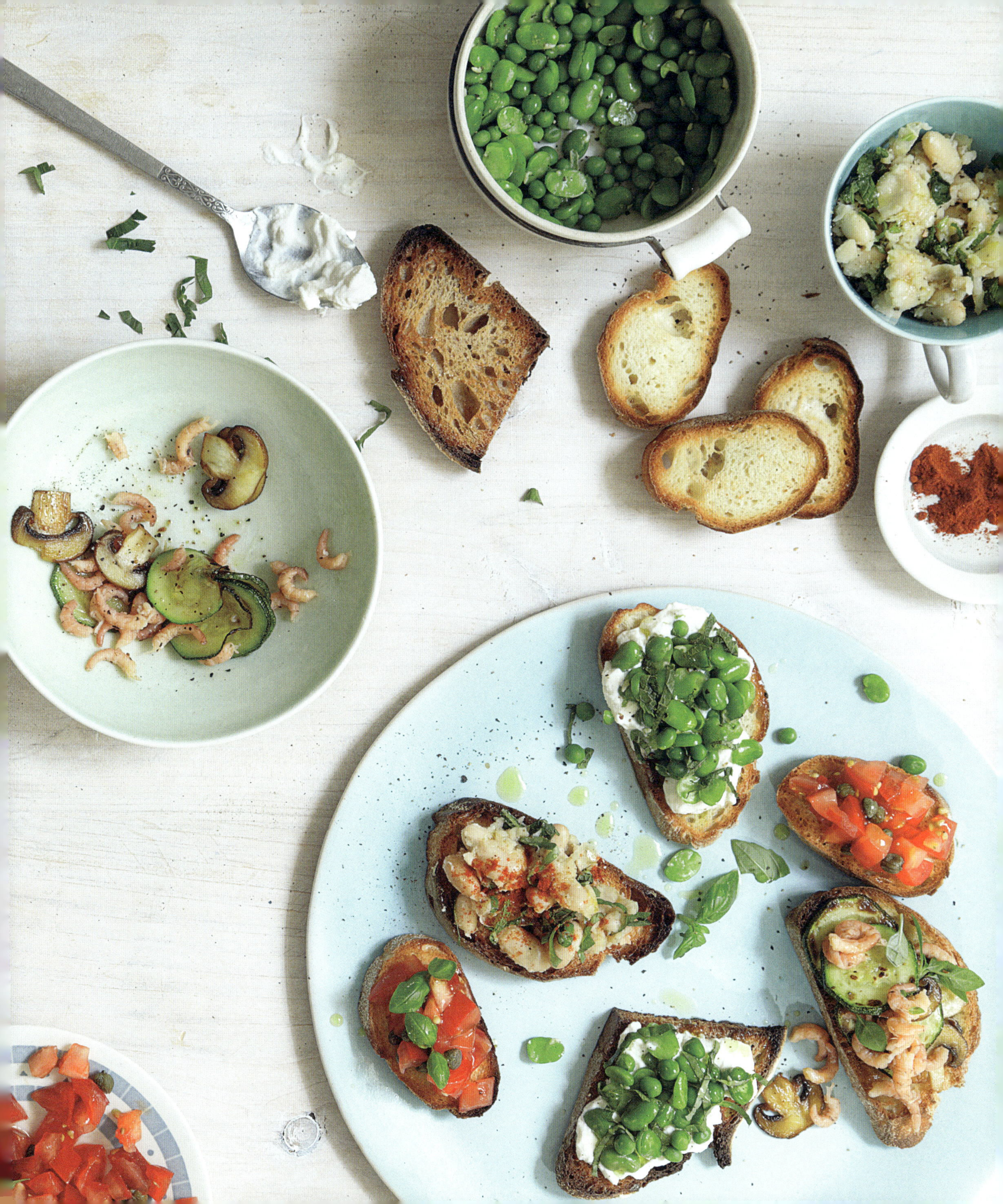

For the white bean and roast garlic topping:
1 head of garlic, *cut in half horizontally*
1 tablespoon olive oil
400g (10½oz) can cannellini beans, *drained and rinsed*
1 tablespoon mint, *chopped*
1 tablespoon basil, *chopped*
½ teaspoon smoked paprika
Salt and freshly ground black pepper

To make the white bean and roast garlic topping, preheat the oven to 200°C/gas mark 6/400°F. Take a sheet of foil large enough to make a parcel around the garlic. Put the garlic, cut-side up, on the foil and drizzle with half the olive oil. Form the parcel around it and put on a baking tray. Roast in the oven for about 45 minutes, until the garlic is soft.

When cool enough to handle, squeeze the flesh of the garlic into a small bowl and discard the skin.

Roughly mash the beans. You want the mixture to be quite textured, so don't overprocess and leave some of the beans in quite large pieces. Add the roasted garlic and season with salt and pepper. Stir in the mint and basil and drizzle in the remaining olive oil. Pile onto the prepared bruschette and sprinkle over the smoked paprika.

For the tomato and basil topping:
4 very ripe tomatoes, *diced*
Handful of basil leaves
1 tablespoon capers *(optional), rinsed and drained*
2 tablespoons olive oil
Salt and freshly ground black pepper

To make the tomato and basil topping, put the diced tomato in a bowl with the basil and capers, if using. Mix thoroughly and drain slightly if very wet – you don't want the bruschette to get soggy, but you do want some of the juices to soak in. Pile the tomatoes onto the toasted bread slices and drizzle with olive oil. Season with salt and pepper.

Bruschetta only – one bruschetta:
Energy 69 kcal/292 kJ **Protein** 3.1g **Fat** 0.9g
Sat. Fat 0.2g **Carbohydrate** 12.9g **Fibre** 2.2g

Broad bean, mint and ricotta – topping per bruschette:
Energy 102 kcal/421 kJ **Protein** 4,2g **Fat** 7.7g
Sat. Fat 2.0g **Carbohydrate** 4.3g **Fibre** 3.2g

Courgette, mushroom and shrimp – topping per bruschette:
Energy 99 kcal/417 kJ **Protein** 15.4g **Fat** 3.9g
Sat. Fat 0.7g **Carbohydrate** 0.9g **Fibre** 0.9g

White bean and roast garlic – topping per bruschette:
Energy 134 kcal/564 kJ **Protein** 8.5g **Fat** 3.5g
Sat. Fat 0.5g **Carbohydrate** 18.2g **Fibre** 7.7g

Tomato and basil – topping per bruschette:
Energy 64 kcal/267 kJ **Protein** 0.6g **Fat** 5.7g
Sat. Fat 0.9g **Carbohydrate** 2.5g **Fibre** 1.1g

SMOOTHIES

There are two smoothie options here. The first is almost a complete meal in itself, as it is quite carbohydrate rich and has soluble fibre from the oats and a low GI. The green smoothie is a great way to kickstart the day, but don't use it as a breakfast replacement. If you are worried about getting enough fruit and vegetables, then this smoothie is perfect as it is packed with beta-carotene and vitamins C and E.

The method for all of these is exactly the same: blitz in the blender until smooth! Makes 1 glass.

Banana, Oat and Honey Smoothie

Energy 454 kcal/1915 kJ **Protein** 12.5g **Fat** 10.4g
Sat. Fat 3.9g **Carbohydrate** 84.4g **Fibre** 7.9g

1 ripe banana
3 heaped tablespoons oats
1 teaspoon honey
Pinch of ground cinnamon *(optional)*
100g (3½oz) blueberries *(optional)*
150ml (5fl oz) milk

A Green Smoothie

Don't be put off by the thought of kale or spinach in a smoothie – the taste is still pleasantly sweet!

Energy 130 kcal/554 kJ **Protein** 2.8g **Fat** 1.0g
Sat. Fat 0.1g **Carbohydrate** 29.4g **Fibre** 7.5g

50g (2oz) kale or spinach leaves *(tough stems removed)*
1 celery stick
100g (3½oz) grapes
1 apple or pear, *cored*
Juice of 1 lime
½ teaspoon grated ginger
Handful of icecubes

FALAFEL

400g (10½oz) can of chickpeas, *rinsed and drained*
½ onion, *finely chopped*
3 garlic cloves, *chopped*
2 teaspoons ground cumin
½ teaspoon turmeric
½ teaspoon ground cinnamon
1 teaspoon salt
¼ teaspoon cayenne *(optional)*
1 teaspoon dried mint
50g (2oz) cooked and mashed butternut squash
2 tablespoons plain flour
3 tablespoons parsley, *finely chopped*
Freshly ground black pepper

Nutritional information before cooking:
Energy 172 kcal/727 kJ
Protein 9.8g
Fat 3.7g
Sat. Fat 0.4g
Carbohydrate 27.8g
Fibre 7.5g

These aren't, strictly speaking, falafel – they are a softer, less dense version. Stuff into pita bread with salad and some yogurt, which has had some dried mint stirred into it. The basic ingredients for these falafel make a low-fat snack that is high in soluble fibre and a good source of iron, beta-carotene and other nutrients including calcium. Limit the amount of oil used for cooking – each tablespoon of oil will add 11g of fat to the whole recipe.

Serves 4 as a healthy-sized snack

Put all the ingredients, except the butternut squash, flour and parsley, into a food-processor and blend to a fairly smooth paste. You could also put everything in a bowl and use a stick blender.

Stir in the butternut squash, flour and parsley. Chill until you are ready to cook.

Form small, flattish patties the size of golf balls – about 30g (1oz) each. Pour a 5mm layer of olive oil in a frying pan and heat. Fry the patties for 3–4 minutes on each side until they are a rich golden brown – or you can deep-fry them, if you prefer.

TIP

- You can keep the mixture in the fridge for a few days or in the freezer. They will also store very well once cooked. If freezing, open-freeze and then, when solid, transfer to a plastic food bag or container.

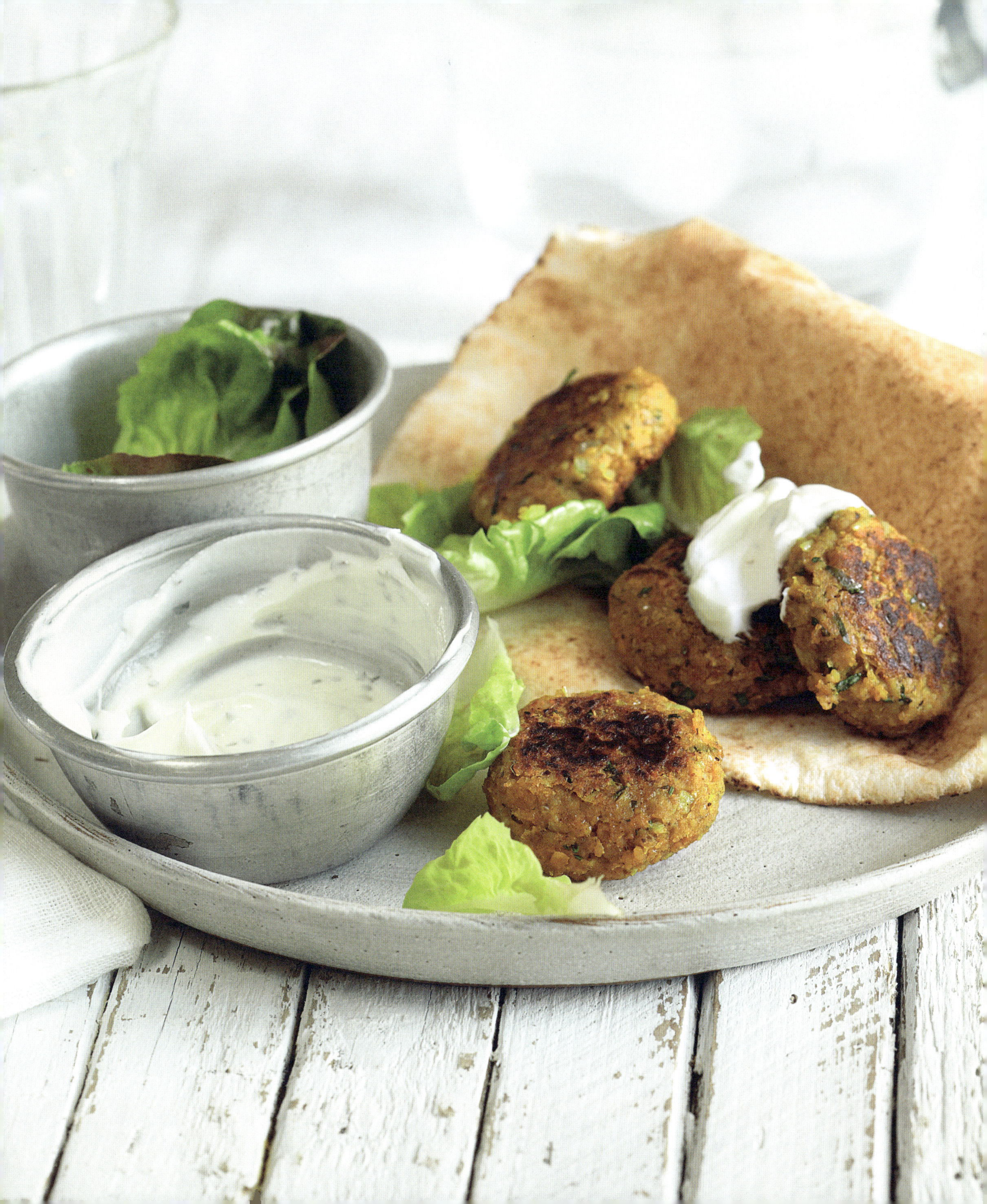

Liz Earle's REFRESHING GREEN

Small handful of parsley
Generous handful of baby spinach leaves
1 celery stick
1 tangerine, *peeled*
2cm (¾in) slice fresh pineapple, *peeled, to garnish*

'Although this is a green juice, it is sweet and full of flavour that everyone will like, including children, so it's a great juice for a boost of vegetables.'
Liz Earle

Juice all the ingredients – it helps to put the parsley and spinach into the juicer first and then push through with the celery and fruit. Serve poured over ice and with a slice of pineapple to garnish.

Energy 75 kcal/317 kJ **Protein** 3.5g **Fat** 1.0g
Sat. Fat 0.1g **Carbohydrate** 13.8g **Fibre** 0g

FRUIT LEATHER

Extra virgin olive oil, *to grease*
300g (10½oz) sweet apples or pears
(peeled and cored weight)
300g (10½oz) soft fruit – berries, plums, peaches or mango
(peeled and stoned weight)

Nutritional information for 1/15 of recipe:
Energy 55 kcal/234 kJ
Protein 0.5g
Fat 0.1g
Sat. Fat 0g
Carbohydrate 13.8g
Fibre 3.0g

This is wonderful stuff – pure fruit, reduced down to a rollable form. Add a bit of honey after you have made the purée if you want to make it slightly sweeter, but you shouldn't need to. This is an excellent way to eat fruit when you need a quick snack and a sweet taste. All the dietary fibre is still present.

Preheat the oven to its lowest setting. Line a baking sheet with greaseproof paper and oil it very lightly.

Dice the apples or pears and the larger of any soft fruits you might be using. Put in a saucepan with 50ml (1½fl oz) cold water and the lemon juice. Simmer gently until all the fruit is very soft – timing will vary depending on the firmness of the apples.

Purée if necessary, then push through a coarse sieve. Spread the purée as evenly as you can over the baking sheet. Don't worry if it seems very thick – it will reduce down as the liquid evaporates from the fruit.

Transfer to the oven and leave for 8–10 hours, perhaps even longer – overnight is ideal. The fruit leather should be shiny and still very slightly tacky. Remove from the oven and either roll up and cut into rounds or just cut into strips. These quantities should make about 15 strips.

POWER BALLS

50g (2oz) crunchy nut butter
50g (2oz) pitted dates, *finely chopped*
100g (3½oz) honey
25g (1oz) cocoa powder
100g (3½oz) desiccated coconut
25g (1oz) sesame or chia seeds
Pinch of salt
Matcha powder, cocoa powder, sesame seeds and/or desiccated coconut, *for rolling*

Energy 93 kcal/387 kJ
Protein 1.8g
Fat 6.8g
Sat. Fat 4.0g
Carbohydrate 6.6g
Fibre 1.9g

These are packed full of energy-giving ingredients, without tasting remotely worthy. They also could not be easier to make. Perfect wrapped up in a twist of foil and kept in your bag for an instant energy burst when you're on the go. They will keep almost indefinitely in the fridge. If you want a chocolate-free version, just omit the cocoa powder and add ground almonds instead. A teaspoon of Matcha powder wouldn't go amiss either, and it goes very well with the sesame seeds.

Makes 16

Put the nut butter, dates and honey in a saucepan. Melt together over a low heat, mashing the dates with the back of a spoon as you go so they break up as much as possible.

Remove from the heat and stir in the cocoa powder, desiccated coconut, sesame seeds and salt. You should be left with a very firm, slightly sticky mixture. Chill in the fridge for a few minutes just to firm up a little more.

Roll the mixture into walnut-sized balls, then roll in any of the suggestions, or perhaps a selection of all four.

Store in an airtight container in the fridge or keep wrapped in foil so they are always at hand.

INDEX

Note: pages numbers in bold refer to photographs.

First published in Great Britain in 2015. This edition published in 2022
by Kyle Books, an imprint of Octopus Publishing Group Limited
Carmelite House
50 Victoria Embankment
London EC4Y 0DZ
www.kylebooks.co.uk

10 9 8 7 6 5 4 3 2 1

ISBN: 9781804190654

Publisher: Joanna Copestick
Designer: Here Design
Photographer: Georgia Glynn Smith
Food Stylist: Valerie Berry
Prop Stylist: Jo Harris
Recipe Writer and Editor: Catherine Phipps
Copy Editor: Stephanie Evans
Editorial Assistant: Claire Rogers and Emma Hanson
Production: Nic Jones, Gemma John, Lisa Pinnell and Allison Gonsalves

A Cataloguing in Publication record for this title is available from the British Library.

Printed and bound in China